Approaches to Substance Abuse and Addiction in Education Communities

This book is designed to increase the awareness among mental health professionals and educators about the potential sources of support for students struggling with substance abuse, addiction and compulsive behaviors. The book includes a description of the scope of the problem of substance abuse in high schools and colleges, followed by sections describing recovery high schools and collegiate recovery communities. A further unique component of this book is the inclusion of material from the adolescents and young adults whose lives have been changed by these programs.

This book was previously published as a special issue of the *Journal of Groups in Addiction and Recovery*.

Jeffrey D. Roth, M.D., is an addiction psychiatrist and group psychotherapist in private practice. He is a fellow of the American Society of Addiction Medicine (ASAM) and the American Group Psychotherapy Association. He has been a practicing group psychotherapist for 25 years. He has presented workshops on group psychotherapy to diverse professional audiences, including group therapists, addictions treatment professionals, psychoanalysts, employee assistance professionals, attorneys and judges. He has served as director, associate director and consultant in numerous group relations conferences sponsored by the A. K. Rice Institute.

Andrew J. Finch, PhD, currently holds an appointment as Assistant Professor of the Practice of Human and Organizational Development at Vanderbilt University. He is also the School Counseling Coordinator for the Human Development Counseling program. He was a co-founder of the Association of Recovery Schools and from 1997-2006 worked for Community High School, a recovery school in Nashville.

Approaches to Substance Abuse and Addiction in Education Communities

A Guide to Practices that Support Recovery in Adolescents and Young Adults

Edited by Jeffrey D. Roth and Andrew J. Finch

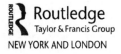

Routledge
Taylor & Francis Group

NEW YORK AND LONDON

First published 2010 in the USA and Canada
by Routledge
270 Madison Avenue, New York, NY 10016

Simultaneously published in the UK
by Routledge
2 Park Square, Milton Park, Abingdon, Oxon, OX14 4RN

Routledge is an imprint of the Taylor & Francis Group, an informa business

Typeset in Times by Value Chain, India
Printed and bound in Great Britain by the MPG Books Group, UK

British Library Cataloguing in Publication Data
A catalogue record for this book is available from the British Library

ISBN10: 0-7890-3696-7 (hbk)
ISBN10: 0-7890-3697-5 (pbk)

ISBN13: 978-0-7890-3696-4 (hbk)
ISBN13: 978-0-7890-3697-1 (pbk)

CONTENTS

Rationale for Including Recovery as Part of the Educational Agenda

Andrew J. Finch, PhD

Vanderbilt University

In recent years, adolescent and young adult alcohol and drug use has garnered attention from scholars, legislators, parents, and the media. There is disagreement as to whether substance abuse by this population is in decline or as problematic as ever. The side one takes depends upon which data is used and how that data are interpreted. While the extent of the issue for adolescents and young adults is in dispute, the existence of problem drug use among this group is not. In 2005, 2.1 million youths in the United States aged 12 to 17 (8.3% of this population) met the DSM-IV (American Psychiatric Association, 1994) diagnostic criteria for a substance use disorder—that is, dependence on or abuse of alcohol or illicit drugs (Substance Abuse and Mental Health Services Administration, 2006). More than 918,000 U.S. college students can be diagnosed as alcohol dependent, and on an average campus of 30,000 students, nearly 9,500 meet the criteria for substance use disorders (Harris, 2006).

For good reason, there has been extensive literature devoted to preventing young people from developing an alcohol or drug problem, early identification and assessment of those who are developing a problem, and evidenced-based interventions and treatment for those who are exhibiting problem use or dependence. The case can be made that investment in prevention and early identification programs can benefit everybody who listens to the message. Some may choose never to drink alcohol or use drugs, others will learn to do so responsibly, and for those who do

Andrew J. Finch, PhD, is in the Department of Human and Organizational Development at Vanderbilt University.

not use substances responsibly, either harm can be reduced or treatment administered.

Far less attention has been paid, however, to those students who have finished treatment. Studies on posttreatment continuing care are growing, but they still are outnumbered by prevention and treatment studies. Programs for students in recovery exist primarily as "aftercare" programs in treatment centers, and these vary in client commitment. Indeed, with less than only about 1% of adolescents and young adults receiving treatment annually (Substance Abuse and Mental Health Services Administration, 2006), it can be difficult to channel funds toward programs that support their recovery.

The data that has been collected on adolescents and young adults after receiving treatment portrays a grim picture. Treatment outcome studies have found first use posttreatment to be 42% in the first 30 days (Spear & Skala, 1995, Table 6), 64% by 3 months (Brown, Vik, & Creamer, 1989), 70% by 6 months (Brown, Vik, & Creamer, 1989), and 77% within one year (Winters, Stinchfield, Opland, Weller, & Latimer, 2000). By 12 months, 47% return to regular use (Winters, Stinchfield, Opland, Weller, & Latimer, 2000). While some of this can be attributed to the quality of the treatment program, much can be attributed to the environmental factors in place after treatment (Godley, Godley, Dennis, Funk, & Passetti, 2002). Adolescents and young adults develop their identities through peer connection and interaction. Once young people have decided to stop using alcohol or drugs, the people with whom they interact and the support systems available will play a major role in determining their success.

This volume is about those systems of support—specifically, systems of support within educational communities. Obviously schools provide a major, if not the main, system of peer interaction and support for adolescents and young adults. According to the U.S. Department of Education, 57% of the U.S. population aged 3–34 is enrolled in a school, and this does not include trade schools or correspondence programs. At age 14 and 15 (the standard age for starting high school), 98.5% of the population is in school. By age 22 through 24 (when many are finishing college), 25% of the population is still in school (Figure 1).

This means that when a person decides to seek help for a substance use disorder, anywhere from a fourth to nearly all of those people—depending on their age—will be involved with an educational community. And young people between ages 14 and 18 will most likely be in a school community every day, seven hours per day. The education community for boarding

FIGURE 1. Percentage of the Population 10 to 24 Years Old Enrolled in School, 2004

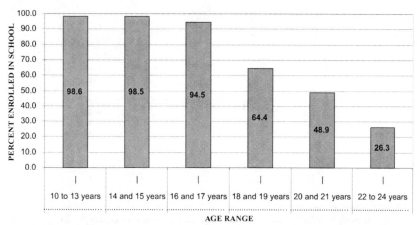

NOTE: Includes enrollment in any type of graded public, parochial, or other private schools. Includes elementary schools, middle schools, high schools, colleges, universities, and professional s chools. Attendance may be on either a full-time or part-time basis and during the day or night. Enrollments in "special" schools, such as trade schools, business colleges, or correspondence schools, are not included. (U.S. Department of Education, 2006, Table 6).

school students and many college students often represents the entire living and social community as well.

Regardless of age or living arrangement, though, education communities provide a powerful source of influence upon adolescents and young adults, and thus there exists both opportunity and risk. The risks have been well documented through substance use and abuse studies and efforts to prevent problem use or reduce the harm of substance "misuse." Efforts to create "social norms" around "responsible" drinking and drug use in order to eliminate "binge" drinking on high school and college campuses have taken root in education communities over the last decade. Though the effectiveness of prevention programs like DARE. (Hallfors & Godette, 2002) and social norms theory (Polonec, Major, & Atwood, 2006) has been disputed, the good news is that the recent reports suggest adolescent substance use and abuse may be in decline (Johnston, O'Malley, Bachman, & Schulenberg, 2007; Substance Abuse and Mental Health Services Administration, 2006). The intense focus on the "teen drug problem" appears to be working.

The number of students ages 12–17 needing and receiving treatment for alcohol or drug use problems or dependence, however, has stayed

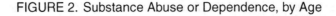

FIGURE 2. Substance Abuse or Dependence, by Age

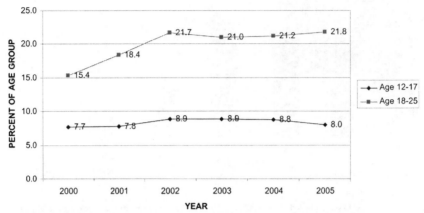

NOTE: Criteria for dependence on or abuse of a substance is based on usage in the past 12 months. Substances include alcohol and illicit drugs, such as marijuana, cocaine, heroin, hallucinogens, and inhalants, and the nonmedical use of prescription-type psychotherapeutic drugs. Classifications are based on criteria specified in the *Diagnostic and Statistical Manual of Mental Disorders*, 4th edition (DSM-IV) (American Psychiatric Association, 1994). According to the NSDUH, dependence is considered to be a more severe substance use problem than abuse because it involves the psychological and physiological effects of tolerance and withdrawal. Although individuals may meet the criteria specified for both dependence and abuse, persons meeting the criteria for both are classified as having dependence, but not abuse. Persons defined with abuse do not meet the criteria for dependence (Substance Abuse and Mental Health Services Administration, 2006).

consistent. In 2000, SAMSHA's National Survey on Drug Use and Health (NSDUH)—formerly the National Household Survey on Drug Abuse—began reporting the number of people with a substance use disorder by age group. From 2000–2005, the percentage of people with a substance use disorder rose from 15.4% to 21.8% for ages 18–25 and hovered between 7.7% and 8.9% for ages 12–17 (see Figure 2) (Substance Abuse and Mental Health Services Administration, 2006).

Since 2002, when the NSDUH began reporting the percentage of people needing and receiving treatment for a substance use disorder in a "specialty treatment center," just under 9% of the population aged 12–17 has needed treatment (see Figure 3), and just under 1% has gotten it (see Figure 4) (Substance Abuse and Mental Health Services Administration, 2006). Policymakers often focus on the obvious "treatment gap," which is the difference between those needing and those receiving treatment—a mean of 8% over the four years. Factors such as treatment availability, cost of treatment, and client demographics and culture impact the size of the "gap."

FIGURE 3. Needing Specialty Treatment for Alcohol or Illicit Drug Abuse or Dependence, Ages 12–17

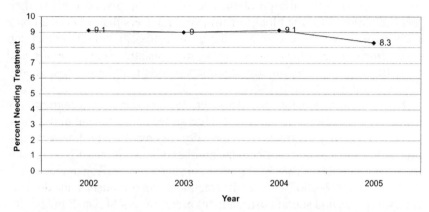

Recovery support programs are concerned with the size of the treatment gap. If people who need treatment—whether it is brief or long-term—cannot get it, they will have no recovery to support. Student assistance programs have existed since the 1970s to identify and assist students at risk

FIGURE 4. Receiving Specialty Treatment for Alcohol or Illicit Drug Abuse or Dependence, Ages 12–17

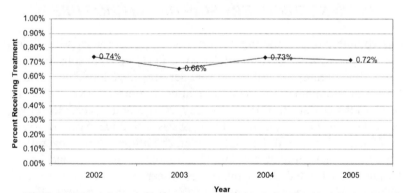

NOTE: SAMHSA defines specialty treatment as treatment received at any of the following types of facilities: hospitals (inpatient only), drug or alcohol rehabilitation facilities (inpatient or outpatient), or mental health centers. It does not include treatment at an emergency room, private doctor's office, self-help group, prison or jail, or hospital as an outpatient. An individual is defined as needing treatment for an alcohol or drug use problem if he or she met the DSM-IV (American Psychiatric Association, 1994) diagnostic criteria for dependence on or abuse of alcohol or illicit drugs in the past 12 months or if he or she received specialty treatment for alcohol use or illicit drug use in the past 12 months (Substance Abuse and Mental Health Services Administration, 2006)

for substance use problems, and these programs have provided a gateway to treatment as well as aftercare for students. Parents may be oblivious to or contributing to the problem, and parents simply do not see their teenage children for the blocks of time around peers that schools do on a daily basis. Once these young adults go to college, parental contact and involvement usually becomes sporadic and episodic. Thus, school-based identification, intervention, and treatment efforts may be the best chance for some students to access services.

Beyond the treatment gap, however, recovery support programs are keenly aware of the data in Figure 4. Though the percentage of high school students receiving treatment at a specialty treatment center has remained under 1% of that population, the raw number of students age 12–17 reveals a range of 168,000 to 186,000 high school students receiving treatment annually from 2002–2005. And as the treatment gap diminishes, the demand for appropriate and sound posttreatment programs could rise dramatically. While not every young person who uses (or abuses) substances requires treatment, hundreds of thousands do. The school environment they return to after that treatment experience will contribute to integration of the "gains" of treatment—or to the reemergence and/or worsening of pretreatment substance use.

EXISTING RECOVERY SUPPORT LITERATURE

This volume will provide the deepest review yet of the existing literature on the continuum of care for adolescent and young adult substance use disorders. Post-treatment continuing care services have long been seen as an "essential" component of the treatment continuum (Brown & Ashery, 1979; Hawkins & Catalano, 1985; McKay, 2001). With some exceptions, however (Godley, Godley, Dennis, Funk, & Passetti, 2002; Spear & Skala, 1995; Winters, Stinchfield, Opland, Weller, & Latimer, 2000), overall research about posttreatment continuing care for adolescents and young adults has been limited. Even thinner is research conducted on recovery schools, which has been limited to theses and dissertations (Doyle, 1999; Finch, 2003; Rubin, 2002; Teas, 1998), single-site evaluations (Diehl, 2002), and unpublished reports (Moberg, 1999; Moberg & Thaler, 1995).

Professional publications have begun to embrace the concept of recovery support in schools as an emerging field. Recovery historian William White recently coauthored a history of recovery schools and has also looked closely at collegiate recovery communities in particular (White, 2001; White & Finch, 2006). Other professional pieces have examined first person perspectives and challenges facing the expansion of recovery schools (e.g., Finch, 2004). Hazelden has also published a startup manual for recovery high schools (Finch, 2005).

One area where school recovery support programs have received more broad support is the popular media. Television, newspapers, and Internet sites have featured many "human interest" stories from high schools and colleges since the early 1990s. While these stories may lack the rigor of a refereed journal, they have also shined a light on programs and provided a forum for testimonials. This has allowed recovery programs in high schools and colleges to garner support, and 25 recovery high schools and six collegiate recovery communities opened across the United States from 1999 to 2005 (White & Finch, 2006).

McKay (2001) outlined a series of future directions in research on continuing care, and, by design, this volume addresses one of McKay's key concerns: characterizing types of continuing care services and documenting how widely available they are. McKay also called for identifying the types of continuing care services that are associated with the best outcomes, and many of the articles here address program outcomes. By systemically describing the impact of education communities upon recovery from substance use disorders, this volume aims to establish the place of recovery support practices across schools.

ORGANIZATION OF THE VOLUME

This volume is designed to be a synthesis of research and practical design methods for implementing programs supportive of recovery in the educational community. The introduction sets the stage by combining material that provides a rationale for this synthesis with the relevant systems theory, coupled with participation of "authentic voices" of students who have participated in this kind of programming. The next three sections of the book follow the classic pattern of the recovering addict telling the story of recovery: (1) "How it was," (2) "How I got here," and (3) "How it is now." Each of these sections therefore begins with the transcript of a Twelve Step meeting of the students whose "authentic voices" are included in the introduction.

CONTRIBUTORS

Researchers, students, and professionals each have a voice in this volume. Authors were invited based on experience and expertise not only with substance abuse but also with educational communities. The continuum of care is represented, as is a range of schooling from secondary through higher education. All the professionals have worked directly with students who abuse substances, who are in treatment, or who are in recovery. The researchers have conducted studies of school programs designed to assist students with substance use disorders. The researchers have been (or are still) active professionals in the field. The student authors either attend or have graduated from a recovery high school or collegiate recovery community. As they are the only people invited to contribute to this work who were asked to openly acknowledge their chemical dependency, we will protect their anonymity by using only their first names and not linking them directly to a particular school.

CONCEPTUAL BASE

We have attempted to insure that this volume is not ideologically driven. Recovery-based programs in high schools and colleges have come from the "grass-roots." They have been efforts to address recovery support needs—as understood by staff and students—that were not being handled by existing treatment and "aftercare" programs. The pioneers in this field did not rely on "evidence-based" programming, because in most instances, no evidence yet existed. This volume is a step toward filling the literature void and beginning to understand the foundations of recovery support in educational communities.

There are many pathways to recovery, and this volume does not promote one form over another. It is intended to tell the story of people helping themselves, developing programs one step at a time, and trying to "keep it simple." The structure for this volume emerges from the classic format for a "lead" in Alcoholics Anonymous, where the speaker talks about "How it was, how I got here, and what it is like now." The reason for this is two-fold. First, the Twelve Step philosophy is embedded in many recovery school communities—in large part because it was the predominate modality as these programs were established, and it remains pervasive. Perhaps more important, Twelve Step and other "mutual aid" programs are rooted in the stories of their participants. This format lends itself to a literary work.

After the introductory chapters of Section I, therefore, Section II opens with an overview of the problem of substance use, abuse, and dependence in the adolescent and young adult population—that is, "How it was." Section II concludes with a description of interventions designed to help students move toward recovery from addiction—that is, "How I got here."[1] Sections III and IV describe high school and college programs, respectively, which are designed to support recovering students in the educational community—that is, "Where we are now."

Following this format, data directly from students representing the programs we are describing are included in each part of the work. In the introductory Section I, students respond to central questions regarding their histories of substance abuse, dependence, and recovery. In Section II, we use a transcript of an online Twelve Step meeting in a chat room conducted by the students, where the topic was the First Step describing the loss of control and unmanageability of their disease (how it was). In the Section II part, as we transition from "How we got here" to "Where we are now," we include a transcript from an online student meeting on the Second Step. And in Section IV, we conclude the volume with a transcript from an online student meeting on the Twelfth Step (carrying the message—what it is like to be in recovery in their own educational community).

OVERVIEW OF THE CHAPTERS

Following the introductory chapters of Section I, Section II has four chapters concerning "How it was" and "How we got here." As mentioned above, this section opens with a transcript from an online First Step meeting. Step One of Alcoholics Anonymous says, "We admitted we were powerless over alcohol—that our lives had become unmanageable" (Alcoholics Anonymous, 2001). This is the focus of the first meeting in Chapter 3. Co-editor Jeffrey Roth has annotated the transcript of each online meeting to help readers understand how this particular meeting corresponds with the traditions, flow, and content of a traditional Twelve Step meeting.

Chapter 4 is titled "The Education Community as a Collection of Groups and Organizations." In this chapter, Jeffrey Roth and Seth Harkins frame adolescent substance use and addiction within systems and organizational theory. They explain how we must approach recovery support as a systemic issue, of which recovery high schools and collegiate recovery communities are one part.

Section II follows with a paper by Keith Russell, "Adolescent Substance Use Treatment: Service Delivery, Research on Effectiveness, and Emerging Treatment Alternatives." Chapter 5 addresses the scope of the problem of adolescent substance use, along with existing and emerging models for treating it.

A key pathway to recovery for adolescents can be recovery support groups. Lora Passetti and Bill White's chapter, "Recovery Support Meetings for Youths," thus concludes Section II's focus on "How we got here." In Chapter 6, Passetti and White review the history of youth involvement in meetings, provide a rationale for enhancing participation, summarizes current research, and discuss issues professionals may want to consider when making referrals. The authors consider research showing how the Twelve Step approach can be effective, but also how it is not the most appropriate resource in every case. While the Twelve Step philosophy undergirds most of the existing recovery support programs in educational communities, new and continuing programs must consider how to best incorporate not only Twelve Step principles but also other paths to recovery to assist a more diverse student body.

Sections III and IV are concerned with "Where we are now." Step Two of Alcoholics Anonymous states, "We came to believe that a power greater than ourselves could restore us to sanity" (Alcoholics Anonymous, 2001). Young people battling a substance use problem or dependence usually come to the belief stated in Step Two while also being part of an educational community. As a transition into the final sections of the work, Chapter 7 transcribes and annotates an online Step Two meeting. The chapters that follow describe recovery in the educational community, first high schools and then colleges.

Chapter 8, "Recovery High Schools as Support for Substance Use Disorders" by Andrew Finch and Paul Moberg, provides data from the first-ever national study of recovery high schools. This descriptive study describes services provided, funding to assure institutional viability, outcome goals, characteristics of the students in terms of substance use disorder, treatment history, comorbidity, socioeconomic status and accessibility. An empirically grounded descriptive typology of programs is also presented.

Chapters 9 through 11 provide first-person accounts from professional teachers and counselors who work in and administrate three different recovery high schools in Minnesota. The first recovery high school, Sobriety High, opened in Minnesota in 1987, and about a dozen recovery high schools are currently operating in the state. Angela Wilcox has taught in both of the first two recovery high school organizations, Sobriety High and PEASE Academy. Her chapter, "TITLE" describes her experience of teaching English in those schools. She also describes her use of "restorative justice," which has spread to many recovery high schools as a way of handling issues that arise with discipline, relapse, dishonesty, and so on.

The first recovery high school to utilize restorative practices was Solace Academy in Chaska, Minnesota. In Chapter 10, "A Secondary School Cooperative: Recovery at Solace Academy, Chaska, Minnesota," Monique Bourgeois explains how this school formed and operates. Solace Academy has a unique institutional basis, operating as a cooperative venture between two counties and seven school districts. In times where collaborations beyond school walls and across community boundaries have become essential for small schools, the story of Solace Academy offers a promising concept for new schools.

Chapter 11, "The Insight Program: A Dream Realized," describes the creation of a "school within a school." The Area Learning Center (ALC) is an alternative school modality established first in Minnesota, serving K-12 students and adults. ALCs offer a broad range of services, including both regular and GED diplomas, as well as child care and remedial programs (Barr & Parrett, 2003). ALCs were authorized by the so-called "second chance law" passed by the Minnesota State Legislature in 1987 (Boyd, Hare, & Nathan, 2002). Any student up to age 21 residing in Minnesota, regardless of his or her "home" district, may attend any ALC, as long as the student meets one of a number of qualifying "at-risk" conditions, including assessment for chemical dependency. The Insight Program was created as a recovery school within the White Bear Lake (Minnesota) ALC, and Bowermaster explains the creation and development of that program.

In recent years, there has been a surge in recovery support services on college campuses as well. Four chapters here focus on collegiate recovery communities. The term "collegiate recovery community" was coined by the Center for the Study of Addiction and Recovery at Texas Tech University, a program begun by Carl Anderson in 1986. In Chapter 12, "Achieving Systems-Based Sustained Recovery: A Comprehensive Model for Collegiate Recovery Communities," the current director, Kitty Harris, and colleagues provide data around the need for and effectiveness of college recovery support programming. The Texas Tech collegiate recovery community has been promoted as a model program by the Substance Abuse and Mental Health Administration (SAMHSA).

Unlike high school recovery support programs, collegiate recovery communities obviously do not enroll full schools of students. For this reason, the extent of services varies from college to college depending on need and institutional design. Rutgers University opened its Alcohol and other Drug Assistance Program for Students (ADAPS) in 1983. Lisa Laitman is the founder of that program, and in 1986 she opened the first "recovery house" on a college campus. The Rutgers program provides services along the full continuum of care, from early identification and intervention through residential recovery support. Laitman and colleague Linda Lederman explain Rutgers' extensive model in Chapter 13, "The Need for a Continuum of Care: The Rutgers Comprehensive Model."

As mentioned earlier, published research and evaluation works on recovery schools are lacking. In Chapter 14, "Assessment and Outcome of a College Substance Abuse Recovery Program: Augsburg College's StepUP Program," Ken Winters provides one of the first published program evaluations of a collegiate recovery community.

The last of the four college-focused chapters is one of the volume's "authentic voice" pieces. In 1977, Classics professor Bruce Donovan was appointed Associate Dean with Special Responsibilities in the Area of Chemical Dependency at Brown University. He served in that role until 2003, and in the process established the first and oldest recovery support program on a college campus. One year after his retirement, Professor Donovan gave an address at the Association of Recovery Schools' third annual conference at Rutgers University. He reflected upon his career and the experience of breaking ground in the area of collegiate recovery support at a prestigious university. Chapter 15 has been developed from the text of his talk on July 10, 2004.

The volume concludes with a final online student Twelve Step meeting. Step 12 of Alcoholics Anonymous says, "Having had a spiritual awakening as the result of these steps, we tried to carry this message to alcoholics, and to practice these principles in all our affairs" (Alcoholics Anonymous, 2001). Ongoing support of oneself and others who may be suffering is the crux of this message. Hence, the online Twelve Step meeting in Chapter 16 focuses on how these students have been supported and "carried the message" to others.

CONCLUSION

This work covers a large swath of territory concerning recovery support in educational settings. We address many issues along the continuum of care in an effort to place attention on this topic. Of course, much ground remains uncovered. Studies comparing recovery school programs to each other and to nonrecovery school communities are needed. The field needs to examine schools within alcohol and drug treatment centers as well as the growing presence of "grass-roots" student recovery support organizations and houses not affiliated with schools. Furthermore, we need to understand the lack of racial and ethnic diversity in specialty treatment programs and recovery school communities. How can schools reach a broader base of students? Should more recovery high schools start providing outpatient treatment services as a precursor to recovery school enrollment? What doors to recovery other than Twelve Step programs are showing promise and wide-spread availability to students? Special needs and barriers to access both deserve more attention. This volume has fired a starting gun we hope will generate discussion, research, and publication in these and other areas relevant to recovery support in educational communities as recovery finally establishes a place on the nation's educational agenda.

NOTE

1. Student Assistance Programs (SAPs), a main source of prevention and intervention in high schools, are not addressed at length in this work. SAPs have existed in the United States since the 1980s, and, while they provide some level of recovery support, many student assistant professionals focus on prevention and early identification/intervention. The scope of SAPs varies from state to state and district to district, and a relevant discussion of these programs deserves its own volume. The National Student Assistance Association (http://www.nsac.info/) can provide more information about the scope and evidence-based practices of SAPs in the United States

REFERENCES

Alcoholics Anonymous. (2001). *Alcoholics Anonymous: The story of how many thousands of men and women have recovered from alcoholism* (4th ed.). New York: Alcoholics Anonymous World Services.

American Psychiatric Association. (1994). *Diagnostic and statistical manual of mental disorders: DSM-IV* (4th ed.). Washington, DC: American Psychiatric Association.

Barr, R. D., & Parrett, W. H. (2003). Alternative Schooling. In J. W. Guthrie (Ed.), *Encyclopedia of Education* (2nd ed., Vol. 1, pp. 82–86). New York: Macmillan Reference USA.

Boyd, W. L., Hare, D., & Nathan, J. (2002). *What really happened? Minnesota's experience with statewide public school choice programs: Center for School Change, Hubert H. Humphrey Institute of Public Affairs.* Minneapolis: University of Minnesota.

Brown, B. S., & Ashery, R. S. (1979). Aftercare in drug abuse programming. In R. L. DuPont, A. Goldstein & J. A. O'Donnell (Eds.), *Handbook on drug abuse* (pp. 165–73). Rockville, MD: Department of Health Education and Welfare, Public Health Service, Alcohol, Drug Abuse, and Mental Health Administration, National Institute on Drug Abuse.

Brown, S. A., Vik, P. W., & Creamer, V. A. (1989). Characteristics of relapse following adolescent substance abuse treatment. *Addictive Behaviors, 14*, 291–300.

Diehl, D. (2002). Recovery high school. In S. L. Isaacs & J. R. Knickman (Eds.), *To improve health and health care: The Robert Wood Johnson Foundation anthology (Vol. V)*. San Francisco: Jossey–Bass.

Doyle, K. (1999). *The recovering college student: Factors influencing accommodation and service provision.* Unpublished Ed.D. dissertation, University of Virginia, Charlottesville, VA.

Finch, A. J. (2003). *A sense of place at Recovery High School: Boundary permeability and student recovery support.* Unpublished Ph.D. dissertation, Vanderbilt University, Nashville, TN.

Finch, A. J. (2004). First person: Portrait of a recovery high school. *Counselor, 5*(2), 30–32.

Finch, A. J. (2005). *Starting a recovery school: A how-to manual.* Center City, MN: Hazelden Publishing and Educational Services.

Godley, M. D., Godley, S. H., Dennis, M. L., Funk, R., & Passetti, L. L. (2002). Preliminary outcomes from the assertive continuing care experiment for adolescents discharged from residential treatment. *Journal of Substance Abuse Treatment, 23*(1), 21–32.

Hallfors, D., & Godette, D. (2002). Will the "principles of effectiveness" improve prevention practice? Early findings from a diffusion study. *Health Education Research, 17*(4), 461–70.

Harris, K. (2006). *Why are recovery communities important?* Retrieved April 13, 2006, from http://www.texastech.edu/news/CurrentNews/display_article.php?id=2081

Hawkins, J. D., & Catalano, R. F. (1985). Aftercare in drug abuse treatment. *The International Journal of the Addictions, 20*(6 & 7), 917–45.

Johnston, L. D., O'Malley, P. M., Bachman, J. G., & Schulenberg, J. E. (2007). *Monitoring the future national results on adolescent drug use: Overview of key findings, 2006* (No. NIH Publication No. [07-6202]). Bethesda, MD: National Institute on Drug Abuse.

McKay, J. R. (2001). Effectiveness of continuing care interventions for substance abusers. *Evaluation Review, 25*(2), 211–32.

Moberg, D. P. (1999). *Evaluation of Chicago Preparatory Charter High School. Final grant report to the Robert Wood Johnson Foundation.* Madison: University of Wisconsin Center for Health Policy and Program Evaluation.

Moberg, D. P., & Thaler, S. L. (1995). *An evaluation of Recovery High School: An alternative high school for adolescents in recovery from chemical dependence.* Princeton, NJ: An Unpublished Report to the Robert Wood Johnson Foundation.

Polonec, L. D., Major, A. M., & Atwood, L. E. (2006). Evaluating the believability and effectiveness of the social norms message, "Most Students Drink 0 to 4 Drinks When They Party." *Health Communication, 20*(1), 23–34.

Rubin, B. T. (2002). *Changing lives through changing stories: A phenomenological study of adolescents in recovery from addiction.* Unpublished Ph.D. dissertation, Vanderbilt University, Nashville, TN.

Spear, S. F., & Skala, S. Y. (1995). Posttreatment services of chemically dependent adolescents. In E. Rahdert & D. Czechowicz (Eds.), *Adolescent drug abuse: Clinical assessment and therapeutic interventions (NIDA Research Monograph 156),* (pp. 341–64). Rockville, MD: U.S. Department of Health and Human Services, National Institute on Drug Abuse.

Substance Abuse and Mental Health Services Administration (2006). *Results from the 2005 National Survey on Drug Use and Health: National Findings.* Office of Applied Studies. Rockville, MD: Substance Abuse and Mental Health Services Administration.

Teas, T. G. (1998). *Chemically dependent teens with special needs: Educational considerations for after treatment.* St. Paul, MN: Bethel College.

U.S. Department of Education (2006). *Digest of Education Statistics, 2005, NCES 2006-030.* Washington, DC: U.S. Department of Education, National Center for Education Statistics.

White, W. L. (2001). Recovery university: The campus as a recovering community. *Student Assistance Journal, 13*(2), 24–26.

White, W. L., & Finch, A. J. (2006). The recovery school movement: Its history and future.*Counselor, 7*(2), 54–57.

Winters, K. C., Stinchfield, R. D., Opland, E., Weller, C., & Latimer, W. W. (2000). The effectiveness of the Minnesota Model approach in the treatment of adolescent drug abusers. *Addiction, 95*(4), 601–12.

Authentic Voices: Stories from Recovery School Students

Andrew J. Finch, PhD

Vanderbilt University

ABSTRACT. One of the central elements of 12-step recovery is the story. Every member of a 12-step group has one and is expected to share it. These stories are told in full "speaker" meetings, but also in increments as people share "experience, strength, and hope." The story of a "newcomer" evolves over time to become the fully developed story of an "old-timer." Gradually, stories stop emphasizing "how it was" and are able to focus more upon the lessons learned and "how it is today." One powerful aspect of recovery stories is that they tend to help the sobriety of both the listener *and* the teller.

This chapter is not a work of research but rather the narration of eight students from recovery schools. Each was posed with a different question to address about their recovery school experience. Each was also asked to share brief pieces of their personal recovery stories as an introduction. These are the same students who participated in the online meetings annotated later in the volume, and last names have been removed in the tradition of AA, of which each student is a member. The intent is to represent an "authentic voice" of recovery schools that is genuine more than analytic. While all eight students believe recovery schools have been integral to their sustained recovery, the point of these stories is not necessarily to draw conclusions. Rather, it is to allow the reader a glimpse inside the walls of a recovery school ... to hear the types of stories staff members and peer

---

Andrew J. Finch, PhD, is in the Department of Human and Organizational Development at Vanderbilt University.

students hear everyday. Indeed, it is stories like the ones that follow that keep many of these staff and students coming back day after day, and they serve as a testament to what recovery schools can be. The editors of this journal could think of no better way to introduce a volume on recovery in educational communities.

STUDENT REPRESENTATION

Students were chosen in an effort to balance the perspectives between high schools and colleges. They are presented here in two sections: first high school students, then college students. Within each section, the student stories are in alphabetical order by first name. The question each student was asked to answer is listed before the response.

The high schools represented include the following:

Archway Academy (Houston, Texas)
Northshore Recovery School (Beverly, Massachusetts)
Sobriety High (Maplewood, Minnesota)
Solace Academy (Chaska, Minnesota)

The colleges represented include:

Augsburg College (Minneapolis, Minnesota)
Case Western Reserve University (Cleveland, Ohio)
Rutgers University (New Brunswick, New Jersey)
Texas Tech University (Lubbock, Texas)

In order to protect anonymity, we have removed the names of schools as directly connected to students.

HIGH SCHOOL STUDENTS

Dena B.

What made you select a recovery high school instead of returning to your former school? Did you think going to a non-recovery high school was an option?

I was eleven years old the first time I got drunk. I have a bar in my basement where my grandpa keeps all the alcohol he hasn't even touched in years. So my friend and I decided we wanted to try it, and we figured he would never notice anything was missing. We snuck a bottle of Jack Daniels over to her house that night, and after I took that first sip and felt my throat and stomach starting to get warm, I knew I liked it. My friend spit it out right away and thought it was disgusting. But I loved it and kept drinking until I started to get really sick, and her mother sent me home. I spent the rest of the night throwing up. After that, I decided that now that I had tried it and knew what it was like, I shouldn't drink anymore.

It was Christmas, and I was thirteen. Every Christmas, my grandparents and I went over to my aunt's house for dinner, and usually after that, my cousins would take me to a movie and then drive around to look at Christmas lights. As we were driving around looking at lights, my cousins started smoking weed in the car, and when it got passed around to me, I just took a hit without thinking—like it was just the right thing to do. I liked the feeling of getting high. So I started smoking a lot of pot throughout eighth grade and the beginning of ninth.

After a while, though, I had to smoke more and more, because it would barely get me high anymore. The summer before 10th grade, I started hanging out with new friends and older guys. I went to a club one night and tried coke for the first time. I loved that, too. That night, I left with two guys that I just met. I didn't call my grandparents or even bother to tell them I wouldn't be coming home.

On the drive to these guys' house, I found out they lived about two hours away from me, but they promised they would give me a ride home in the morning. We stayed up all night partying, and we decided to go swimming in a lake near their house. I almost drowned, but I thought I had the time of my life.

I snuck out of my house again a few weeks later to meet up with the same guys and go to their house again. I tried OxyContin for the first time there, and since then, I was off and running. I would lie, cheat, and steal just to get drugs. My grandparents eventually caught on, and I got arrested a few times, until finally the judge said I could not go home anymore and I needed to get help. They placed me in a DSS shelter until a bed opened up in a rehab. After I completed the rehab, I stayed an extra month because I did not think I was ready to go home yet. Then I went to a halfway house for three extra months, and finally came back home to live with my grandparents again. I've stayed sober since.

In May 2006, when I left the halfway house, I was still only 15 years old, so I was legally not allowed to drop out of high school yet. The courts told me I needed to figure out where I was going to go to school. My first plan was just to not go anywhere until I turned 16, so I could drop out. My only options seemed to be to go back to my old high school or go to a charter school. Neither of those sounded good to me.

I knew if I went back to my old school, I would have to be around all of my old friends who still actively use, and I probably wouldn't have been able to stay sober longer than two weeks. And I just didn't like the idea of going to a charter school at all. Then one day, my grandmother saw an article in the newspaper about a recovery high school that would open in September 2006. Excited about this new possibility, we called every day to try to find more information about it, and eventually I was the first person accepted into the school. After more than six months here, I can safely say that for me, Recovery High is a much better option than any other school.

At Recovery High, I've made good, sober friends with whom I can have a good time without getting high. Also, at my new school, there are always people available for me when I need to talk. At my old school, there were no counselors you could talk to and barely any support. It seemed like people did not want to recognize the drug problem that was right in front of them.

At Recovery High, there are some staff members who are in recovery themselves and look out for the students. They know when to tell us that they are concerned about our behaviors, or when we are doing something that could potentially harm our recovery. In a regular high school, I would not have that option or the support. It's much easier to go to school with other kids my age who have all basically been through the same things and can relate to me if I am having an issue. In return, I can be there to help them if they need me, because sometimes just the fact that you helped another person can make you feel better.

Some non-recovery high schools claim that they have, or are trying to start, anti-drug programs. I know that when I went to regular high school, nobody took these programs seriously at all. People would come and preach about how bad drugs are, but never did they speak about their own experiences, or know at all first-hand what it's like to be sober or in recovery. Now at my school, when people visit we can listen to them and relate to them, because they've been through what we've been through.

I could not see myself at a non-recovery school at this point in my life. I don't think that I am far enough into my recovery to be thrown into a regular school again. It would only be harmful to me. Recovery High is exactly where I'm meant to be right now, and the teachers and students have been nothing but helpful to me.

Jessica S.

What about attending a recovery high school has had the most valuable effect on your life?

There are not enough words to express how much a recovery high school has affected my life. I have been attending a recovery high school for three years, and it has taught me so many things—things that I can take with me for the rest of my life.

Principles, gratitude, and honesty are a few things I have learned, but what I value most and has meant the most is being shown a new way to live. The staff and community at my recovery high school have helped me change my life around by knowing that I want to stay sober. Yes, there have been some ups and downs, times when I did not think I was going to be able to stay sober without the help of my recovery school. During those times, my recovery school was always in the back of my mind. If I [thought about using] drugs or [making] a bad decision, I would think about the consequences that I would have to face and how everyone would feel. They have shown me that my actions affect everyone in my school, not just myself. I always know the staff and my peers are there to fall back on if I need their help.

My recovery high school had a lasting effect on my academic career by teachers going out of their way to help me graduate. It has helped outside of school as well. It has taught me that I am able to handle things without using drugs or alcohol, and it has shown me constructive ways to manage my life. Attending a recovery school has helped change and shape my relationships with other people and my family members. It has shown me that I am able to have a healthy relationship with my peers and authority.

The staff have been there for me through thick and thin. They have always been so understanding of the disease of addiction and everything that it entails. They always have more patience with assignments and lessons. I have a more personal relationship with the staff, which really makes the environment more relaxed and more at home. They know when I'm having a hard time, when I need to talk to them about an issue, or when to be funny. It makes me want to keep coming back day after day.

I have realized that attending a recovery high school has made me grateful for all the things in my life thus far. It has made me grateful for the past and for the things that could come in the future. It has given me so many opportunities that I would never have had attending a normal public high school: speaking engagements, my trip to Washington DC,[1] and speaking at the (state) capitol. It has helped my self-perception so much that I now have the ability to feel grateful about the things that I have.

I do not think I would have stayed sober at a normal public high school after getting out of treatment. My recovery high school has helped me succeed in everything that I have put my mind to. There should be more recovery schools in the United States to help more youth like myself just getting out of treatment, because I know it's saved my life.

J.R.

Describe how being a student in a recovery high school has impacted your relationships (positively or negatively) with people your age who are not in recovery. How has it changed your "out-of-school" time?

It has been almost vital to my recovery to be in a recovery high school. I think that had I gone to my zoned high school I would probably not have stayed sober. It's hard enough to get sober with out being around it, and it's even worse when it's constantly being pushed your way.

I can remember being put in an Alternative Peer Group (APG) against my will. It sucked really bad. That's the least I can say. It really ruined my drugging. Every day I'd be pissed all day at school because I knew I could drug in school, but as soon as I got out of school, I went straight to my APG and would get busted regularly.

Then my parents put me in (my recovery school), and I HATED it. I missed all of my friends from my public school, and I couldn't easily get high at school anymore. Time went on, and I got sent to treatment. After three months there, I went back to (my recovery school), and I continued to get high. To shorten the story, I got desperate enough to ask for help, and (my recovery school) was there to hold a hand out.

Relating to my peers outside of school was nearly impossible for me to do without the use of drugs. I had no social skills on how to make a real friend; the only thing I knew was to get high. I actually came to find out that a lot of the kids I used to think were good friends disappeared as soon as I got sober.

I believe that overall, my relationships outside of recovery with my peers have improved, because I am someone that they can come to when they are ready to get sober. I am also there emotionally, which before was nearly impossible. I have friends at my zoned school that I still talk to occasionally, and they are glad that I am sober because they remember how messed up I was before I got sober.

When I told my story at my zoned school recently, I was amazed to see how many people came up to me and told me that they cared, and that they were glad to see me so happy. That means a lot.

Now, as far as my out-of-school time, I don't have much homework, so I can focus mainly on my recovery. Now, focusing on my recovery is not really a problem; but at first it was vital. I also have met a lot of kids I'm not sure I would have met had it not been for [my recovery school]. I have friends that I would take a bullet for now, and they would do the same for me. These are relationships that will last for as long as I live, and I will always remember them if we split apart.

The only thing that has kind of sucked about recovery high school is that A LOT of the kids who used to go there are gone, either graduated or got high and were removed from school. It sucks but it's all part of the game.

Stefanie K.

Describe how a recovery school has supported your recovery. What challenges would you have faced attending your old school? Do you feel you have "missed out" on anything by attending a recovery high school?

My name is Stefanie. I am an alcoholic and an addict. I have been clean and sober since April 11, 2005, thanks to the recovery high school I attend, my supportive family, the network of sober friends that I have today, and of course the 12-step program for alcoholics and addicts.

As with most other alcoholics and addicts, my story is very similar. I started out using drugs and alcohol at the young age of 12. I used on occasion. As time went by, occasion turned into weekends, to every few days, to daily. I started out just using pot and alcohol, but soon enough the high was not as good as in the beginning, so I moved on to so-called "bigger and better" drugs, such as pain killers, ecstasy, acid, mushrooms, Adderall, coke, etc.—basically anything that I could get my hands on that would give me that feeling of escaping.

Once I was about 13 or 14 years old, I started to get put into drug abuse programs because I started to ditch school and not care about my family or myself. I was constantly on the run from home, just trying to find that next high. I did have some legal consequences, such as minor consumptions and assault charges.

After a while it got to the point where I was on the run [15 years old] not knowing where I was going to stay that night and not really knowing what was going on around me. I felt so horrible inside, and all that I could possibly want was to die. I wanted to stop using drugs and alcohol, but I had tried many times before, and I couldn't. I was completely hopeless. I knew that I needed help!

I finally ended up in the hospital and went into an inpatient program. After facing all of those emotions of first getting sober, I found some hope in the program of Alcoholics Anonymous.

Now my life is amazing. I am 17 years old and couldn't be happier. I have regained the broken relationships with my family. I go to AA meetings on a regular basis and talk to my 12-step sponsor. Though I had a few slips after treatment, I have gotten right back on the path of my recovery. I can actually enjoy life being sober. I have a connection with a Higher Power. My life is saved, and I owe it all to the program of the 12 steps.

I have come to realize that my sobriety is a journey rather than a destination. In my journey of sobriety, I have found that I have needed much support. As a teenager with the disease of alcoholism and addiction, recovery high schools have enabled me to receive my education and maintain my sobriety. Though there are some things I feel I have missed out on by not attending my old high school, there is no way that I would have stayed sober if I had gone back.

I have attended (my recovery high school) for three years now. I continued to stay in a recovery high school because it has helped support my sobriety as well as enable me to receive an education. Some may ask how does a recovery high school support your recovery? Through my experience, I have found many ways that a recovery high school has supported my sobriety and recovery. The first and most important way that a recovery high school has supported me is the simple fact that you need to remain clean and sober to attend. That means that all the students are drug and alcohol free, therefore students don't have to go through the challenge of having drugs or alcohol in front of them in a school environment.

Also at my recovery high school, they require you to attend one 12-step meeting a week and have contact with a 12-step sponsor once a week. (A sponsor is someone who helps you to work the 12-step program.) They enforce this by having each student sign a contract agreeing to follow these requirements.

In the beginning I didn't understand meetings and sponsors; I thought that meetings were some kind of a cult, so the contract helped to force me to go and find out what they were really about—and meetings are not by any means any form of a cult!

Being at a recovery high school and having to attend these meetings and have contact with a 12-step sponsor has helped my sobriety a lot.

I now do not have to be told to attend meetings. I do so on a regular basis as well as contacting my 12-step sponsor. Having a sponsor and attending 12-step meetings is a very important thing in my journey of recovery. It is something that I will always need to do. The recovery high school's requirements, therefore, have helped me to learn a lot of things about my disease of alcoholism and addiction by requiring that I attend these meetings and have a sponsor. They helped to set me on my path to recovery.

Another way that attending a recovery high school has helped me is that when most kids get out of treatment, it is hard for them to get back in the habit of going to school, as some, such as myself, didn't attend while in treatment. Also, when I was using drugs and alcohol I did not do much—if any—of my homework, and I didn't attend school on a regular basis. At a recovery high school, the teachers and staff understand this and help you get back into that regular habit of going to school and doing homework. They help you re-learn how to become a successful student again.

The teachers at recovery high schools from my experience are very special people. They understand the disease of addiction and alcoholism and are willing to help students in any way possible. Whether it be educational, personal, or recovery needs, they have been there for me. Examples of the teachers being there for me are family issues, struggles in math class, and my relapse. The teachers all hold a special place in my heart.

Fortunately the class sizes in a recovery high school are smaller than a normal high school, so students are more likely to have their educational needs met. There is also a lot more one-on-one communication with the teachers in a recovery high school. Since the class sizes are much smaller, you are able to build a better relationship with students as well as staff.

This brings me to the next topic of meeting amazing sober peers. Getting a large sober network that you can receive from attending a recovery high school is extremely important to have when in recovery. When I got out of treatment, I thought to myself there was no one out there who is my age and trying to be sober. I thought that all teenagers were supposed to be experimenting with drugs and alcohol, so why would anyone want to be sober? Soon after applying to go to a recovery school—with the help of my parents—I was shocked; there were about 40 kids, and they were all trying to live a life of recovery. My experience with students at a recovery high school is that all the kids are really accepting. No matter your race, religion, age, sexual preference, or looks, they still accept you for who you truly are. I still to this day have some of my friends that I first met at (my recovery high school) three years ago. Going to a recovery high school has helped me to form a sober network of friends.

Relapse is something that can happen in sobriety/recovery. I have relapsed a couple times, but my recovery high school students and staff were very supportive and helped me jump right back on my path to recovery.

Finally, one of the most amazing and helpful things that a recovery school has is called "group." It consists of all the students for an hour once a day. Students get the chance to talk about how their recovery and sobriety is going. They can share things that may be a struggle in their everyday life as well. Then, after sharing, the student gets a chance to get feedback. Feedback is advice, strength, or experiences that other students have to offer and share. I find group extremely helpful, because I am able to talk about problems or struggles in my recovery, and there are students my age who can relate to me and offer me advice on similar situations they may have been in. Those are only a few of the ways a recovery high school has supported my recovery.

I would have never been able to attend my old high school and get the same support I do at a recovery high school. I feel that I would have faced many social and academic challenges if I had decided to return to my old high school. The most challenging thing about returning to my old high school would be seeing my old friends every day that I used to use drugs and alcohol with. It would be extremely hard for me to face my old friends and hear them talk about, "Oh! Remember that time we got high?" and about parties that are going on. I wouldn't be able to stay away from the peer pressure.

I personally would not know where to begin finding sober friends at my old high school. It would be difficult to find a sober network at my old high school, because all the friends I know there use drugs and alcohol. And being able to find friends that understand my disease of alcoholism and addiction would definitely be a struggle. There is not much support for teenagers trying to stay sober at a regular mainstream high school. I know that there are chemical dependency counselors, but from my experience most of the kids that talk to them are forced by probation and don't want to be sober.

If I were to relapse and use drugs or alcohol, who would call me out on it? And help me jump back on the path of recovery? I honestly do not think that I would be sober today if I went back to my old high school.

I would have faced academic struggles as well. Teachers at a mainstream high school do not necessarily understand that I basically need to relearn how to become a successful student. These are just some of the challenges I would find most difficult if I were to return to my old high school.

There are, though, a few things I feel I have missed out on by not attending my old high school, such as the variety of electives, sports teams, physical education, and the guidance counselors. A mainstream high school offers electives, such as photography, ceramics, wood shop, small engines, foreign languages, etc. Most recovery high schools, from my experience, do not offer very many choices. I also feel that I miss out on sports teams and physical education. In my old high school they had a variety of sports you could try out for. My recovery school has none. Also in a mainstream high school, they have a variety of physical education classes. My recovery high school has had some in the past, but they cannot afford to hire physical education teachers and are not certified in physical education. I think that every growing teenager needs some sort of exercise regularly.

Also, we have no guidance counselors at my recovery high school. It was nice to have someone there to speak with about college and other things. We do have teachers that listen at my recovery school, but there is not always someone available as they have to teach classes. Unlike in a mainstream high school, there are counselors that are there for only your needs. Though I feel I have missed out on some opportunities by not returning to my old high school, my hope for the future is that they [my recovery school] will be able to offer those activities.

In the end, attending a recovery high school has helped to support my recovery in so many ways. I have only I mentioned a few. I am very grateful that I did not have to return to my old high school and face the challenges that I would be going through. Though I felt I missed out on some opportunities, I am so pleased that recovery schools exist, because they have helped me to become a successful student again, maintain my sobriety, and to begin my life-long journey of recovery. Recovery high schools have saved my life.

COLLEGE STUDENTS

Andrew C.

Describe how recovery-based housing has supported your recovery. What challenges would you have faced attending a college without a recovery house?

I was born 19 years ago as the second of five children, with an older sister and three younger brothers on Long Island in New York. My family has been very supportive, and we have always gotten along well. I went to local public schools through eighth grade, after which I went to a private, Catholic, all-male high school. I went into this high school knowing very few people and just feeling generally uncomfortable and lonely.

I knew my dad was sober but I knew very little about alcoholism. I only knew that, as the son of an alcoholic, I was more likely to be one myself, but this knowledge helped me very little. I had my first drink at a keg party during my third year in high school. I didn't drink very much, and I remember feeling just as uncomfortable that night as I usually did around groups of people. I also remember people smoking weed in the garage and thinking I would never do that. Later that year I drank on occasion, but not very frequently. Also later that year, I smoked pot for the first time. At this time I had started spending time in school with a few kids I shared a free period with. We would sit in the library and talk about music, but they often talked about hanging out with one another outside school and getting high. I began to like the sound of it more and more. This is why I smoked my first time, at a friend's house one night after a rock concert.

Around this time, one of my brothers, who is a year younger than I am, started drinking and smoking with his friends. During that year we smoked and drank together frequently. I also started spending a lot of time with the friends I had met in the library in school, and we would smoke whenever we saw each other and drink on occasion too. By the end of my junior year, I was smoking every day, usually by myself. I noticed some effects of this, but they didn't bother me much. I was lying to my parents about what I was doing, where I was going, and who I was spending time with. My grades started to suffer. I stopped spending time with other friends who I used to occasionally see but who didn't use. Using became a mental obsession; it was all I thought about.

This continued through my senior year of high school. As I got my driver's license and had some more freedom, I was using more and more. I could get weed and alcohol easier because I could drive to pick it up. I could stay over at people's houses and drink because I could drive myself home the next day. My grades continued to slip and at graduation I missed the four-year honor roll award by a tenth of a point, dropping about five percent from my first year. Due to my slowly declining grades, most of the colleges I applied to rejected me or placed me on waiting lists. One school called me up after the application deadline, even though I had not applied or even visited there. They encouraged me to apply anyway, so I did, and

I was accepted and offered a scholarship. I visited the school and liked it, so I decided to enroll there.

I partied through the summer before college, and my parents even encouraged me to get a fake ID in New York City before I went away to school. My sister was in college at the time and they knew she often went out to bars with her friends, so they thought I might want to do the same. I went off to college, 17 years old, with my fake ID and a big bag of marijuana. I didn't know anyone at the school, but I quickly found people interested in using like I was, and we were smoking in my dorm room during orientation. I took advantage of the new freedom college offered me. I rarely went to class, choosing instead to stay up all night and sleep all day. I partied with other people, but during the week I was often just smoking with my roommate or another friend or, many nights, by myself. Since I had a fake ID, I went on beer runs with fellow students, buying huge amounts of alcohol at a time and stashing it in our dorm rooms. We took my closet door off the hinges and used it as a beer pong table. I started to get in trouble with the RAs and with campus security. I got in trouble for drinking and other things. I also started to isolate. I was calling home very infrequently and lying about how things were going at school. I was going out less and less, choosing instead to stay in the dorm room alone or with a few other people. At the end of my first semester, I had a 1.3 GPA. My parents knew something was wrong, but I managed to convince them that drugs and alcohol were not the problem.

I returned to school after winter break. I knew using was causing problems and I was determined to improve that semester. I decided I would cut down on drinking and smoking and go to class. Within a week I was using just as much, and I was written up for my first drug violation. I was smoking pot in my room one afternoon, and someone called security. An officer banged on my door with his flashlight and confiscated my weed and some of my paraphernalia as well. A hearing was scheduled. I started ordering marijuana online at this point, having it sent to me through the mail from Canada. I didn't see the huge risk involved in this, and I was ordering pot in huge amounts. I was high all day, every day. I sealed up the cracks around my door with tape so that whenever I closed my door, I had an airtight seal. I was totally isolated whenever I wanted to be. Before my hearing came around for my drug violation, I was written up again and again. I set off the smoke alarm in my room late one night, and soon afterwards I was caught carrying alcohol across campus. Finally, I met with the judicial board, who decided that I would have to meet with a counselor on campus who specialized in drug and alcohol abuse. If I didn't comply with her recommendations, I would be kicked out of school housing.

I met with the counselor and was dishonest in my conversation with her as well as my responses to a written evaluation I filled out. Nevertheless, she realized that I had a problem with alcohol and marijuana, and she pointed this out to me. She recommended that I go to a rehabilitation program, so I agreed, realizing there was no way I could get out of it. I signed a release so she could speak with my parents and figure out the best course of action. I called my parents that night and told them what I had to do, but I was still unwilling to take responsibility. I blamed the counselor and the school for my problems. I was told I would be withdrawing from school on a medical leave and that I would be going to a rehab somewhere. I had one more week to wait at school, so I continued to use for that week. I figured I would have to go to a rehab program somewhere and at the end of the summer, I could go back to school and party again. I did not want to be sober. The first day of spring break came, and my dad came out to pick me up. My last use was on March 11th, about an hour before my dad arrived to pick me up. We drove home for what was the most uncomfortable eight hours of my life. I sat at home for a few days and, due to my health insurance, I was to go to an outpatient program for the rest of the summer instead of a 28-day inpatient. My parents said the only reason I didn't go to an inpatient was the physical change they saw in me after just a few days sober.

I was finally totally honest at the intake for the outpatient program. I started there the next day. At that program I learned about the disease of alcoholism and the importance of AA. I still didn't want to be sober for the first few weeks there, but I was willing to stay sober for the program and check it out. They forced me to start attending AA meetings and get a sponsor or I would not move on to the next group, which met only twice a week with a different counselor. I started going to meetings, a couple a week, but I didn't talk to many people and I didn't really want to be there. As I kept going back, I saw how happy people were when they were sober, and I realized how much better I felt. I looked back on how unmanageable my life was when I used. I finally got a sponsor and started to call him every day. I met many people in meetings who I related with and started to really want to be sober. I was in contact with the counselor from my school, who told me that the school had a recovery house, one of only a few in the country, for students just like me. I decided I would go back to (my college) that fall and move into the recovery house. I finished the outpatient program at the end of the summer. My employers pointed out to me how much of a helpful worker I was that summer. They had not told me what a great job I did in past years before I was sober. People were noticing a change in me.

I went back to school in August of 2006 and moved into the recovery house. There I met students in the same position as me. We started going to meetings together, a meeting just about every day. Recovery-based housing has been essential to my recovery. I probably would not have been able to return to college without such an opportunity. The support of the recovery house comes in many forms, and the challenges I would have faced if I attended a college without a residential recovery program would have been immense. The benefits of the recovery house include sober living, sober friends, recovery meetings, and helpful staff.

The first and most obvious benefit of the recovery house is a substance-free living and learning environment. University dormitories house some students who are using alcohol and other drugs, sometimes very frequently. Living in the recovery house affords me the opportunity to avoid being around alcohol and other drugs. Without this sober living and learning environment, returning to college in early sobriety would have been very difficult. Being in the presence of students using would be a constant temptation to relapse. Removing me from this dangerous environment has been one of the major benefits of the recovery house.

Along with this sober housing comes the support of other sober students in the recovery house. Attending college sober can be intimidating and lonely at times, and this would surely be so without the support of the other members of the recovery house. We have fun together doing things like taking trips to (a local) Amusement Park, spending time together after meetings, and going to parties together. More importantly, however, is the everyday support that comes with living with sober people. We talk to each other about how we are doing and we help each other with any problems we are having. We can also hold each other accountable, something which I have found very helpful in my recovery. Attending a college without a recovery house, I would have less contact with sober people and, therefore, less supportive help in staying sober.

Another example of the support of the recovery house is the help I receive through meetings each week. My treatment plan as a recovery house member includes attending a number of different meetings. There is a meeting each Monday in the recovery house with all the residents, the Resident Coordinator, and a counselor from University Counseling Services. I also attend a meeting Thursdays at University Counseling Services which is open to the whole campus, to anyone recovering from any dependency. The recovery house members share dinner in the House each Sunday, and we take turns cooking Sunday dinner. In addition, I attend 12-step meetings with other members of the recovery house. We even hold two such meetings in the recovery house on Friday and Saturday, which are open to the recovering community of (the local city). All of these meetings are essential to my recovery. While 12-step meetings are central to my recovery program, the other meetings I attend as a member of the recovery house also help to keep me focused and allow me to share with other people as well as to listen to them. Without the recovery house, I would have fewer opportunities to do this each week.

Another helpful element of the recovery house is the involvement of staff members. This includes counselors from University Counseling Services and College Behavioral Health and the Resident Coordinator, as well as members of the Advisory Board. Counselors take an active role in my recovery, facilitating the Monday recovery house meeting and the Thursday University Counseling Services meeting. They are extremely helpful in these meetings as well as outside of them. The Resident Coordinator lives in the recovery house and is always around to talk to or to help with anything. Another way the counselors and Resident Coordinator have helped me is through advocacy. After my first semester in the recovery house, I was placed on academic separation due to my poor academic performance. I had done poorly before I was sober and didn't make enough improvement in early sobriety to reverse this. I appealed this decision and, with the help of those involved in the recovery house, I was welcomed back to school to continue my education. This form of support is another one of the many examples of how the recovery house has helped me.

Without the recovery house, returning to college as a sober student would have been very difficult. The challenges of living in the dormitories, not having sober friends on campus, having less access to recovery meetings, and being without the help of staff members would have proven difficult. The support of the recovery house and the residents and counselors was essential—I would not have been able to return to (my college). I got a sponsor in (the local city) and started working the 12 steps with him. I got involved in meetings and met lots of sober people in (the local area). My first semester back was an improvement, but I still fell short of how I hoped to do academically. Now, in my second semester sober, I am doing really well in school. I still get to a meeting almost every day. I am able to show up in class and be a productive student. I can help out other people—even just by driving them to a meeting. I have a great relationship with my family again. I have met tons of friends in sobriety. I am truly happy and content with myself. On March 12, 2007, I celebrated a year of sobriety. It has been amazing looking back over the past year and seeing all the changes I have been through.

Dana O.

Describe how being a student in your school's program has impacted (positively or negatively) your relationships with students on campus who are not part of that program.

Hello, my name is Dana. I am a 22-year-old college student (in a collegiate recovery community). I was born just north of the Twin Cities in White Bear Lake to a very loving family. There was always incessant pressure that I felt from my parents to be involved in activities, get straight As, be in shape, and work out regularly. At one point in my life I was involved in nearly every sport possible—soccer, basketball, softball, competitive gymnastics. You name it, I tried it. There was a point when I got sick of the constant whirlwind that had become my life; I just wanted to stop. I was never good at communicating with my teammates. In all of the years I was involved in sports and activities, I had never made any friends. They had stayed "teammates" for all those years.

There was a point when I started not to care what my parents thought anymore, and I started to do what I wanted to do. I wanted to drink and get high. I wanted to go to parties and kiss boys. I loved the attention! When I was drinking and partying, I felt like I finally had friends. I was always invited to parties, always made people laugh, and the guys I hung out with were starting to find me attractive. I felt like I was on top of the world. By this point, I had gotten into trouble with the school, being restricted from involvement with any activities that were school related, including sports. I was in heaven, but I cannot say that my parents approved; yet this behavior continued throughout middle school and high school. I experimented with a lot of different drugs, but found my favorite had become cocaine, which came to an end when I discovered meth; meth's high was much better, lasted longer, and the drug itself was much cheaper. This "wonder drug" that I had discovered brought me several possession charges, helped me total two cars, got me arrested, and sent me through court—which finally led me to a choice I had to make: Did I want this for my life?

After deciding this was not the path I wanted to take in my life, I pled out in court and agreed to go to treatment. I soon entered a 28-day treatment program at (an adolescent residential treatment center). Directly following, I was sent to an all-woman's extended care facility. After completing four months of extended care, I returned to (the state where I had received treatment) to a halfway house, where I stayed an additional four months. This halfway house was more of a transitional period, where we were given more responsibilities, allowed to have a job and attend AA meetings on our own, with a few mandatory house meetings each week. After the four months at (my halfway house), I moved in with my parents for a month, until I could move into the (collegiate recovery community) at (my college).

In May 2004, I became a part of the (collegiate recovery community). I started taking classes that summer, worked a part-time job, and hung out with new friends I had found through the (collegiate recovery) program. Through (my collegiate recovery community), I learned to open up to and have substantial relationships with people, especially women. I learned to trust and to be honest and to share myself with others in the program. I never really knew who I was, and I was ashamed of whom I was; I learned that I was okay. (My collegiate recovery community) gives you access to licensed counselors, which we meet with weekly. It holds a Circle Meeting, which is a chance for everyone in the program to get together. Each week one individual tells his or her personal story, as a chance for us to get to know each member on a more personal level. We announce our anniversary/birthday dates to acknowledge personal victories, along with struggles within the group where extra support may need to be focused. There is also the CLASS office on campus, which helps us with our academics, by setting aside specific time increments each week to work on our studies. The CLASS office has tutors available for any additional help you may need. All of these aspects within the program concentrate on dealing with the mental and emotional stability and the academics of each individual student.

The only difference between a student in the (collegiate recovery) program and any other student at the college is that as a (collegiate recovery community) student, I live with people who are also in recovery. No student in any one of my classes would ever know I was in the program unless I told them. I still make friends, study, get coffee, and converse with students in my classes, experiencing the same college experiences as any other students. I just have additional resources/outlets on campus that are recovery-based and focus more on my mental/emotional needs.

I am in my fourth year at (my college); I will be graduating this winter, in December. I have been a part of (my collegiate recovery community) for the entirely of my time at the college. It has been such a great experience, and I have made such great friends that I just do not want to leave.

Ryan U.

As an alumnus of a university with a collegiate recovery community, how do you feel your experience at your college prepared you to live a clean and sober lifestyle after college?

My story is similar to many people's and begins in high school. My freshman year of high school I played soccer and refused to even smoke cigars with my friends. That quickly changed however by the time my sophomore year came around. At that point, I started drinking after school alone and with friends. I felt like the void of insecurity began to be filled and like I was fitting in. However, it didn't take long before I stumbled into my parent's friend's house in a blackout, and in another incident I was arrested for underage possession of alcohol. Eventually, it seemed easier to get and use marijuana, so I switched to using that particular substance during my junior year.

The toll my actions were taking on my family was felt immediately. There was constant arguing between myself and my mother and step-father. The cycle continued through my senior year, only growing in intensity and severity. Fortunately I did well enough to graduate and attend college; however my parents gave me an ultimatum: if I messed up in college, I would return home and go to rehab.

I'm grateful now, as that's exactly what happened. From the moment my parents dropped me off at college, I used. Eventually, I was kicked out of the dorms for possession and consumption of marijuana. I thought my life was completely ruined and that everything I worked hard for was destroyed. I attended an outpatient program, graduated, went to 12-step meetings, and after a period of several relapses finally now have six years of continuous recovery. With recovery I was able to get an Associate's degree from (a local college) and a B.A. from (a four-year college), study overseas, and just recently I have been accepted to a graduate school program at Johns Hopkins University in China. Besides being able to successfully go back to school, my relationship with my family is excellent, and most importantly I feel good about the person I am becoming.

While working on my B.A. degree, I lived in the recovery housing that's offered by (my college). The recovery house is administered and run through a division of the health services of (the university). The director of the program works in cooperation with Resident Life to oversee the housing. The program is a college dorm open only to students of the university with recovery-related issues. The program staff oversees admittance to the program, which can house 20-plus male and female residents.

The recovery house is run largely by the student residents. There are monthly "house" meetings where the staff and students meet to discuss house-related issues. A senior member of the house is also chosen to be the Resident Assistant, who works directly with the program's administration as well as Resident Life on campus.

Living in the recovery house did wonders for my recovery. First of all, as soon as I moved in, I immediately had a whole group of peers who I could identify with, hang out with, and have fun in recovery with. Having a network of people my own age in recovery, especially in a college environment, made it much easier for me to adapt to the college scene and do well in school. Many of the people became and still are my best friends, including my girlfriend who has been with me for the past four years. Also, I had the distinction of serving as the Resident Assistant for the recovery house for one semester.

Living in the recovery house also afforded me the opportunity to live on my own, take care of myself and have people who supported me in that process. That experience proves more valuable everyday as I continue to live a clean and sober life beyond my college experience.

While I was working on my B.A., I was really fortunate to be able to study abroad with a friend I met in the recovery housing. I started studying Chinese after the first semester I went to [this university] and was able to receive two scholarships to study in Taiwan the summer after my junior year. Once I graduated, my recovery house friend and I lived in Taiwan for a year, where I studied and taught English. We were able to stay clean and take a little piece of the recovery house with us to the other side of the world.

In all, my college experience would have been radically different if it weren't for the recovery house and the network of people I met there. It's something I'm extremely grateful for and has helped me live clean and sober, both in college and for the rest of my life.

Austin M.

What made you select a college with a collegiate recovery community instead of a college without one? Did you think going to a college without a collegiate recovery community was an option?

I was born November 7, 1982, in Oklahoma City, Oklahoma. My parents, Greg and Debbie, have been married for over 30 years now. I have one younger brother Ben. I was born into an upper-middle-class, Lutheran, Caucasian family. We lived in the suburbs of Oklahoma City my whole life. Family life was great. Both of my parents were very hard working and very passionate about their children. They both gave Ben and me the love that we needed as children. My childhood was great until about middle school.

When I started sixth grade, I was treated differently than most of the other kids. I wore glasses and was pretty smart. This made me an outcast of sorts, and eventually I began to socially isolate and slip into a state of depression. Depression is the word that would best characterize my mood for the next six years. I hated life, hated school, just plain hated. High school felt like a new start for me. I started by joining the debate team, which led me to both some of the worst and best outcomes of my early adolescence. I began to emulate the older debate students who drank and smoked cigarettes. I immediately became addicted to cigarettes and then started drinking. I remember vividly the first time I got drunk. I felt as if I would never have another negative emotion and would always be loved by everyone. The night promptly ended when I threw up in front of the whole party, right next to the keg.

My addiction was born on that night. I learned quickly that chemicals can fix the way I feel. If I feel depressed, I can smoke some pot. If I need to be able to interact socially, alcohol will bail me out. This cycle continued until it became one of the centralizing themes of who I was. I eventually got into harder drugs; cocaine, specifically, quickly brought me to my knees. I went from being an "A" student with much potential to a juvenile delinquent, constantly in trouble with my parents, the school, and eventually the police. My parents finally discovered my cocaine usage one summer night, and I was sent to a juvenile rehabilitation center promptly afterward.

In treatment, I learned a new way to live and a new reason for living. I discovered that masking negative emotions with chemicals just makes it that much worse. Processing emotion, I would say, was the greatest lesson I received from the treatment center. I left treatment after six months and headed to Dallas to try living on my own for a while before I went to school. I flourished there, learning much about being an adult and life in general.

The decision to go to school was one I intended to make but led me to a host of fears. The primary fear was that I would begin drinking again because I would have to enter into the world of my peers again. I feared that if I didn't somewhat assimilate back into my peer group, I would feel isolated and alone again. It was somewhat of a double bind in that I felt I was damned if I went to school and damned if I didn't. Additionally, I was damned if I joined my peer group and again damned if I didn't.

I learned about [my collegiate recovery community] when I first arrived in [a nearby city]. News of the program had spread by word of mouth. I knew once I heard of the [collegiate recovery community] I was going to go to school at [that college]; there were simply no other options in my mind. I knew that if I could get hooked into a group of my peers in recovery, I would have a chance to make it. I know myself very well, and because of that wasn't willing to trust myself in another environment. This was especially pertinent, since that I was so fragile in my recovery at the time. I was by my own account still quite immature and in the process of adolescent development—identity-wise—during this transition period. I believed that the collegiate recovery community would enable me to have a safe recovery environment to use as a springboard back into the world of my peers.

Now life is great. I am currently working on my Master's degree in Marriage and Family Therapy, and I hope to pursue a PhD when I'm finished with that. I've been clean and sober for over six and a half years now. I have transitioned well and feel that I am a very well-adjusted and socially secure person.

NOTE

1. This is in reference to the 2007 Joint Meeting on Adolescent Treatment Effectiveness (JMATE), at which all eight of the students represented here presented their stories and question responses as part of a panel.

Twelve Step Meeting—Step One

Recovery School Students

Jeffrey has entered Young People's Twelve Step Meeting

andrew has entered Young People's Twelve Step Meeting

Jeffrey says Hi, Andrew!

andrew says Hi

andrew says Looks good for the meeting tonight

Jeffrey says Thanks for your help. I am grateful that this chat room is functioning today.

andrew says Me too, it's my pleasure

Jeffrey says If you are OK with me staying in the room as a silent observer, that would help me collect the transcript.

andrew says No problem

Jeffrey says Thanks. Please let the others know when the meeting is happening that I am not responding so as to keep the meeting for all of you.

andrew says sure

Jeffrey says So I will stay in the room (unless, as sometimes happens, I am booted out, and then I will return.)

andrew says sounds good

Jeffrey says Fantastic. I hope you have a great first meeting!

andrew says Thanks. I'll be logging back in a little before 10:00 EST. See you then.

Jeffrey says I am leaving my computer now. I will be back at 10. Bye for now.

andrew has logged out

Jeffrey D. Roth, MD is present in the chat room to facilitate collection of the transcript. His presence at the meeting also provides an immediate representation of the readers' virtual presence here, since the members are aware that this transcript will be published. The process of the meetings being held is also challenged by some dysfunction of the chat room technology.

austinm62 has entered Young People's Twelve Step Meeting
austinm62 has logged out
austinm has entered Young People's Twelve Step Meeting
Andrew has entered Young People's Twelve Step Meeting
S_K_11 has entered Young People's Twelve Step Meeting
S_K_11 says Am I late?
Andrew says nope
austinm says how many more are we waiting for?
Andrew says hopefully 3 more
S_K_11 says Just making sure didn't know if EST was an hour ahead or behind me
Andrew says but we'll start in about 2 mins
austinm says k
Andrew says so Austin did you want to take the lead in setting up the next meeting?
austinm says sure, we should do this time again.
Andrew says this seemed to be the best time for everyone
S_K_11 says Yeah this time works out best for me as well
austinm says Hopefully everyone shows up and we can set a time for sure
Andrew says Yeah I hope
Andrew says Well we may as well get started for now
austinm says k
Andrew says Welcome to the Young People's 12 Step Meeting
Andrew says Jeffrey is here as an observer and to copy the meeting transcript.
Andrew says The topic for the meeting is Step 1
Andrew says Step one says We admitted we were powerless over alcohol-that our lives had become unmanageable.
Andrew says This meeting is not affiliated with any particular fellowship so feel free to comment about drugs or alcohol or anything else.
Andrew says To comment, type an ! and when you are called on you can comment.

Stef indicates her awareness of time boundaries, which is so often impaired during active addiction, and is often restored during recovery. Austin similarly indicates his awareness of group boundaries of membership.

Andrew exercises his authority as chair of the meeting to determine the starting time, and demonstrates his respect for the Tradition of rotating leadership of the meeting by offering to transfer authority for the next meeting to Austin.

Austin agrees to perform this service for the group, since service is understood to be useful as part of the process of recovery.
The group then effortlessly agrees on the boundaries of their next meeting, and proceeds to open the formal meeting with a welcome.
Andrew announces the presence of an observer, again indicating an awareness of group boundaries, and then sets the group task for this meeting, which is Step One. He continues with another boundary concerning the task; since this meeting is not an AA meeting or any other specific Twelve Step meeting, the discussion of Step One may relate to any area over which the member is powerless and which generates unmanageability.

Andrew says Type a couple sentences at a time and hit send so that we can read as you continue to type.
Andrew says Does anyone care to begin sharing on anything related to Step 1?
austinm says !
Andrew says Austin
austinm says I guess I'll start
austinm says I was sent to a treatment center on Aug. 24, 2000 by my parents. I was 17
austinm says I fought very hard when I first got there, I didn't think that anything that the treatment center was trying to sell applied to me.
austinm says I was miserable in the confines of the treatment center for about 3 months when I became very suicidal
austinm says At that time I decided that it was not normal that I was fighting to use cocaine again so bad taht I was willing to kill myself rather than be sober
austinm says That was when I first admitted that I was powerless over cocaine.
austinm says I began working the steps with a sponsor and also with the therapists at the treatment center.
austinm says They helped me to realize that my life was unmanagable way before I started cocaine
austinm says That realization really floored me, because I was such an egotistical prick that I thought that everyone else was my problem and I wasn't responsible for the state my life was in
austinm says Admitting that I was powerless over cocaine really helped me to put life back into perspective and turn my life around
austinm says I've been sober for about 6 1/2 years now thanks to that treatment center getting me started on my way
austinm says I guess I'll stop for now so I can give someone else a chance to talk, I'll speak more later if we have time
S_K_11 says thanks austin
Andrew says thanks Austin
Andrew says !
austinm says HI ANDREW!!!

Andrew concludes with some procedural boundaries, and then invites the group to participate.

Austin volunteers to open the sharing section of the meeting. He eloquently describes the unmanageability of his addiction in terms of his inability to accept help and support, either from his parents or from the treatment center, and his powerless over his addiction in terms of his willingness to die rather than stop using.

Austin them alludes to surrendering to a power greater than himself (Step 2) in working with a sponsor and his therapists.

Austin shares that he suffered from one of the typical defenses of the practicing addict, projection.

Note that 6 1/2 years later, Austin remains committed to sharing his story with others in the service of maintaining his recovery.

The group acknowledges Austin's contribution in the usual Twelve Step meeting fashion, and then welcomes Andrew to share.

S_K_11 says Hi andrew!
Andrew says I first got sober in a similar situation
Andrew says After basically destroying my opportunity at success in my first year of college
Andrew says I was written up a bunch of times
Andrew says I was sent to see a school counselor who specializes in drug and alcohol abuse.
Andrew says I had done really poorly my first semester, never going to class, skipping homeworks and tests, and so on
Andrew says So i figured for my second semester that I would just cut down on my use of drugs + alcohol and stick to just weekends
Andrew says Well, as soon as I started using, I couldn't stop
Andrew says Within a few days I was back where I had left off the month before
Andrew says After the writeups that followed and the meeting with the counselor, I had to start a treatment program or be kicked out of University housing
Andrew says I figured I would take an extended summer break and stay sober for a while and then go back to what I wanted to do, which was use
Andrew says I started an outpatient program last year in March and after a couple of weeks, the physical changes I began to notice was amazing
Andrew says I had to start going to meetings and I began to relate with other people there
Andrew says I saw that my life was totally unmanageable
Andrew says I started to realize I am powerless not over drugs and alcohol but a lot of things in my life
Andrew says That was really the beginning of my recovery.
Andrew says So with that I'll pass.
S_K_11 says thanks andrew
S_K_11 says !
austinm says thanks andrew, hi S K
Andrew says hi S K
S_K_11 says Hi my name is Stef I am an alcoholic and an addict

While commenting directly on what another members shares is discouraged, identification by offering similar experiences is an important part of the process of the Twelve Step group.

Andrew first offers a list of the ways in which his academic career was sabotaged by his addiction, and then indicates his powerless over his disease by his inability to cut down on his use, and his inability to stop.

Andrew is also honest about a common strategy among all addicts, which is to "go on the wagon" with the implicit intention to resume using.
He then offers his insight into how recovery took hold in his life by giving him the opportunity to experience a different physical, psychological and social way of being.

Andrew says Hi stef
austinm says hi stef
S_K_11 says Step on for me is similar to the both of yours, though I am younger
S_K_11 says I first started to use drugs and alcohol when I was in middle school, around age 12
S_K_11 says I would use only ocassionally on the weekends, but it slowly progressed into every other day to every day
S_K_11 says I went into my first out patient treatment program at age 14, I didn't understand why they didn't want me to experiment with drugs and alcohol after all I thought that was what teenagers were suppose to do
S_K_11 says Between 14 and 15 I attended 3 treatment centers, I didn't take anything seriously and continued to use
S_K_11 says untill the summer of 2005 I was a complete mess. I was 15 years old and was running away from home to get drugs and only caring about getting that next high
S_K_11 says I was then put into a impatient treatment center and I started to realize how powerless I was over drugs & alcohol
S_K_11 says I also became suicidal and didn't want to live. I felt there was nothing to live for. Once I got out of treatment I went to meetings.
S_K_11 says I began to see that the people at meetings were happy and had many things in common with me. I started to talk to people and got a sponsor, whom have helped me to get to 2 years sober coming up on 4/11
S_K_11 says I to have to remember that I am powerless over other things besides just drugs and alcohol such as, people places and things. I guess I will pass for now, thanks
Andrew says Thanks Stef
austinm says thanks stef
austinm says !
austinm says Hi, Austin I'm an addict
Andrew says Hi Austin
S_K_11 says Hey Austine
S_K_11 says austin* sorry
austinm says I guess some other things related to step 1 I could talk about is that recovery and step 1 in general apply to behavior after being sober as well as to drugs

Stef opens our eyes to a situation that most of us would like to deny: that drug and alcohol use may begin early and progress insidiously. How, at the age of 14, she received the idea that teenagers were supposed to be using alcohol and drugs is an important foundation for this book. Her continued use despite three treatments underscores the importance of integrating recovery into the educational community. She shares her identification with Austin's suicidality, and the relief that she received by attending meetings.

Since this is a small meeting, Austin offers to share again.

Stef's slip of the keyboard may represent a wish to have another female member of the meeting. She apologizes for the slip without interpretation.

austinm says I have gone through periods while in recovery in which my life was again unmanagable

austinm says I think it has everything to do with how I react to the world when I get depressed.

austinm says I've had many bouts of serious depression for my whole life

austinm says This pattern of depression continued on through my sobriety

austinm says I would sometimes go through a period of depression and act out in unhealthy ways that made my life unmanageable againn

austinm says One example of this was about 3 years ago.

austinm says I was having a major bout of depression coupled with an existential crisis in which I didn't know what I wanted to do for a career anymore or what I wanted to do with my life

austinm says I fixated and obsessed about poker during that time

austinm says I have always enjoyed poker and it seemed to be the only avenue that gave me any joy at that time

austinm says The poker made life even worse and I ended up dropping out of school for 2 semesters in a row

austinm says There were many other issues and extenuating circumstances goinng on at the time, for example obsessing abbout my girlfriend at the time and our horrible and chaotic relationship, but gambling was a big piece of the puzzle

austinm says I sort of had an epiphany with that situation when I realized that I needed to seek real help for my situation

austinm says I started goinng to therapy again and life really started to turn back around

austinm says I stopped playing poker for a while and eventually the girlfreind situation dissolved for good

austinm says I was close to using during this time

austinm says I realized that recovery and the first step does not just apply to using, it also applies to living.

austinm says For me to be in recovery, I need to be living a qualitatively differnent lifestyle than the one I had before

Austin takes up the implicit invitation from Stef to examine another area of powerlessness in his life, his use of gambling associated with periods of depression. Like alcohol and drugs, the impact of gambling and other compulsive behaviors on students may be minimized and underappreciated in our educational communities.

Austin's story indicates that even after sobriety from drugs and alcohol, the need for continued recovery extends into other areas of the recovering addict's life, including relationships. The unmanageability from these other areas may affect the addict's ability to remain sober. Fortunately, many recovering addicts recognize the need for and availability of help.

austinm says I still play poker today, but have learned when it is appropriate and healthy to do so.

austinm says I was frustrated because everyone labeled me a compulsive gambler at meetings and other recovery communities

austinm says I however have learned much about a healthy lifestyle and balancing fun with responsibility

austinm says I guess I'll stop rambling now

austinm says thanks

Andrew says Thanks Austin

S_K_11 says thanks austin

S_K_11 says !

Andrew says Hi Stef

austinm says hi stef

S_K_11 says Hello, well i liked what Austin had to say about how step one is not just for staying sober and not using, and about how it is used in living

S_K_11 says Step one is somethinG I have to remind myself of daily

vijay has entered Young People's Twelve Step Meeting

S_K_11 says The powerlessness over not only drugs and alcohol but people places and things

vijay says Hi everyone – sorry I'm late, I just got back from my homegroup, forgot we had a business meeting

S_K_11 says When I am at work, school, around family, and friends I always have to remember that I am powerless over them and their actions

Andrew says it's ok

S_K_11 says I can really work my self up when I want to control outcomes of situations or the way that people act

S_K_11 says I also have to accept that I am powerless.

S_K_11 says Well I feel like I am rambling [img id=em-10] so i will pass. thanks

Andrew says Thanks Stef

vijay says thanks for sharing!

austinm says thanks stef

Andrew says !

S_K_11 says hi andrew

vijay says hi andrew

austinm says hi andrew

Significantly, Austin chooses a different "bottom line" for his poker playing than for his alcohol and drug use. He does not see himself as a compulsive gambler. He demonstrates to us the importance of humility and maintaining an open mind with respect to the process of recovery. When he says he will "stop rambling for now," he does not indicated whether he is aware of the play on words, "rambling" and "gambling," but the effect seems to achieve his balance of fun with responsibility.

Vijay's name has been changed to protect his anonymity. Note how his late arrival does not disrupt the flow or the process of the meeting. As Stef notes, those in recovery from addiction engage in the group process, they accept their powerlessness over people, places and things in addition to their addiction. Therefore, the group accepts its powerlessness over a member who shows up late. Andrew, who chairs the meeting, uses his authority to welcome Vijay, and the meeting proceeds seamlessly.

Andrew says Thanks for your comments so far, I like what has been said about remembering I'm powerless over lots of things and about remembering Step 1 every day

Andrew says For me, remembering I'm powerless over other people, places and things is essential

Andrew says I often find myself trying to control situations and people that I'm powerless over

Andrew says My support group, especially my sponsor, is helpful in pointing this out.

Andrew says I try to get to a lot of beginner's meetings and talk to new people to remind myself that I'm powerless over drugs + alcohol

Andrew says I often hear people say that step 1 is the only step I have to work perfectly

Andrew says Because if I forget I'm powerless then why not take that first drink

Andrew says So thanks again, I'll pass

S_K_11 says thanks andrew

austinm says thanks andrew

Andrew says Any further comments? We still have a bit more time.

Note that Andrew makes space for Vijay to share, but no one pressures Vijay.

austinm says I'm good

S_K_11 says I think thats all for me tonight

Andrew says Ok then, if you could please join me in (saying, not typing) the serenity prayer:

Andrew turns over leadership of the next meeting in advance.

Andrew says Thanks for coming tonight, thanks for your comments, and I believe Austin is taking the lead in the next meeting, so check your email for more info i guess.

austinm says Ill email everyone that didnt make it, lets do 10 EST next sunday

austinm says That Vijay?

Again, the group includes Vijay in the group conscience, whether or not Vijay chooses to participate.

austinm says work for you I meant to type

S_K_11 says Sounds good to me. Thanks a lot guys. I enjoyed the meeting

austinm says K see you all next sunday at 10 est

Andrew acknowledges my presence at the very end of the meeting with regard to the task of recording the transcript. Note that Vijay has not yet logged out.

Andrew says ok, later all

S_K_11 says sounds good Thanks. Take care

austinm has logged out

Andrew says DId you get the transcript Jeffrey?

S_K_11 has logged out

Andrew has logged out

Schools as a Collection of Groups and Communities

Seth Harkins, EdD
Jeffrey D. Roth, MD

ABSTRACT. When viewed as social systems, schools are a collection of groups and communities. An effective way to understand schools is from the vantage point of social systems theory. The concepts of boundaries, boundary managers, roles, authority, splitting, projection, and projective identification are particularly useful in understanding schools as dynamic systems. From this perspective, the school board defines policies and procedures, which set forth the boundaries that govern behavior by students, parents, and community members. Administrators set forth the procedures that regulate these boundaries and provide authority and leadership for the academic, social-emotional and behavioral growth of students. Where school personnel model healthy behaviors and effective, rational problem solving, schools have the capacity to be embracing and inclusive. Where school personnel model addictive behavior, students learn addictive behavior through the hidden curriculum, which covertly teaches the values, beliefs, and defense mechanisms associated with addictive behavior. Within each school community are behavioral expectations, and when these expectations are violated, systems split off the violating behavior into alternative structures. Some students who violate these norms may require specialized settings in which to address such complicated and complex behaviors. This is particularly the case with students with social-emotional and behavioral problems

Seth Harkins, EdD, is in the Illinois Department of Human Services, Chicago, IL 60634.

Jeffrey D. Roth, MD, is in Working Sobriety, Chicago, IL 60602.

and addiction, which cannot be addressed within the traditional school setting. For these youth alternative schools are required. Effective alternative schools function as benevolent holding environments, which are structured enough to contain problems and flexible enough to facilitate growth and recovery through relationship-based intervention models. These programs are effective if they are operationalized from a systems and organizational perspective and linked to partnerships within a broader system of care within the larger community.

INTRODUCTION

In this chapter we set forth five arguments about schools and addiction. First, we contend that schools can be understood from a psychoanalytic social systems approach, the Tavistock group relations model. From this perspective, schools are open systems and are a collection of groups and communities. Second, we maintain that addiction is "any substance or process that has taken over our lives and over which we are powerless" (Schaef & Fassel, 1988). From this vantage point, almost anything can be addictive and may be practiced by individuals, groups, or organizations. Third, we hold that it is a myth that youth learn about drugs, alcohol, and addiction primarily from their peers. It is our position that schools caught up in the addictive process model addictive thinking and behavior. Fourth, schools systems are like family systems when dealing with addiction. Where families enforced covert family rules to further denial and the addictive process, schools do similarly through a hidden curriculum that covertly teaches the values, beliefs, and behavior necessary for addiction to thrive but go unnoticed. Lastly, we hold that alternative schools offer hope for schools and communities and that if recovery is to be effective, it must occur organizationally.

Schools as Complex Social Systems

Educational systems are a collection of groups and communities that can be described as having defined inputs and outputs accomplished by individuals with designated boundaries, roles, authority, and tasks. The explicit input of an educational system is its student population; the output consists of its graduated students. The boundaries of the system are defined in terms of time (duration of the educational process) and space (the physical campus of the educational environment). The roles within an educational system include student, teacher, administrator, and support personnel. Authority generally flows from administration to teachers and to support personnel, with students occupying the role of followers. The explicit task of the educational system is learning for the students, and professional employment for the teachers, administrators and support personnel.

However, as in any complex system, implicit tasks may enhance or interfere with the primary task, which is learning. The major implicit task in an educational system is socialization, and this task affects all members of the system from the top down. We suggest that addiction in its various forms represents the most important obstacle to functional socialization in the educational system, and that recovery from addiction is a powerful support to this process of socialization. Ironically, popular culture supports the myth that the culture of addiction is learned by the student in the educational system from the peer group, rather than imported into the educational system through the families in the educational community, including those in authority (administrators, teachers and support personnel). This mythology leads to the assumption that the student population consists of two groups, winners and losers, and that the strategy of optimal socialization involves joining the winners and shunning the losers, who are the unsuccessful addicts. Powell, Farrar, and Cohen (1985) conceptualized schools as a shopping mall in which there were winners and losers in the educational marketplace. The shopping mall metaphor suggests that school policy, curriculum, and instructional practices involve appealing to competing producers and consumers of knowledge. The producers involve the board of education, administrators, faculty, and nonprofessional staff. The consumers involve students, parents, and community groups. Products important to these producers and consumers involve policies, curriculum, instruction, and cocurricular activities relating to a wide range of students, including mainstream students, talented and gifted students, vocational technical students, special-education students, athletes, band and orchestra students, fine arts students, world language students, and others. These authors do not mention one implicit product of the educational system, which is the system's support for the practice of addiction. Indeed, the assumption that producers' and consumers' competing, rather than mutually supportive interests, may underlie the justification for the continued practices of addictive behavior.

To understand schools as a marketplace, it is important to understand schools as a collection of groups and communities from the vantage points of systems and organizational theory. Social systems theorists (Berttalanfy, 1969; Miller & Rice, 1978; Stapley, 2006) maintain that all systems are dynamic and interactive in which change in any part of the organism or organization results in change to some degree or another in other parts of the system. According to this theory, the whole is greater than the sum of the parts, and human growth and development is viewed from an ecological perspective, integrating psychological and sociological dimensions of reality. Note this theory provides the basis for an interdependent model of functioning, where the entire system needs to be involved in problem solving if dysfunctional dynamics are to be successfully addressed.

Central to systems theory is the notion that systems and subsystems are bounded entities, operating along a continuum of open to closed. Open systems are said to be permeable, while closed systems are nonpermeable. Boundaries between systems and subsystems do two things. First, they provide definition and identity, and, second, information is exchanged within and across the boundaries. Boundary management is important to this flow of information and serves to establish the steady state of the system, or homeostasis. In schools, boundary management is represented in a number of ways. The board of education develops policy that gives definition and importance to values, roles, and behavior in the system. A superintendent and principals carry policies into professional practice, as do teachers, who translate curriculum policy into instructional practice. Counselors, social workers, school psychologists, and para-educators are also boundary regulators in their support of the primary task of the system, which is the care, intellectual growth, and social-emotional development of students. In short, boundaries and boundary management define the roles of professionals, students, groups, and communities.

In an open system, recovery from addiction becomes a process that the entire system embraces. Boundary management is accomplished with the cooperation of all the parts of the system that exercise authority. This principle has far-reaching implications for the educational system that wishes to provide opportunities for recovery from addiction to its students; the most important of these implications is the necessity for those in authority to be aware of and actively engaged in their own processes of recovery from addiction.

Psychoanalytic social systems theory (Bion, 1961; Miller & Rice, 1975; Rioch, 1975a; DeBoard, 1978; Kets de Vries & Miller, 1984; Hirschhorn, 1988; Stapley, 2006) is particularly useful to the study of educational systems as collections of groups and communities, especially in understanding how addiction and its concomitant anxiety, fear, and affect influence schools and their relationships with various groups and communities. This perspective incorporates the psychosocial life of schools. Addiction and denial, its primary defense mechanisms, profoundly influence schools, as systems. Anxiety, fear, or affect experienced in any one subsystem has an impact in all others subsystems, and thus maintenance of individual, group, or organizational balance relates directly to how emotional life is expressed, mobilized, and harnessed. A teacher working with a particular student or group of students may have his or her teaching or behavior management affected by anxiety over the students' sense of adequacy, which is often colored by addiction in the student or the student's family. Conflict between rival student groups, which often serves as masks for addictive behavior, may color the emotional life of the school as a whole or a certain grade level. Anxiety within a classroom may make instruction particularly challenging. Political advocacy can influence the tone and progress of a board of education meeting. Those things that are disruptive to the homeostasis tend to be regarded as threatening, deviant and throwing the system out of balance. Like individuals, schools maintain defense mechanisms to protect against being overwhelmed by addiction and its attendant anxiety, fear or suppressed affect.

Psychoanalytic systems theory also helps us to understand the overt and covert processes in a school system, or the rational and irrational aspects of the system. The formal curriculum, for example, represents the rational technical dimension of the school. The unspoken values and beliefs employed in the teaching-learning process constitute the hidden curriculum. This is often seen in the treatment of class, race, ethnicity, gender, and sexuality in school curriculum and instruction. It is also evident in addiction in schools, as the modeling of compulsive, addictive behavior is learned through the hidden curriculum. By design, schools are intended to be rational institutions. However, school systems are human enterprises, and the personalities of individuals and groups, and how they employ conscious and unconscious behavior, strongly influences the extent to which boundaries are open or closed or functional or dysfunctional. Responses to addiction run the gamut from rigidly controlling to permissive and boundariless. Some administrators, teachers, and support personnel are rigid, while others are permissive, and still others operate between these poles in the realm of creative and flexible. This accounts for one of the reasons why schools, as systems, often have distinctly different cultures, for the norms of the boundary managers differ from school to school, if not classroom to classroom, or community to community. Students and student groups are expected to fit within these norms or risk being defined as deviant, which may be the label applied to those with addictions.

Central to this theory are the concepts of splitting, projection, introjection, and projective identification. According to these notions, all individuals and groups manage the pain of anxiety and affect by splitting off uncomfortable or unwanted feelings and projecting them onto or into others. Projection is common to the human condition because individuals, without adequate social support, cannot completely contain anxiety and affect without becoming overwhelmed and self-destructive. This process of splitting and projecting develops as the infant differentiates and separates from his or her mother or primary caretaker, and sometimes mother is the "good mother" and sometimes the "bad mother," depending on whether primary needs are met within a safe holding environment. How an infant develops is dependent on what kind of holding environment the parents create for the child. A healthy holding environment permits the child to experience a wide range of thoughts, feelings, and fantasies, including those that are unpleasant. Unfortunately, the holding environment that is struggling with its own intolerable addiction may not be available to support the healthy emergence of the child's needs.

It is through this process that personality emerges and ideas about authority, leadership, and groups evolve. At the most primitive, infantile-level anxiety, love, or hatred is projected onto neutral screens or into receptacles. Infants, for example, project anxiety, fear, and hatred onto mothers, who may be perceived as "good" or "bad depending on how the infant perceives maternal or caretaker responses. When an individual acts on the projection, projective identification occurs. Since splitting and projection is the vehicle by which individuals first interpret external reality, caretakers can be internalized as "good" or 'bad" depending on how dependency needs are met or not met. As the infant matures, fathers, teachers, and other authority figures, groups, and organizations become receptacles for projection of anxiety, fear, hatred, envy, greed, or jealousy. It is through this process that the infant differentiates himself or herself from primary caretakers or from the "me" and the "not me." Splitting the world into "good" and "bad," the infant establishes a sense of self and nonself.

In schools school systems, functional classrooms operate as holding environments similar to that established by the child's mother. Optimal learning occurs in safe and nurturing learning environments. Administrators, teachers, students, parents, or groups may be the object of projections and thus "good" or "bad." Similarly, when anxiety, fear, and so on are accepted by the projection object, they are said to be introjected and internalized as subjective reality. Individuals or groups who internalize negative perceptions of themselves and then act on them through projective identification are vulnerable to isolation and scapegoating. Some student groups come to perceive themselves as damaged, defective, or otherwise deviant because the source of the projection cannot tolerate holding an unwanted part of himself or herself. Individuals or groups that promote such perceptions relieve themselves of the anxiety, fear, hatred, or envy that is stimulated by individual or group differences. When this is generalized, scapegoating occurs. In schools, there may be any number of scapegoats, from the disruptive student in the class to students in the lower curriculum tracks to "freaks," "druggies," "burnouts," "bandees" or "speds." Importantly, adults model this process of splitting, projection, and scapegoating, whether they are adults in the families or in the schools. The modeling of addictive behavior by school personnel has significant implications for the hidden curriculum, which covertly teaches students values, beliefs, and addictive behaviors, including denial, rationalization, and suppression of affect.

Case Studies of Adult Models of Addictive Behavior in Schools

It is often said that schools are the reflection of the community. School personnel and students reflect a community in which addiction thrives in the schools. Addictive behavior within the community is this imported into the school system. Schools and addiction function very much like families and addiction. Regardless of the addiction of choice, schools are profoundly impacted by the addicted adults' attitudes, behavior, and performance, which are reflected in the hidden curriculum. The modeling of compulsive, addictive behaviors forms the foundation for denial within schools, blinding school personnel and families to the impact of addicted school personnel and addiction within the student body. The dynamics of denial of addictive behavior and manifestation of maladaptive defense mechanisms are evident in the following case studies. These case studies are based on an accumulation of experiences. The school district and characters are fictitious.

1. The Case of Janice McNamara and Grand Prairie Middle School

The Grand Prairie School District serves five thousand students with six hundred staff. Grand Prairie educates children K-12 from three communities, two of which are economically advantaged and one of which is ethnically diverse. The district's elementary, middle, and high schools are well recognized for educational excellence. The board of education consists of five men and two women. The superintendent, Dr. Gerald March, has a national reputation as a leader committed to both excellence and innovation.

Grand Prairie Middle School (GPMS) is a school of one thousand students in grades six through eight. The building is led by a very able principal, Dr. James Hoffman. The GPMS middle school community is considered a difficult community from the standpoint that parents have high expectations and make it known with considerable frequency. Often this is evident in the volume of telephone calls and e-mails to faculty and administrators with requests for special accommodations for their children.

In a community of upwardly mobile professionals, who have relatively easy access to medical and legal resources, the special education program takes on particular significance, as many families with disabled children move to Grand Prairie for its fine special education services. Many parents believe their disabled children should be enrolled in Janice McNamara's special educational class. Many families pursue private, independent evaluations and employ special education advocates and attorneys to ensure that their children receive all the services to which their children are entitled by federal and state law and then some. Enrollment in Ms. McNamara's class is governed by Grand Prairie School District guidelines for special education eligibility, Individual Education Program (IEP) development and placement. The entry boundary is regulated by the Grand Prairie Student Services Team (SST), a multidisciplinary group consisting of the principal, school psychologist, school social worker, special education teacher, and other professionals as necessary to understand the needs of a given student. Although there are entrance criteria, admission to the special education program sometimes yields to parental pressure and influence.

Ms. McNamara, an intelligent and articulate instructional leader, is widely regarded as a creative instructor. A large woman with a reputation for a quick wit, McNamara also has a reputation for excessive drinking, particularly at faculty gatherings. On Friday nights, for example, McNamara and a small cadre of disaffected GPMS faculty retire to the Cozy Restaurant and Tap, where McNamara binges and the participants trade gossip and complain of administrators and "pushy" parents.

Within the community, Ms. McNamara developed extensive relationships with private practitioners, clinical psychologists, licensed clinical social workers, and psychiatrists. Families eager to get their children enrolled in Ms. McNamara's class frequently approached her for advice. This set up a collusion between McNamara, parents, and private providers regarding eligibility and educationally related services, such as school counseling. This codependent relationship between McNamara and parents angered the Grand Prairie administration because it blurred professional boundaries and was role inappropriate.

Within the faculty, Ms. McNamara was a formidable force. Her sharp intellect and quick wit were ever apparent in faculty meetings. She was adept at derailing established agendas and "going off" on administrators or fellow educators. An imposing physical presence, Ms. McNamara frequently attacked administrators as insensitive tools and lackeys of the district administration. When unsuccessful at attacking the building administration, Ms. McNamara directed her verbal assaults on district administrators as the "them" that controlled the school district and fostered mediocrity and suppressed teacher creativity. She was also known to openly question the competency of teachers in faculty forums, such as building or district-wide committees. Ms. McNamara was feared by her teaching colleagues, as she was a master of gossip who did not hesitate to "put people in their place" if they questioned or opposed her. Through an insidious use of humiliation and sarcasm, Ms. McNamara raised scapegoating to an art form.

Ms. McNamara's power was buttressed by three factors. First, because the special education program was high-profile and sought by many parents, McNamara cultivated a reputation in the community as a strong advocate for special needs students. Second, McNamara managed to hold together an alliance with articulate but disaffected teachers who enabled her acting out and her compulsive and addictive behavior. Third, she was successful in getting administrators to bow to her will. Administrators managed Ms. McNamara by giving in to her demands and thereby further enabling her. They often allied with her as a way of deflecting her covert and overt attacks on their authority.

Dr. James Hoffman, the principal of GPMS, broke ranks with his predecessors and attempted to limit Ms. McNamara's acting out in faculty meetings. After one of Ms. McNamara's particularly bombastic assaults on authority, Dr. Hoffman suspended Ms. McNamara from faculty meetings. Furious, McNamara escalated her covert activity within the faculty and the community. Believing Ms. McNamara to have undue influence regarding admission to the special education program, Dr. Hoffman reduced her teaching load in the special program, assigning her to several general education classes and assigning another teacher to work part time in the program. Enraged at this move, Ms. McNamara began a whispering campaign to influential parents, who appealed to Superintendent March to intervene on her behalf. When Dr. March refused, parents flooded board of education members with telephone calls and e-mails regarding their concerns. The board president agreed to provide time during the public comment section of the board meeting for parents to be heard. The parents usurped the public comment session and railed for most of the night about administration diluting excellence and promoting Ms. McNamara as the savior of special needs children.

In view of the intense pressure, Dr. March reluctantly urged Dr. Hoffman to reconsider his position regarding Ms. McNamara's teaching assignment. The upshot was that Dr. Hoffman was forced to reverse himself. Within the year, Dr. Hoffman resigned to assume a principalship in another district. In the end, no one addressed Ms. McNamara's addiction, codependency with faculty and parents, and the pattern of authority problems. The dysfunctional relationships and dynamics were repeated with Dr. Hoffman's successor.

2. The Case of Martin Williams and Grand Prairie Elementary School

Grand Prairie Elementary School (GPES) is located in one of the most affluent areas of the district. Students are bright and score very high on state and local achievement tests. As principal, Martin Williams was known to be a powerful force in his community and influential within the district administrative team. A man of two hundred and fifty pounds, Mr. Williams's addiction of choice was food and compulsive overeating and workaholism. He prided himself as a gourmet cook and often brought exotic dishes to the school's teacher lounge. Mr. Williams's addiction was also marked by compulsive behavior, which was particularly evident in the numerous times during the year when he rearranged his office furniture. His compulsivity was most evident in his attention to detail and controlling behavior. Williams worked excessive hours and his car was parked in the school parking lot on weekends. A perfectionist, Mr. Williams was intolerant of the smallest errors. He held his faculty and staff to high standards, which many regarded as beyond reason, such as his penchant for expecting non-tenured teachers to work beyond the hours stipulated in the Grand Prairie Board of Education and Teachers Association Agreement. A principal with a steel-trap mind, Mr. Williams used his tongue to lash teachers, who left his meetings feeling demeaned and humiliated. He was also well known for talking behind their backs about teachers he considered troublesome.

A man who had a gift for charm, the staff often experienced him as manipulative, controlling, and seductive. GPES teachers strongly felt that he played favorites within the faculty, which made them leery and fearful of teacher evaluations. Despite the fact that Mr. Williams had an excellent grasp of curriculum and instruction, teachers did not see his instructional advice as helpful. Particular angst was raised when Mr. Williams would take over a teacher's class and conduct a demonstration lesson.

Mr. Williams' addiction was also apparent in his difficulty managing interpersonal boundaries. Teachers felt that parents had the run of the school, as there were few controls on parents entering the building and going to their children's classes to drop off lunches, lunch money, or just "pop in" to briefly chat with their child's teacher. This left teachers feeling unsafe and vulnerable to having their classrooms micromanaged by "helicopter" parents, who attempted to micromanage their child's teacher and classroom. Insecure about his position and having an intense desire to be liked, Mr. Williams cultivated relationships with key parents, whom he openly regarded as his form of tenure.

The physical arrangement of the principal's office made the boundary management problems further evident. The waiting area outside Mr. Williams's office had a workstation for the school secretary. The work area had no counter or workspace demarcation. Consequently, students, teachers, and parents seeking attention from Mr. Williams frequently overwhelmed the secretary. Despite the loose boundary regulation, Mr. Williams could suddenly shift into control mode, giving curt directions and orders.

Mr. Williams's boundary management and interpersonal problems were especially manifest in GPES faculty meetings. Mr. Williams maintained tight control over the meeting agendas. Although he provided for faculty input regarding certain issues, he managed to lay the groundwork for orchestrated input, which the faculty experienced as inauthentic. Beneath the surface of the faculty was a strong current of resentment. A subgroup of disaffected teachers mobilized to challenge Mr. Williams' control. Faculty meetings became tense and a subgroup of teachers acted covertly to sully Mr. Williams's reputation in the district by complaining to teacher union leaders about his management style.

Mr. Williams' controlling personality was still further evident in district administrative team meetings. He was quick to criticize district administrators within meetings and follow his critiques with telephone campaigns to principals after meetings. Superintendent March admired his intellect but was wary of his influence with GPES parents, who were quick to mobilize when there was an objection to the implementation of policy. Dr. March was further concerned about Mr. Williams' mental state, as he frequently appeared to March to be highly anxious and stressed by his staff and community. As the relationship between Williams and his faculty deteriorated, Dr. March was made aware by the union leadership of the poor morale at GPES. By this time, parental concern and discontent over GPES morale was bubbling up to the superintendent. Dr. March believed an administrative intervention was necessary to address the morale problem and hired Dr. Elizabeth Schaeffer, a clinical psychologist from Metropolitan University, to serve as a consultant and help GPES improve its climate and morale. It was March's hope that Mr. Williams and the GPES faculty could work out their differences with Dr. Schaeffer as mediator.

Dr. Schaeffer met weekly with Mr. Williams and attended faculty meetings. Through counseling and coaching, she provided management consultation to Mr. Williams and the faculty. Dr. March and Dr. Schaeffer agreed that if the relationship between Mr. Williams and his staff did not improve, a radical intervention would be necessary. That intervention was to not renew Mr. William's contract and to transfer the most disaffected and acting out staff to different buildings.

Things came to a head when a third-grade class spun out of control. The third-grade teacher had poor classroom management skills. Bright and articulate students consistently challenged the teacher's authority, which prompted disciplinary interventions by the teacher and principal. Unfortunately, these were short-lived interventions and the morale of the classroom deteriorated, as had the morale of the faculty building wide. As things worsened, Mr. Williams came under siege by parents and his faculty. Dr. Schaeffer was unable to mediate the differences between Williams and his faculty and ultimately Dr. March took action, not renewing Williams' contract and transferring oppositional teachers to other buildings within the district. In the end, things settled down as a new principal took over a reconstituted faculty. Unfortunately, no one addressed Mr. Wlliams's addiction, his codependent relationship with parents, and the parallel process that occurred between faculty and student behavior.

3. The Case of Dr. Harold Carson and Grand Prairie High School

Grand Prairie High School has a national reputation for excellence in education. The vast majority of its students are college bound for prestigious colleges and universities. The principal, Dr. Harold Carson, was principal for 10 years. In the early years of his principalship, Dr. Carson hired a number of young, energetic, and talented teachers. In each of the core content and elective departments, Dr. Carson created a first rate faculty with excellent departmental instructional leaders. Dr. Carson also built an administrative team that was equally talented. It was also deeply loyal to Dr. Carson. A charismatic leader, Dr. Carson also earned the loyalty of his faculty. He was renowned for providing acknowledgments and rewards for teaching excellence. Within the community, he was extremely popular. Indeed, he had more power and strength in the community than Superintendent March.

However, Dr. Carson was not without his flaws. The tremor in his left hand was emblematic of his alcoholism. With a partiality for fine scotch whiskey, Dr. Carson had high blood pressure often associated with alcoholism. Further, Dr. Carson's thinking and behavior reflected the obsessions and compulsions of an addicted person. Dr. Carson was charismatic, but he was also grandiose. He could grand stand with the best of leaders. To be sure, he could tell an off-color joke in almost any audience and get away with it. "That was just Harry Carson" people would say. He was obsessed with detail and vacillated between micromanaging and over delegating. Things were expected to go well or there was hell to pay with Dr. Carson's wrath. With biting criticism, sarcasm, and harshness, Dr. Carson could reduce an administrator or teacher to tears, and then praise and stroke the very same administrator or teacher. Although one could argue that building a school of excellence required a high degree of accountability, it was Carson's tendency to be overbearing and menacing with employees about their performance that was at issue.

Carson's problems with alcohol colored his approach to students struggling with addiction. It was not uncommon for GPHS parents to hold prom and turnabout dance parties where liquor was freely served under parental supervision. While publicly Carson was critical of such parties, he turned a deaf ear when it came to working with groups like the Grand Prairie Alliance Against Drug Abuse. Faculty frequently expressed concern about student leaders and athletes who were known to be drinking and substance abusing. Alcohol- and drug-related vehicular accidents were well known within the faculty and student body. The deaths of several intoxicated students mobilized school and community concern for a short period of time and then student practicing of addiction returned to normal.

In an affluent community, students had ready access to illegal substances. Dr. Carson was frequently at odds with Georgia Beatty, the assistant principal for guidance services, over student addiction. Dr. Carson

encouraged Beatty and her staff to refer substance-abusing students to rehabilitation hospitals and then, upon reentry, placement into special education. In Beatty's view, Dr. Carson wanted to sanitize regular education and
split off addicted students into the special education subsystem. The special
education administrator, Dr. Brent Morgan, staunchly resisted Dr. Carson's
position. Georgia Beatty found herself riding an uncomfortable boundary
between special education, her guidance counselors, and Dr. Carson. Guidance professionals were particularly frustrated because they had nothing
significant to offer students returning from rehabilitation facilities. In their
view, the special education alternative school seemed to be a reasonable
outlet for dealing with substance abusing youth. Blocked by the special
education administrator, who did not believe substance-abusing students
were disabled within the meaning of state and federal law, counselors
were frequently bitter and felt powerless. They often found themselves negotiating arrangements with teachers when recovering students reentered
midway through the academic quarter or semester and then witnessed them
crash and burn academically and socially. Moreover, they were powerless to
challenge addiction as a family disease and community problem. Although
a Student Assistance Team was established at GPHS, it was primarily a
pipeline to rehabilitation facilities. The tension between special education
administration and Beatty and her counselors increased, with conflict playing out in the building's Student Services Team, a multidisciplinary group
that reviewed students with multiple failures, need for special education,
or return from psychiatric or rehabilitation facilities. Special education
administrators and counselors were at loggerheads, unless the recovering
student could be shown to be emotionally disturbed and a candidate for the
district's special education alternative school. Tired of riding the boundary
between his guidance staff, Dr. Carson, and special education administration, Georgia Beatty resigned her position and returned to her former role
as a social studies teacher.

As Carson became closer and closer to retirement, he became increasingly less physically and emotionally available to his administrators, department chairs, and faculty leadership. It was not uncommon for
Dr. Carson to arrive at school at ten o'clock in the morning and leave before
three. His administrators covered for him and rationalized his abbreviated
school day as necessary because of the evenings he spent working in the
community. As he became increasingly isolated, these loyal, codependent
administrators picked up the leadership slack. The assistant principal for
curriculum and instruction stepped in and effectively ran the building. The
other assistant principals kept up a positive image and skillfully managed

school–community relations. At age sixty-five, Dr. Carson retired. Accolades abounded for his leadership. Unfortunately, Carson's alcoholism and his codependent relationship with his administrative team were never addressed.

These case studies illustrate the impact of addiction on school climates and cultures. The principle defense mechanisms employed by these schools involved denial, splitting, and projection. As with families in denial of an addicted parent and enabling spouse and/or children, school leaders struggling with addiction often go unchallenged. The result is that addicted adults model addictive behavior for students, setting up an unfortunate parallel process, which often is mirrored in the community. This modeling also sets up a hidden curriculum in which students are covertly socialized to accept compulsive, addictive thinking and behavior as the norm. This creates a school climate for student addiction to which school leaders turn a blind eye because to address the problem as a school and school community would unconceal the "family secret" and the covert "family rules" that enable it.

Alternative Schools and Addiction

Organizational theory is yet another way to make sense of schools as a collection of groups and communities and addiction. This is particularly true when considering alternative learning environments such as special classrooms or alternative schools. Skrtic (1991), Weick (1976), and Boleman and Deal (1997) maintain that there are three paradigms of organizations. The first is the rational machine bureaucracy, which addresses needs and behavior through uniform or standard knowledge and procedures. The rational machine bureaucracy is most evident in the way students are processed through the educational system. Things are done "by the book" and the curriculum is standardized. This is particularly the case when students are identified and referred to special programs. Students who do not fit the standard curriculum are squeezed into alternative structures because the system lacks the skills necessary to embrace such students and include them in the mainstream of school life. Thus, the more rationalized the machine bureaucracy the more difficult it is for schools to handle difference and diversity, and addiction, splitting it off into separate educational structures.

The second organizational paradigm is the professional bureaucracy. This involves the infrastructure necessary for organizations to train and socialize its members. In schools, the professional bureaucracy is important in building the teacher's instructional repertoire to deal with a wide range of student needs. The degree to which students are included in the mainstream of school life is predicated upon the skill sets of the faculty to meet a wide range of student needs and learning and behavioral styles. When the school system lacks a professional development bureaucracy with which to socialize faculty into accepting diversity within the student body, the teachers lack an adequate professional tool kit to address the diverse needs of the student body. Schools that lack an effective professional development bureaucracy resort to reliance on the rational machine bureaucracy to deal with diversity. In other words, students who do not fit the skill span of the faculty are systematically split off and located in separate structures such as special classes or alternative learning environments and schools.

The third paradigm is the adhocracy, which is best conceptualized as a flexible problem-solving team. Skrtic contends that, even within specialized learning environments, schools are nonetheless bureaucracies and there are invariably complex student needs that can only be addressed in alternative structures. Indeed, Skrtic argues that bureaucracies squeeze out "differentness" ("unwanted parts" in psychoanalytic systems terms) when student needs go beyond the skill set of general educators. The knowledge and skills needed to effectively educate the most challenging learners is not standardized but emergent. Flexible instructional teams are required to invent the knowledge to work with complex individual students and their families. Skrtic contends the Individualized Education Program team as initially conceptualized is the hallmark of the adhocracy. Effective ways of working with very challenging youth are thus invented and customized to meet the unique needs of the students.

The rational machine bureaucracy, professional bureaucracy, and adhocracy have significant implications for how schools interact with groups and communities and addiction. Application of the machine bureaucracy to diverse learning needs means that not just individual students are projected into or squeezed into separate structures but whole subclasses of individuals are. This results in deviance labeling, which is introjected and students may act in accordance with the projection, setting up self-fulfilling prophecies for failure. Not only do the students become deviance-labeled but so too do their parents and teachers. The implication of the professional bureaucracy is seen in the degree to which the system can flex its boundaries and include individual students, special student groups and families in the mainstream of school life. An adhocracy is a flexible problem solving team, which creates a benevolent holding environment for challenging learners, who require highly individualized approaches to learning.

As collections of groups and communities, schools have the challenging task of educating all learners, including those challenged with addiction. Acceptance of the disparate parts of individuals, groups, and communities is essential if schools are to be truly inclusive. To return to the shopping mall metaphor, schools, as producers, have the awesome task of tailoring curriculum and instruction to meet a wide variety of competing consumer needs. The key question is: How can these many needs be met, given the competition for scarce resources? And can this be done in ways that enhance and promote the esteem, respect, and dignity of all students, their friends, families, and communities? It falls to school leadership and the community to support schools in their quest to serve the diverse needs of the school community. The humanity of the school is demonstrated in the ways it educates and makes room for its most challenging individuals, groups, and communities in the educational marketplace.

As systems, schools cannot tolerate behavior that goes beyond the permissible deviation range, and thus must split off and project out individuals who violate this norm. This is especially true with behavior associated with social-emotional disorders and addictive behaviors. School districts throughout the country have policies that address behavior challenges that are potentially dangerous to self and others. When it comes to addictive behaviors, school districts often take a "zero tolerance" stance. Any use, distribution, intent to distribute, or distribution of alcohol, drugs, or look-alike drugs are swiftly dealt with through suspension, or the temporary removal from school, and expulsion, the cessation of educational services by an act of the board of education. The expectation of zero-tolerance policies is that the punishment is severe enough to discourage alcohol or drug use at school and may spur the youth and his or her family to seek appropriate medical intervention. Zero tolerance policies constitute a machine-bureaucracy approach to the problem of student addiction.

Unfortunately, zero-tolerance policies simply keep the offender out of the school system. They do not necessarily invoke families to seek treatment. Often, the problem is simply moved from the school to the family and community, where it continues to cycle to the detriment of the expelled youth, family, and community members. Enlightened school districts, such as those with Student Assistance Programs (SAP), identify and refer students struggling with addiction to appropriate treatment programs and collaborate with an array of community medical and mental health agencies. Such districts do not strictly adhere to zero-tolerance practices. Instead, enlightened school districts find ways to use the process of suspension and expulsion to leverage students and families in denial to seek treatment.

This is accomplished by invoking suspension and expulsion procedures and then offering lesser punishments if the student goes into treatment, completes a course of treatment, and maintains acceptable behavior upon reentry to school. Some school districts favor a tiered approach, utilizing degrees of suspension. This leveraging gives school administration and SAP personnel the authority and power necessary to protect the student body on the one hand, while providing some serious consequences on the other.

In school systems with safe schools, which are alternative schools for youth whose primary problem is not a disabling condition, students may be expelled to them and work their way back to the regular school campus and community. Support for this approach may be found in the 2004 Individuals with Disabilities in Education Act (IDEA), which permits school districts to place students who violate drug and alcohol policies in a 45-day interim alternative interim educational setting (AIES). While in this interim service, the youth undergoes a comprehensive case-study evaluation to consider special education eligibility. Students who are disabled and addicted may be provided services within the special education continuum. Depending on the severity of the problem, this can involve referral to a public or private therapeutic day school. However, addictive behavior alone does not constitute a disability within the meaning of IDEA. For these youth, some states, school districts, and regional service agencies have created safe schools as effective alternatives and an alternative to special education. Those who are not determined to be disabled may be referred to safe schools. Importantly, enlightened approaches to dealing with student addiction and promotion of recovery require a professional development bureaucracy to increase the faculty's understanding of addiction and strategies to maintain students within the mainstream of school life.

The current Recovery Schools movement is an effort to create alternative, safe school settings for students struggling with addictive behavior. It reflects the adhocracy in action. These schools reflect the growing understanding that addictive behaviors must be dealt with from a multisystemic vantage point that involves a small school setting where individualized academics and social-emotional challenges can be addressed within the context of a therapeutic milieu. A school setting of this sort can be referred to as a benevolent holding environment, providing the structure necessary to address serious academic, social-emotional, and behavioral difficulties, while at the same time providing the structure and flexibility to provide effective, individualized interventions. Just as parents establish benevolent holding environments in which children can experience the full range of emotions and integrate parental boundaries, the alternative school does similarly with adolescents. Alternative schools of this sort recognize that students who receive treatment inpatient or outpatient programs require considerable support to simultaneously work toward sobriety and reentering school. Without a well-defined support structure, these students often return to school, only to find themselves significantly behind in academic work, have difficulty making up the work, and then relapse, beginning the cycle of addictive behavior all over again.

Students with addictive behaviors often are challenged by comorbid mental health conditions such as depression, impulse control disorders, opposition defiant disorders, anxiety disorder, attention deficit disorders, and bipolar disorders, to name a few. Since these problems are beyond the scope of the traditional school environment and support services, alternative schools become benevolent holding environments in which the trained teachers, social workers, psychologists, administrators, and community mental health professionals work with the youth to maintain stable behavior and consolidate gains made in treatment facilities. The term benevolent holding environments is used here describe an alternative educational structure that is organized and mobilized around the unique needs of the student challenged with addictive behaviors, because the structure is firm enough to contain behavior, while flexible enough to deal with problems that occur in the here and now. To borrow from Skrtic, the alternative school is an adhocracy in which a team of professionals and paraprofessionals invent interventions to help the youth toward recovery. Since alternative school staff stands *in loco parentis*, they act as educators but also as parental authority figures assisting the youth in developing and integrating the skills necessary for behavioral and attitudinal change necessary for discharge and transition back to the regular educational setting. This is accomplished through the creation of a therapeutic environment and milieu in which the system of adult authority is clear, student and faculty roles are clearly defined, and behavioral boundaries are explicit. A critical element here is the training of staff in strategies to address problems as they arise in the here and now. Milieu therapy can be thought of as the therapy of the here and now, as staff is trained to intervene early in a disruptive behavioral cycle, to deescalate it, and to teach the youth about the triggers that set off the behavior, gain insight into the relationship of their thinking, and find ways to more responsibly self-manage their behavior. In some alternative settings, staff are trained in approaches like life-space crisis intervention (Long, Wood, & Fecser, 2001), which is a systematic approach to problem solving that empowers the youth to take up his or her own authority for his or her behavior. This model, and those like it, contains behavior, while at the same time engaging the youth the identify triggers, reflect on the events as they occurred, examine alternative ways of managing, adopt a more effective behavioral strategy, and test it out. It is within this context that staff and youth engage in a collaborative approach to problem solving in which ownership of behavior is central to the process. Further, it is within this context that the youth begins to internalize healthy boundaries and see adult authority as helpful rather than simply controlling.

To operationalize a therapeutic milieu, a number of things must be in place. First, the entire staff has a systems mindset. In other words, staff believes that no single individual can provide for all the needs of the recovering student and that each staff member makes a valued contribution to the students' success. Second, staff also adheres to a collaborative approach to teaming in which student boundary and role transgressions and challenges to adult authority are viewed as symptoms of the problems that brought the youth to the alternative school. Third, within this view, administration and supervision is arranged to address staff ambivalences regarding their own authority and leadership in addressing student behavior. Seen from this vantage point, the therapeutic milieu model sees parallel processes within the staff as symptomatic of program disregulation. Therefore, team meetings become important venues for examination of professional practices and compulsive behaviors or processes that interfere with effective teaching and learning. Just as the staff must establish a benevolent holding environment for students in which to work, administration and supervisors establish a benevolent holding environment for staff. This is particularly important to the effective operation of the milieu because the intensity of the interpersonal work often awakens unresolved unconscious issues, complicating the transferences and countertransferences that occur within the milieu. Clinical consultation is often available to administration and staff in dealing with particularly complicated dynamics. Since addiction is ultimately a family problem, family therapy is a vital dimension of the alternative school. Further, student recovery cannot effectively occur without recovery occurring within families and within the alternative school staff.

The therapeutic milieu cannot sustain itself without a systems perspective that goes beyond the alternative school setting. To effectively support students in their recovery, the school itself must be part of an ongoing system of care. In other words, the school requires interorganizational relationships within the broader community to support students in their recovery and return them to the community school. Partnerships between the school, local mental health agencies, hospitals, and faith communities are critical in creating an expanded holding environment that assists the recovering youth in adapting to community life. Like the school as a collection of groups and communities, the system of care is also a collection of groups and communities, which can be mobilized to support, monitor, and treat students as they reintegrate into community life.

SUMMARY

When viewed as social systems, schools are a collection of groups and communities. An effective way to understand schools is from the vantage point of social systems theory. The concepts of boundaries, boundary managers, roles, authority, splitting, projection, and projective identification are particularly useful in understanding schools as dynamic systems. From this perspective, the school board defines policies and procedures, which set forth the boundaries that govern behavior by students, parents, and community members. Administrators set forth the procedures that regulate these boundaries and provide authority and leadership for the academic, social-emotional, and behavioral growth of students. Where school personnel model healthy behaviors and effective, rational problem-solving, schools have the capacity to be embracing and inclusive. Where school personnel model addictive behavior, students learn addictive behavior through the hidden curriculum, which covertly teaches the values, beliefs, and defense mechanisms associated with addictive behavior. Within each school community exist behavioral expectations, and, when exceeded, systems split off the violating behavior into alternative structures. Some students who violate these norms sometimes require specialized settings in which to address complicated and complex student behavior. This is particularly the case with students with social-emotion and behavioral problems and addiction, which cannot be addressed within the traditional school setting. For these youth, alternative schools are required and effective. Alternative schools function as benevolent holding environments that are structured to contain problems and are flexible enough to facilitate growth and recovery through relationship-based intervention models. These programs are effective if they are operationalized from a systems and organizational perspectives and linked to partnerships within a broader system of care within the larger community.

REFERENCES

Bertalaanffy, L.V. (1969). *General systems theory: Foundations, development, applications.* NY: George Braziller.

Bion, W. R. (1961). *Experiences in groups and other papers.* New York: Basic Books.

Boleman, L. G., & Deal, T. E. (1997). *Reframing organizations: Artistry, choice, and leadership.* San Francisco: Jossey-Bass.

De Board, R. (1978). *The psychoanalysis of organizations: A psychoanalytic approach to behavior in groups and organizations.* London: Tavistock.

Hirschhorn, L. (1990). *The workplace within: Psychodynamics of organizational life.* Cambridge, MA: MIT Press.

Kets de Vries, M. F., & Miller, D. (1984). *The neurotic organization: Diagnosing and revitalizing unhealthy companies.* San Francisco: Jossey-Bass.

Long, N. J., Wood, M. M., & Fecser, F. A. (2001). *Life space crisis intervention: Talking with students in conflict.* Austin, TX: Proed.

Miller, E., & Rice, K. (1975). Systems of organization. In A. D. Coleman & W. H. Bexton (Eds.), *Group relations reader* (pp. 43–68). Sausilito, CA: A.K. Rice Institute.

Powell, A. G., Farrar, E., & Cohen, D. K. (1985). *The shopping mall high school: Winners and losers in the educational marketplace.* Boston: Houghton Mifflin.

Rioch, M. J. (1975a). All we like sheep—Followers and leaders. In A. D. Coleman & W. H. Bexton (Eds.), *Group relations reader 1.* Washington, DC: A.K. Rice Institute.

Rioch, M. J. (1975b). The work of Wilfred Bion on groups. In A. D. Coleman & W. H. Bexton (Eds.), *Group relations reader* (pp. 11–33). Sausilito, CA: A.K. Rice Institute.

Schaef, A. W., & Fassel, D. (1988). *The addictive organization.* San Francisco: Harper.

Skrtic, T. M. (1991). *Behind special education: A critical analysis of professional culture and school organization.* Denver: Love Publishing.

Stapley, L. F. (2006). *Individuals, groups, and organizations beneath the surface.* London: Karnac.

Von Bertalanffy, L. (1968). *General systems theory: Foundation, development, applications.* New York: Braziller.

Weick, K. E. (1976). Educational organizations as systems. *Administrative Science Quarterly, 21,* 1–19.

Adolescent Substance-use Treatment: Service Delivery, Research on Effectiveness, and Emerging Treatment Alternatives

Keith C. Russell, PhD

ABSTRACT. Adolescent substance use remains a persistent and serious problem in society despite use patterns showing consistent declines in alcohol and other illicit drug use since 2000. This paper provides an overview of the somewhat confusing landscape of substance-use treatment options available to families and professionals seeking treatment services. A case study is presented illustrating one treatment option, termed *outdoor behavioral healthcare*, to highlight one example of alternative treatment and educational program that has developed in recent years to meet increased demand for services. Conclusions developed from a review of treatment service availability and research conducted on the effectiveness of treatment suggest that alternative treatments for adolescents should continue to be identified, developed and evaluated using suggestions put forth by researchers in the area of substance-abuse treatment research to increase the likelihood that adolescents who need treatment services are getting those services in a timely, effective, and safe manner.

Keith C. Russell, PhD, is Associate Professor, Recreation and Youth Development, 1900 University.

INTRODUCTION

Adolescent substance use remains a persistent and serious problem in the United States despite use patterns showing consistent declines in alcohol and other illicit drug use since 2000. The Substance Abuse and Mental Health Services Administration (2006) publishes an annual survey of drug use and health, which is considered to be a primary source of information on adult and adolescent use patterns in the United States. In 2005, SAMHSA reported that illicit drug use among adolescents ages 12 to 17 had steadily declined since 2002, when a 12% overall rate of use was reported. In 2005, the rate was reported at just below 10%. Declining use patterns are good news to parents, teachers, youth workers, mental health practitioners, researchers, and agency personnel involved in the prevention and treatment of adolescent substance use in the United States. Similar trends are also noted when examining use reduction in specific substances. For example, marijuana use was 8.2% in 2002 in this same age group and has significantly fallen to 6.8% in 2005. Despite these trends, substance use among American youth continues to remain sufficiently widespread to merit concern. According to the Monitoring for the Future Study (2006), which annually surveys 8th-, 10th-, and 12th-graders, 50% of youth in 12th grade have tried an illicit drug by the time they finished high school. Of particular concern was the finding that nearly a third (30%) of 8th graders had tried inhalant drugs (one of three drugs, along with OxyContin and sedatives that showed signs of increased use in past years). The use of prescription drugs was also noted as a serious concern because they have become more easily available to youth because of their increased prescriptive use in the general population. Another notable trend for youth was reported "past-month" and "binge drinking rates" that have remained unchanged and are still considered alarmingly high. For example, 30% of all youth reported drinking in the past month, and 20% of those (nearly 7.2 million youth) were characterized as binge drinkers. The conclusions generated from both of these reports are not meant to be alarmist, but rather to highlight that, although use trends have slowed in some categories, substance use among adolescents is still a persistent and costly problem in the United States that requires effective prevention and treatment programs that are suitable for adolescents' developmental needs.

The purpose of this paper is not to focus on prescriptive prevention strategies designed to help adolescents better understand the risks and costs of substance use. These prevention strategies, which are literally being forced to strategically develop drug by drug, and use pattern by use pattern, address the determinants of drug use and are based on the perceived benefits and risks that adolescents have regarding specific drugs. The development of prevention strategies across cultural and socioeconomic strata are of paramount importance (see Asherey, Robertson, & Kumpfer, 1998; Faggiano et al., 2006; Foxcraft, Ireland, Lowe, & Breen, 2006) but this paper addresses what happens when these strategies do not work and an adolescent requires a treatment intervention. The goal is to provide an overview of the somewhat confusing landscape of substance-use treatment options available to adolescents and to discuss challenges faced when parents, schools, and mental health practitioners try to determine the most suitable treatment model, given the adolescent's use history and likely mental health disposition. A detailed case study of one treatment option, what has been termed "outdoor behavioral healthcare" (Russell, 2003), is then presented to (a) shed light on the private-pay, demand-driven market for services that has developed in recent years due to perceptions that readily available services were not sufficient for adolescent dispositions, (b) illustrate the types of issues with which adolescents who are seeking these types of services present at admission, and (c) present the outcomes from such treatment to highlight transition and aftercare issues that are often overlooked in discussions of treatment outcome. The case study will be presented in the context of synthesized findings from the relatively few studies on adolescent substance-abuse treatment (Williams & Chang, 2000).

NEED FOR AND ACCESS TO ADOLESCENT SUBSTANCE-ABUSE TREATMENT

Currently, demand outweighs the supply of appropriate and effective behavioral healthcare services for adolescents and their families seeking substance-abuse treatment. In a report by McManus (2003) funded by the William T. Grant Foundation, behavioral healthcare services, including substance-abuse treatment, were examined in four major U.S. cities. Significant barriers were identified in each of the four cities, indicating that most adolescents requiring treatment were not being adequately served. The two most significant barriers to behavioral healthcare services were provider shortages and inadequate reimbursement rates. The authors state that "severe shortages of mental health and substance-abuse providers trained to care for adolescents were reported in all four cities" (p. 16). In addition, the authors concluded that few inpatient psychiatric and substance-abuse beds are available for adolescents and families in need. Adolescents who are deemed to have mental health "crises," including an immediate need for substance-use treatment, are often hospitalized for extended periods of time awaiting more appropriate services. Those less fortunate typically end up in the criminal justice system where their chances for adequate treatment services are limited, and recidivism becomes a significant and very real possibility (Latessa, 2004). Indeed, the criminal justice system is responsible for the largest percentage of growth in a steady rise of substance-use treatment referrals since 1995. Between 1995 and 1998, the number of substance-abuse treatment admissions for adolescents in the United States rose by 46%, to 138,000 admissions of 12- to 17-year olds (Morral, McCaffrey, & Ridgeway, 2004). According to SAMSHA (2006), 50% of all adolescent substance-use treatment admissions and 55% of all adolescent admissions to long-term residential treatment programs were made by the criminal justice system. Recent alarming estimates suggest that 70.9% of adolescents in the juvenile justice system warrant a mental health diagnosis, and of these, 60.8% also meet the criteria for a substance use diagnosis (Shufelt & Cocozza, 2006).

When families are actively seeking substance-use treatment services, several barriers present themselves that make the goal of finding appropriate interventions difficult, meaning on an annual basis millions of youth requiring services do not receive them. According to the Public Health Services Office, in a report by the Office of the Surgeon General (2000) referencing research conducted on the broader mental health service utilization (of which substance-use treatment services were a part), a high proportion of young people with a diagnosable mental and/or substance use disorder do not receive any mental health services at all (Burns, et al. 1995; Leaf, et al. 1996). These findings follow a report conducted in the 1980s by the Public Health Services Office (1986), which also indicated that approximately 70% of children and adolescents in need of treatment do not receive the services they required. In the 1990s, Burns et al. (1995) concluded that only one in five children with a serious emotional disturbance utilized mental health specialty services, and the majority failed to receive any services at all. The most likely reasons for underutilization of mental health and/or substance-use treatment services are defined as 'barriers,' and include: a) perceptions that treatment was not relevant or was too demanding, b) an associated stigma with needing and utilizing mental health services, c) the reluctance of parents and children to seek treatment, d) dissatisfaction with services when they do seek treatment, and e) the prohibitive cost of treatment (Pavuluri, Luk, & McGee, 1996;

Kazdin & Crowley, 1997). These barriers are reinforced in the suggestion that that most adolescent treatment approaches for substance use disorders (SUD) are adaptations of adult models and may not be appropriate for youth (Winters 1999; Winters, Stinchfield, Oplans, Weller, & Latimer, 2000).

In summary, the "continuum of care" talked about by behavioral health-care experts that consists of services in schools, outpatient, inpatient, day treatment, and accessible residential facilities appears to be nebulous and extremely difficult to navigate for most adolescents and their families seeking treatment. The demonstrated historical demands, current lack of services, and barriers to treatment make it highly likely that innovative or alternative programs, and, more important, effective programs, will be increasingly utilized by families in search of help for their children. This increased demand also creates the likelihood that programs with little or no protective oversight could also be utilized by desperate parents and their children seeking treatment. If and when parents and families identify an appropriate treatment alternative, questions remain as to whether the intervention will be effective in helping to alleviate the problems warranting treatment. Research on adolescent substance treatment outcome has increased in the past years, lending insight into treatment models and interventions that are promising; yet convergent interpretations of the literature suggest more research is needed.

RESEARCH ON ADOLESCENT SUBSTANCE-ABUSE TREATMENT OUTCOME

There are comparatively fewer studies on adolescent substance-abuse treatment when compared to the over 1000 studies conducted on adult treatment (Miller et al., 1995). The limited research and, in many cases, poor methodological quality of studies make it difficult to draw distinctive conclusions as to which type of treatment programs are most suitable for adolescents. Despite these shortcomings, most reviews suggest that treatment is better than no treatment, but no conclusions can be made as to which treatment type may be better than others (Catalano, et al., 1990). In a detailed review of over 50 studies on substance-abuse treatment outcome, Williams & Chang (2000) state that "there is no evidence concerning the relative merits of treatment setting, treatment length, treatment intensity, treating homogeneous or heterogeneous populations, or whether certain types of adolescents are best treated by certain programs" (p. 159). More research is needed to better understand treatment types and models to address these concerns, and Williams and Chang recommend several strategies for researchers to address the shortcomings in the literature, including providing detailed descriptions of the treatment services being researched, using improved and consistent substance use assessment procedures, and using common follow-up periods in research (6 and 12 months posttreatment). Recent research has begun to address the limitations outlined by Williams & Chang through evaluation of existing treatment and aftercare and transition programs using more rigorous research methodologies that shed light on current promising interventions and strategies (Kaminer, Burleson, & Goldberger, 2001, 2002; Godley et al., 2005).

One of the most comprehensive efforts to identify characteristics of adolescents in treatment and to evaluate outcomes across multiple settings is the Drug Abuse Treatment Outcome Studies for Adolescents ((DATOS-A), see www.datos.org). In one of several studies resulting from this project, Hser et al. (2001) found that substance-abuse treatment for adolescents is effective in achieving many important behavioral and psychological improvements, including reductions in marijuana use, heavy drinking, positive adjustment and school performance. When examining treatment outcome for adolescents with comorbid diagnoses, Grella, Hser, Joshi, and Rounds-Bryant (2001) found that comorbid youth (64% of sample) reduced their drug use and other problem behaviors after treatment. However, the study also noted that they were more likely to use marijuana and hallucinogens and to engage in illegal acts in the 12 months after treatment, as compared with the noncomorbid adolescents. The study concluded that integrated treatment protocols need to be implemented within drug treatment programs to improve the outcomes of adolescents with comorbid substance use and mental disorders.

Coupled with the limitations noted above are the conclusions by some researchers that most of the studies on adolescent treatment services have evaluated interventions that are described by Weisz, Weiss, and Donenburg (1992) as being *research therapies*. These therapies are reasoned to be theorized, manual driven, resource intensive, and implemented in research settings that offer intense training, supervision, and monitoring. Many of these treatments have been shown to be efficacious (see Winters, 1999, for discussion of proven strategies), yet few are implemented across the country by treatment centers and other service delivery providers because of diverse client needs, staff background and experience, resources and funding, and because most programs subscribe to a "multimodal model" of delivery, drawing on various treatment approaches and behavioral strategies to effectuate change (Lamb, Greenlick & McCarty, 1998). Recent research addressing the implementation of research therapies has found mixed results. The Cannabis Youth Treatment study (Dennis et al., 2004) tested treatment conditions across multiple settings (a combination of motivational enhancement and cognitive behavioral treatment compared with a family support network model), found similar results across the three conditions, and concluded that outcomes may have been driven more by general helping factors beyond the specific treatment approaches tested. Godley et al. (2006) examined the critical role that aftercare plays in transitioning adolescents from brief intensive therapeutic settings to home environments in evaluating the effects of the assertive continuing care (ACC) program, and noted that ACC predicted superior early abstinence for adolescents with diagnosed substance use disorders. Despite these results suggesting successful research therapy implementation, challenges to providers still exist, leading to many promising interventions not being used by practitioners.

Treatment approaches that primarily draw on self-help principles based on experiential knowledge implemented by staff and counselors who have a history of drug and alcohol dependence and recovery have been termed 'community-based treatment' approaches (Morral et al., 2004). These community approaches typically fall into one of two broad types: a) Minnesota model treatment, a residential outpatient or residential approach utilizing recovery steps from Alcoholics Anonymous, and b) therapeutic community treatment, an approach using behavioral consequences inherent in group living and phases to move participants through the program. Very few studies have been conducted on the effectiveness of community-based treatments that use "gold standard criteria" of controlled pretreatment conditions and random assignment of participants to treatment services. The primary reasons for this are ethical issues of randomizing control and treatment groups from consumers in need of treatment services, interruption of on-going service delivery, prohibitive costs of assessment and follow-up, because many private-pay consumers, educational consultants, and probation officers responsible for the care of adolescents are unwilling to agree to randomization because they want to have a say in what is best for the youth. Williams and Chang (2000) found just four studies that examined community-based treatment services and only one that used random assignment. The one randomized study contained only 73 subjects and found no difference in drug-use outcomes at 1 year between a group that received a residential psychoanalytic approach compared with a group that received outpatient probation supervision and basic follow-up services (Amini, Zilberg, Burke, & Salasnek, 1982). More recently, Latimer et al.

(2000) evaluated youth receiving residential, outpatient, or no treatment (not randomly assigned) at a large community-based program and reported no significant differences between pretreatment characteristics and post-treatment outcomes. In a second analysis of this study, the authors conclude that youths who received at least some treatment were less likely to report substance use at 12 months than the no-treatment group (Winters et al., 2000).

In one of the most comprehensive community-based treatment studies to date, Morral et al. (2004) compared outcomes from adolescent probationers who received treatment in the Phoenix Academy (a therapeutic community for adjudicated youth in probationary court-referred substance-use treatment) with those who received treatment in alternative probation dispositions using a case-mix strategy to control for pretreatment characteristics. The average length of stay at the Phoenix Academy was 162 days, while the average length of stay at the alternative dispositions was 169 days. These control groups were represented by six group homes not ascribing to the therapeutic community approach. The authors conclude that the Phoenix Academy "is associated with better outcomes than the average expected outcomes had the same youths received alternative probation dispositions" (p. 265). Reported outcomes included reduced substance use and improved psychological functioning, with the Phoenix Academy youths reporting outcomes that represented small to medium effect sizes. Two findings of particular interest were noted in this study. The first is that the Phoenix Academy participants reported steady reductions in psychological distress, with the authors suggesting that this is due to the development of effective coping strategies and the development of internal resources through the intense group-living model representing the approach. The second was the reported *increase* in tobacco use by the subjects, suggesting that therapeutic communities represent a recovery environment that facilitates tobacco use.

This review of treatment service delivery and the relative effectiveness of such delivery clearly indicate a lack of treatment services for adolescent in the United States, a stigma associated with current treatment options that present formidable barriers to families seeking treatment. "Research therapies," as they are referred to in the literature, are not being widely implemented in communities in the United States, which are implementing interventions based on experience and resources available. These findings suggest the following regarding treatment services for adolescents in the United States. First, little research using rigorous research designs that include randomized assignment and control groups have been conducted on community-based approaches, the primary delivery of substance-use abuse treatment in the United States. Several barriers to implementing these research designs were noted, including ethics of no treatment options, cost, difficulty in having parents and other custodial authorities agree to such a process, and the myriad pretreatment factors that can confound results. Moreover, what may be of particular interest to researchers and policy makers is how adolescents find programs and seek out services, which is lost in random assignment and is simply not the way the process works for families. Second, research has shown that there are little or no treatment differences between control and treatment groups in the few studies that did use appropriate designs, making it difficult to ascertain which approaches may be more appropriate for adolescents. Lastly, the study on the Phoenix Academy by Morral et al. (2004) represents potential outcomes from models that employ similar treatment approaches, namely the potential of programs that develop coping strategies and social skills in treatment through a social living milieu that is less restrictive and inherently motivating. Williams and Chang (2001) also suggest in their review of studies six guidelines for treatment providers in providing effective treatment options for families. They include: (a) readily available programs for large numbers of consumers, (b) procedures that minimize treatment drop-out and maximize treatment completion, (c) a concentration on posttreatment aftercare, (d) provision of comprehensive services other than treatment (e.g., school curricula, social skill development, health and wellness, family), (e) a focus on the family system through family based therapeutic approaches, and (f) aftercare plans that include parent and peer support (p. 160).

CASE STUDY: OUTDOOR BEHAVIORAL HEALTHCARE TREATMENT

Using these recommendations, and findings from the Morral et al. (2004) study, a case study is presented that highlights the ways in which private programs are meeting some of these needs and adhering to these recommendations. These programs number in the hundreds and remain largely underevaluated and a mystery to stakeholders in the area of substance-abuse treatment. The case study also highlights pretreatment characteristics of adolescents seeking these services and what likely outcomes may be a result of such treatment.

Outdoor behavioral healthcare (OBH) is an emerging treatment modality in mental health practice for adolescents with emotional, behavioral, psychological, and substance-use disorders. The term *outdoor behavioral healthcare* refers to programs that subscribe to a multimodal treatment approach within the context of wilderness environments and backcountry travel to facilitate progress toward individualized treatment goals (Russell, 2003). The approach incorporates individual client assessment, individual and group psychotherapy conducted and/or supervised by licensed clinicians, and the development of individual treatment and aftercare plans. While incorporating these core elements of established psychotherapy and substance-abuse treatment, OBH programs apply principles of wilderness therapy, which contain the following key elements that distinguish it from other approaches: (a) extended time in a wilderness setting that provides for removal from cultural influences, immediate and natural consequences, and the promotion of self-efficacy and personal autonomy through task accomplishment; (b) implementation of an individualized treatment plan facilitated by a treatment team utilizing a wilderness context measured by tangible and concrete indicators of success, (c) a restructuring of the therapist-client alliance and development of a unique therapeutic relationship through shared experience between client and staff; and (d) complete immersion in a social/peer group focused on long-term positive change and working toward common goals. OBH programs have become popular because they combine psychotherapy, family work, and traditional drug and alcohol treatment approaches with elements of a wilderness challenge to provide an alternative for resistant adolescents unwilling to commit to traditional treatment. This is especially relevant given current reported demands for behavioral healthcare services.

Depending on definitions, there are over 150 programs currently operating in the United States that fit the description presented above for an OBH program. OBH programs appear to be moving toward professionalization and have begun to form national associations, such as the National Association of Therapeutic Schools and Programs. According to a recent national survey of programs, almost 90% of these programs are licensed by state agencies, and over 60% are nationally accredited by the Joint Commission or the Council on Accreditation (COA) (Russell, 2007). Combined, they treat thousands of adolescents a year, a conservative estimate based on actual adolescent admissions of known programs. Estimates have ranged from 30,000 to 50,000 clients a year (Cooley, 2000). The growth and popularity of these programs underscores the need for such services and highlights the critical need to provide outcome and safety assessment of these private programs to inform parents and consumers of their relative safety and effectiveness. Though some research and evaluation has been conducted (see Behrens and Satterfield, 2006; Russell, 2002, 2003, 2005) more research is needed to determine which types of adolescents are most suitable for treatment, and to compare the relative effectiveness of the intervention to other traditional treatment types. OBH programs were chosen as an illustrative case study for this paper because the intervention reflects the Phoenix Academy approach in focusing treatment on the development of coping, resiliency and social skills outlined by Morral et al. (2004) through the use of group living in natural and wilderness environments.

An assessment of five OBH treatment programs was launched in 2003 and included a census of all adolescent clients admitted to treatment during one calendar year (2003–2004) in five programs operating in Oregon, Utah, Arizona, and Illinois that averaged 45 days in length. All five programs (Anasazi, Aspen Achievement Academy, Catherine Freer Wilderness Therapy, RedCliff Ascent, and OMNI Youth Services) are licensed by their respective state agencies and accredited by a national accreditation agency. The goal of the assessment was to better understand the pretreatment substance-use characteristics of adolescents entering these programs and to conduct a basic assessment of substance-use frequency outcome at 6 months posttreatment.

Specifically, the assessment focused on: a) the readiness and motivation to change problem behaviors of adolescent clients at admission and discharge, including treatment satisfaction at discharge; and b) clients' substance-use histories and the prevalence of substance-use disorders at admission, discharge, and follow-up. Assessing motivation to change was based on studies that suggest that most adolescents who enter treatment do so through coercion by parents or other authorities (Winters and Stinchfield, 1995) and that coercion into treatment is a significant barrier to change (De Leon et al., 1994; De Leon et al., 1997; Melnick, De Leon, Hawke, Jainhill, & Kressel, 1997). Assessing substance-use prevalence and outcomes was based on a desire to better understand client-use histories seeking these services and to identify OBH treatment outcome on adolescents with diagnosed substance-use disorders (SUD).

PROFILE OF OBH CLIENTS

A total of 872 clients entered treatment in these five programs during the study recruitment period. A total of 774 agreed to participate in the study, yielding an 89% recruitment rate. The median treatment length was

49 days, which was used to describe the typical treatment length because of severe outliers in the sample. The treatment length ranged from 2 days to 300 days, with nine clients spending over 200 days in treatment. No data are available on the 112 subjects who declined participation in the assessment. This was because study protocols dictated that no demographic data would be collected on subjects who did not agree to participate. Of the 774 clients who agreed to participate in the study, 53 did not complete treatment, a 93.2% rate of treatment completion (successfully completing the program based on the individual treatment plan and being discharged to parents and or other custodial authorities).

Results are presented by analyses associated with each specific aim, including (1) client characteristics, (2) motivation to change illustrated by cluster profiles, (3) discharge stages of change illustrated by cluster profiles, (4) psycho-social factors surrounding substance use and substance use frequency characteristics, and (5) 6-month follow-up results.

CLIENT CHARACTERISTICS

The study population was predominantly male (68%), Caucasian (81%), between ages 16 and 17 (67%) and are reasoned to be from middle-class socioeconomic backgrounds (see Russell, 2003), though this study did not collect data on socioeconomic status. The average age of the OBH client was 15.9; only 3.4% were under the age of 14. More than 90% of all OBH clients were either diagnosed or entered treatment with an existing diagnosis (as specified by the DSM-IV). One fifth were diagnosed with only a mental health diagnosis (21%), one quarter with a substance-use diagnosis (25%) and one half were concurrently diagnosed with both a substance-use and a mental health diagnosis (50%).

Most clients in OBH treatment have tried prior treatment services before making the decision to enter OBH treatment. This is an important finding and suggests that most adolescents had tried other forms of treatment that were not successful. Three-quarters of all clients in this sample had tried at least some form of outpatient counseling, defined as a periodic visit to a mental health professional to help address problems the adolescent was experiencing while still residing in a home environment. A much smaller percentage (23%) had tried inpatient treatment services, defined as some type of clinical residential setting to address any problems the adolescent was experiencing. A total of 160 clients had tried both types of services before OBH treatment (21%).

CLIENT MOTIVATION: STAGES OF CHANGE

It is reasoned that most adolescent clients in OBH treatment have been at least partially coerced into entering treatment by external influences, such as parents, mental health professionals, or school officials, which likely impacts their likelihood of treatment success (Pompi, 1994; Pompi & Resnick, 1987; Winters, 1999a). This study assessed the adolescent's motivation to change using the University of Rhode Island Change Assessment Scaler developed by Prochaska and Di Clemente (1983). The URICA assesses readiness to implement major lifestyle changes across four well-supported factors that are defined as (1) precontemplative, (2) contemplative, (3) action, and (4) maintenance (Belding & Iguchi, 1996; Pantalon & Nich, 2002). Clients do not fall into one discrete category on the URICA (e.g., precontemplative) indicative of a specific stage. Rather, Prochaska and DiClemente (1983) developed "profiles" based on their scores in each of the stages were used as templates in this study to create similar profiles. This study assessed participating clients' willingness to change as they entered OBH treatment and again at discharge and then "clustered" these into profiles using an analytic strategy that consisted of two types of cluster analysis. After data cleaning, omitting partial responses, and screening for outliers, a total of 665 of the 774 URICA assessments was analyzed (85.9%) at admission, and a total of 624 (81%) at discharge.

Hierarchical cluster analysis produced three distinctive cluster profiles *that were evident at admission*, defined using supporting characteristics and terminology from McConnaughy and Prochaska (1983) as (1) *Uninvolved*, (2) *Reluctant*, and (3) *Participating*. At discharge, three clusters were again identified and defined as (1) *Reluctant*, (2) *Participating*, and (3) *Maintenance*. After clusters were developed, k-means cluster analysis was performed to categorize each client into one of the clusters based on his or her standardized scores on each of the four subscales.

The profile with the highest frequency ($N = 293$ or 44%) was the *Uninvolved* profile, that is characterized by average scores across all four URICA subscales (see Table 1). Clients are theorized to demonstrate a lack of action on addressing any of their problems and are not actively thinking about their problems. They are merely going through the motions and maintaining the status quo. The second most represented profile was the *Reluctant* cluster, which consisted of 29% of the sample with higher than average scores on the Precontemplation subscale, and lower than average scores in Contemplation, Action and Maintenance. This group is characterized as being reluctant to take action on a problem, although

TABLE 1. Cluster Names, Definitions, and Number of Clients
Classified Based on Hierarchical and K-means Cluster Analysis
Techniques for a Sample of OBH Participants at Admission

Cluster Name	Definition	Frequency	Percent
Uninvolved	Not contemplating change Not engaging behaviors to change Maintaining the status quo	293	44.1%
Reluctant	Reluctant to take action on a problem A sense they might be thinking about it No commitment to change	191	28.7%
Participating	Not ignoring the presence of a problem Engaged in thinking about the problem Taking some action in changing the problem Maintaining some of these actions	181	27.2%
	Total	665	100%

they have begun to think about it to some degree. However, there is no commitment on the part of the client to want, or need, to change any behavior.

The third cluster, represented by 27% of the population, was termed the *Participating* cluster and is comprised of clients that have higher than average scores on Contemplation, Action, and Maintenance and lower than average scores on Precontemplation. This group consists of clients who are directly engaged in addressing a known and understood problem and have begun to take action to change and to help them maintain that change. These clients are considered to be highly motivated to want to change. In summary, at admission time, almost three quarters (73%) of all OBH clients were not participating in treatment and either were ignoring that a problem might be present and not thinking about change or had just begun to think that a problem exists. Only one quarter of this sample was actively participating in the process and would be considered motivated, suggesting that significant barriers were in place at the initial stages of treatment.

DISCHARGE STAGES OF CHANGE CLUSTER PROFILES

Clients' readiness to change was also assessed at discharge to test the hypothesis that the majority would have moved to a *Participating* or *Maintenance* profile. This hypothesis was largely supported, with over 90% of all clients being in the *Participating* or *Maintenance* profiles, the absence of the *Uninvolved* cluster completely, and small percentage remaining in the *Reluctant* profile (9%). Thus, though these clients were very unmotivated at admission to treatment, the majority had shifted to an awareness of problem issues in their lives and had begun to actively work on these problems.

ASSESSING SUBSTANCE USE FACTORS AND FREQUENCY

The Personal Experience Inventory (Winters & Henley, 1989). was utilized to create a comprehensive and standardized self-report inventory of substance-use history. The PEI consists of two primary sections, as well as several validity indices. The first section is called the Chemical Involvement Problem Severity section and is the focus of this case study; it consists of 153 questions that are organized into five basic scales and five clinical scales. A follow-up assessment used a shorter version of the instrument to assess specific aspects of substance use posttreatment and certain psychosocial issues surrounding use. As with any self-report assessment involving adolescents, there is a risk of over- or underreporting of behaviors given the nature of the questions and the respondent issues. The PEI has been shown to be an excellent instrument to assess substance use and associated psychosocial factors (see Winters & Henley, 1989, for detailed overview of the development and psychometric qualities of the PEI).

Results will be presented based on these three classifications of clients: (1) those who were diagnosed with only a substance-use diagnosis (reasoned to be more frequent users), (2) those who were concurrently diagnosed with at least a substance-use diagnosis, and (3) those who were not diagnosed with a substance-use diagnosis (those who had no diagnosis are included in this group for simplicity).

RESULTS FOR CHEMICAL INVOLVEMENT PROBLEM SEVERITY

The Basic Scales in the PEI contain five subscales that assess (a) Personal Involvement with Chemicals (PICS), (b) Effects from Drug Use (Effects), (c) Social Benefits of Drug Use (Social Benefits), (d) Personal Consequences of Drug Use (Consequences), and (e) Polydrug Use (Polydrug). The normalized scores used in this descriptive analysis are from a

TABLE 2. Key Scales of the Personal Experience Inventry (PEI)

Chemical Involvement Problem Severity Section

Basic Scales

Personal Involvement with Chemicals
Effects from Drug Use
Social Benefits of Drug Use
Personal Consequences of Drug Use
Polydrug Use

Clinical Scales

Social Recreational Drug Use
Psychological Benefits of Drug Use
Transituational Drug Use
Preoccupation with Drugs
Loss of Control

Drug Use Frequency, Duration and Age of Onset
Alcohol beverages, Marijuana or hashish, LSD and Psych, Cocaine, Amphetamines, Quaaludes, Barbiturates, Tranquilizers, Heroin, Opiods, Glue, Age of Onset

sample of adolescents developed by Winters and Henley (1989) to detect differences in PEI scores for a variety of adolescents in different settings and serve as benchmarks with which to compare OBH client scores. The *Residential Treatment Sample* (RT) ($N = 141$) resembles adolescents referred to residential drug clinic treatment, and the *No Treatment Sample* (NT) ($N = 47$ respectively) reflects adolescents from "normal" school settings. OBH scores on each subscale are presented based on diagnosis at admission to treatment for comparison purposes.

Table 2 shows that for each subscale the three diagnosis groups used to categorize subjects in this study (Substance, Mental Health, and Concurrent) differed significantly ($F[2, 654] = 27.58$, $p < 0.001$). Post hoc analyses showed that the Substance and Concurrent groups reported significantly higher scores (and thus have more serious issues in these domains) on these subscales than the Mental Health group. Finally, the Mental Health group was not shown to be statistically different from the RT sample noted above on all five scales. The OBH Substance group scored significantly higher than the normed RT group ($t = 4.34$, $p < 0.001$), indicating that the OBH sample may be more psychologically and behaviorally involved in drug-use than this sample. These results suggest that OBH clients have significant use histories with substances and present to treatment with

TABLE 3. Scores on PEI Subscales for a Sample of OBH Participants Compared to Samples of Typical Adolescents and those Referred to Residential Treatment using ANOVA

Scale	Group[1]	Frequency	M	SD	F	P	M No Treatment[2]	M Residential Treatment[2]
PICS							53.47	78.54
	Substance	152	73.92	20.23	27.58	<.001		
	Concurrent	270	72.78	21.35				
	Menial	127	49.91	24.13				
Effects							15.70	21.54
	Substance	152	19.95	7.24	12.20	<.001		
	Concurrent	270	20.53	7.24			7	
	Mental	127	15.30	6.65				
Social benefits							12.84	17.42
	Substance	152	15.59	5.67	1.91	<.001		
	Concurrent	270	16.12	5.94				
	Mental	127	11.87	4.98				
Consequences							14.32	19.68
	Substance	152	18.97	5.98	14.90	<.001		
	Concurrent	270	18.76	6.28				
	Mental	127	14.20	4.99				
Poly Drug							11.20	15.52
	Substance	152	17.63	5.98	12.99	<.001		
	Concurrent	270	16.00	6.25				
	Mental	127	12.72	5.51				

[1] These groups are based on whether the client was diagnosed with a substance use diagnosis, a concurrent dignosis of substance and mental health, or just a mental health diagnosis.
[2] The no primary treatment and residential treatment samples were used by Winters and Henley (1989) to discriminate PEI scores for adolescents found in different settings.

symptoms that are similar to adolescents being referred to residential drug treatment.

CLINICAL SCALE RESULTS

The Clinical Scales contain five subscales that assess (a) Social Recreational Use (Social Use), (b) Psychological Benefits of Drug Use (Psych Benefits), (c) Transituational Drug Use (Trans), (d) Preoccupation with Drugs (Preoccupation), and (e) Loss of Control (Loss of Control). Similar normalized scores were used to compare OBH clients to those of Winters and Henley (1989). Table 3 shows that for each subscale the three groups also differed significantly as evidenced by high F values and significant statistical differences between groups ($p < 0.001$). Post hoc analyses showed that the Substance and Concurrent groups also scored significantly higher than the Mental Health group on the Clinical Scales. The Mental Health group reflected the NT referral group on all five of the clinical scales. An illustration of these findings compares high and low scorers on the Psych Benefits scale, which pertains to the use of chemicals to reduce negative emotional states, such as loneliness, depression, boredom, anxiety, and use related to promoting positive emotional states, such as happiness or tranquility. The OBH group scored consistently higher on this scale, suggesting frequent use to manage undesirable emotional states and/or to enhance or bring about pleasurable states. Lower scorers do not report use to influence their emotional states. (For further descriptions of the PEI and its subscales, see Winters and Henley, 1989).

DRUG USE FREQUENCY

The PEI scale also measures the use of a variety of drugs in the adolescent's lifetime, in the last year, and in the last 3 months prior to enrollment in treatment. Results showed that on average alcohol, marijuana, and to a lesser degree cocaine and amphetamines were the most-used substances presented by the three diagnosis types in the previous 3 months prior to entering treatment. Consistent with diagnosis, Concurrent and Substance groups reported significantly higher rates of substance use in the previous year than the Mental Health diagnosis group. When asked a specific question about alcohol (*On the occasion that you drink alcoholic beverages, how often do you drink enough to feel pretty high?*) three quarters of substance and concurrent diagnosis OBH clients' responded "most of the time," and "nearly all the time." Half the Mental Health group responded that they drink alcohol to feel high half the time or more. On average the substance and concurrent diagnosis group began using alcohol regularly in Grade 7 and marijuana regularly in Grade 10.

SIX-MONTH FOLLOW-UP RESULTS

A 6-month follow-up assessment was conducted on a random sample of clients who agreed to participate in the study upon admission into OBH treatment. A sample size of 257 was required to test the equality of mean treatment scores across relevant outcome domains that could yield a power of 0.90 at a 0.01 significance level (Cohen, 1988). A total of 260 parents and youth were randomly selected from the initial database of clients, contacted across the participating programs, and asked to participate in the follow-up assessment. This was done using therapists who were responsible for the client while in treatment and also responsible for making follow-up contacts with clients and families posttreatment. Parents were first contacted and asked if they would participate and then provided the therapists with adolescent contact information. The clients were then contacted and asked if they would participate. After receiving permission, identifying participation, data cleaning and management, including screening for outliers, a final sample of 243 clients was obtained across the five participating programs.

OUTCOMES AT 6 MONTHS

Specific outcome variables were analyzed at 6 months: (1) URICA stages of change scores cluster analyzed into sample profiles at 6 months; (2) depression, anxiety, and stress scores at 6 months compared with discharge scores; (3) substance use frequencies scores at 6 months; and (4) psychosocial indicators of substance use (assessed through a modified and significantly abbreviated Personal Experience Inventory measure).

URICA T-scores were again cluster-analyzed using the same methodology reported in the previous sections. Two clusters emerged from the analysis indicating two distinct profiles of the 229 clients for whom complete URICA assessments were useable after data cleaning and screening. Two profiles were developed and defined as (1) Participating ($n = 182$) and (2) Reluctant ($n = 47$). Both profiles reflected earlier profiles developed at admission and discharge. The Participating cluster is defined as those clients who scored higher than average on contemplation, action, and maintenance and lower than average on the precontemplation subscale. The Reluctant profile illustrates those who scored higher in precontemplation and lower in the other three scales. This analysis suggests that most clients were in the participating stage, actively addressing problem issues identified in the initial treatment process and acting on them in their aftercare environments, whether home or residential.

To examine changes in depression, anxiety and stress scores, a two-way within-subjects ANOVA was conducted on the three subscales across three time periods (see Figure 1). The time main effect and gender-by-time interaction effect were tested using the multivariate criterion for Wilks's lambda (λ). The time main effect was significant at $\lambda = 0.799$, $F(2, 207) = 25.98$,

FIGURE 1. Average DASS Scores at Admission, Discharge, and Six-month Follow-up for Males and Females.

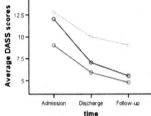

Average DASS scores at admission, discharge and 6-month follow-up for females

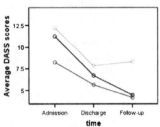

Average DASS scores at admission, discharge and follow-up for males

$p < 0.001$. Post hoc pairwise comparisons showed significant differences between pre- and posttreatment for all three subscales for males and females ($p < 0.01$). From post to the follow-up period, females showed significant differences on the stress subscales, with depression and anxiety not showing significant change (although Figure 1 illustrates a real reduction in scores, which also reflect continued improvement in these areas; however, they were not statistically significant). Males showed a significant increase in stress from post to follow-up, coupled with significant reduction in depressive symptoms. No significant differences were found between post and the follow-up in anxiety for males. Gender by time was not significant, meaning that score changes across the three subscales were similar for males and females. Analysis of real changes in scores shows that Stress increased slightly for males and did not continue to improve at the same rate for females but remained in the mild categories for both genders. All three subscale scores remained in the mild category for both genders at 6 months, suggesting maintenance or continued improvement in these domains after treatment. No significant differences were found between those who utilized inpatient or outpatient services for aftercare across these three domains.

Seven of the original subscales were utilized in the 6-month follow-up to assess related psychosocial indicators and effects of substance use, as well as the actual use frequencies across a wide range of substances. Table 4 shows scores for the five basic subscales at admission and at the 6-month follow-up from treatment for the three diagnosis groups, and those not diagnosed, used in the initial analysis of PEI scores. For the PICS scale, which measures an individual's psychological involvement with chemicals,

TABLE 4. Scores on the Basic Scales of the PEI for a Sample of OBH clients, Including Results from a Pairwise Comparison of Pretreatment to Posttreatment Scores Presented by the Three Diagnosis Groups

Scale	Group[1]	Frequency	M_1	M_2	t	P
PICS						
	Substance	56	75.64	52.57	−4.66	<.000*
	Concurrent	98	70.94	54.86	−4.73	<.000*
	Mental	43	55.49	57.40	.401	.690
	None	21	56.09	51.95	−.504	.620
Total		218				
Effects						
	Substance	56	21.48	16.55	−3.43	<.001*
	Concurrent	98	20.49	17.07	−3.07	<.003*
	Mental	43	17.09	17.56	.308	.759
	None	21	16.71	16.95	.092	.927
Total		218				
Social Benefits						
	Substance	56	16.13	12.09	−3.56	.001*
	Concurrent	98	14.86	12.78	−2.36	.020
	Mental	43	13.86	14.33	.342	.734
	None	21	12.57	11.86	−.359	.723
Total		218				
Consequences	Substance	56	19.19	15.64	−2.89	.005*
	Concurrent	98	16.95	14.86	−.471	638
	Mental	43	15.02	17.37	1.70	.096
	None	21	15.19	17.10	.795	.436
Total		218				
Poly Drug	Substance	56	19.36	12.52	−5.27	<.001*
	Concurrent	98	16.54	13.53	−3.14	.002*
	Mental	43	14.37	13.77	−.418	.678
	None	21	16.09	13.29	−1.34	.194
Total		218				

* Significant differences between pre-treatment and 6-month follow-up scores at $p < .01.1$. Groups refer to categorized diagnoses classes at admission, being either substance only, mental only, or a concurrent diagnosis with each.

both the Substance and Concurrent diagnoses group showed significant changes in scores from pre- to posttreatment. The Mental Health and No Diagnosis groups showed no significant differences in scores from admission to follow-up and also showed a real increase in scores across all five scales. This increase in real scores, though in each case not statistically different from admission scores, was evident in each of the five subscales for the Mental Health and No Diagnosis groups. The Substance group showed

TABLE 5. Results from a Pairwise Comparison of Pretreatment to Posttreatment PEI Scores according to Three Diagnosis Groups for OBH Participants

Diagnosis Group	Frequency	Percent Never		Percent Once or Twice		Percent More than Three Times	
		Pre	Post	Pre	Post	Pre	Post
Alcohol							
Substance	56	9.1	43.5	21.8	14.5	69.1	39.4
Concurrent	98	15.1	47.2	25.6	14.2	59.3	38.7
Mental	43	35.0	34.0	12.5	21.3	52.5	44.7
None	21	30.0	38.1	20.0	14.3	50.0	47.6
Total	218						
Marijiuana							
Substance	56	24.1	41.9	13.0	22.6	63.0	35.5
Concurrent	98	19.3	53.8	12.5	19.8	68.2	26.4
Menial	43	55.0	46.8	7.5	25.5	37.5	27.6
None	21	38.1	52.4	4.8	9.5	57.1	38.1
Total	218						

significant reductions in each of the five subscales, while the Concurrent diagnosis group showed significant reductions in the PICS, Effects, and POLYDRUG subscales, which measure the immediate psychological, physiological, and behavioral effects of chemical use, most of which refer to negative or aversive states and feelings. Once data were cleaned and screened for outliers, 218 of the 243 follow-up clients provided assessments (89.7%).

The abbreviated PEI used to assess substance-use frequency at the 6-month follow-up period contained items that asked respondents to rate the frequency in which they utilized a variety of substances. Table 5 shows the percentage of respondents, classified by diagnosis type, who stated that they had not used alcohol or marijuana in the past 3 months, had used once or twice, or had used more than three times. (The percentage of respondents who reported use in the more severe drug categories was very small, with the majority reporting no use). An ANOVA comparing the average use between the three groups at the 6-month follow-up period showed no differences in alcohol or marijuana use frequency. The percentages also illustrate: (a) the percentage of respondents who reported not using increased significantly for the Substance and Concurrent groups for both alcohol and marijuana use and decreased slightly for the Mental group;

(b) the percentage of those who used more than three times in the previous 3 months decreased as a result of treatment for the Substance and Concurrent groups, but not necessarily for the Mental group; (c) lower marijuana use by all groups was a trend at the 6-month follow-up period; (d) approximately one third of all respondents at the six-month follow-up period reported no use during the previous 3 months; (e) over 50% of all groups reported using alcohol three or more times in the previous 3 months at follow-up, (f) all groups (Substance 54%; Concurrent 53%; Mental 66%, and No Diagnosis 62%) report between 53% and 66% had used alcohol at least once in the previous 3 months; (g) Almost 60% of all Substance and 55% of the Concurrent group respondents had used marijuana at least once. Pairwise comparisons of average responses for all respondents showed a significant reduction in the use of both alcohol ($t = 3.42$, $p < 0.001$) and marijuana ($t = 8.63$, $p < 0.001$), which was consistent for all groups as evidenced by no differences found in a three-way ANOVA of average responses to these two items.

LIMITATIONS

There are several limitations to this study presented as a case study of adolescent treatment. First, no random assignment was used and there was no control group identified. To help address this issue, a large sample size was drawn and standardized instruments were used to compare treatment outcome. Some clients did not agree to participate in the study ($N = 98$ of the 872 clients), potentially biasing the results, though this group only represents 11.2% of the total study population. No further data was available on the clients who did not agree to participate in the study. There also were clients who entered treatment and did not complete all the assessments. These small samples (percentages of noncomplete data sets varied from time to time) were checked against complete data sets for significantly distinguishing characteristics. Any significant findings will be reported along with other results from the study. It has also been suggested that the majority of the study sample may have been coerced into treatment. Though this was not directly asked (e.g., were you coerced into coming to treatment?), the URICA assessment did allow a check of this factor to determine its relationship to outcome. In essence, this dynamic has been integrated into the study to explore its potential effect. It is therefore possible that study participants may have minimized their self reports of alcohol and other drug use history at admission assessment (Hesselbrock, Babor, Hesselbrock,

Meyer, & Workman, 1983). To address this issue, the assessment asking adolescents to describe their previous drug use prior to entering treatment was taken at the midpoint in treatment and was used as a therapeutic tool by each program to help them focus treatment goals and aftercare plans. Program staff reported that clients used the assessment and it was a valuable treatment tool to assess historical use of substances. Some concerns about self report are alleviated by a growing body of literature that suggests drug use self-report is a valid assessment strategy (Stinchfield, 1997; Winters, Stinchfield, Henley, & Schwartz, 1991), despite findings that not all individuals will validly self report (Johnson et al., 1986; Winters et al., 1991).

DISCUSSION

This paper presents an overview of challenges facing adolescent substance-abuse treatment delivery in the United States. The good news is that adolescent substance use continues to decline, which will likely put less stress on a seemingly overburdened delivery system. The challenges are that most adolescents requiring treatment are not receiving treatment, and that more easily identifiable direct services in home communities are needed. Also needed are new and innovative treatment strategies to address hard-to-reach adolescents who are not successful in more traditional community-based interventions. The challenge comes in developing efficacious interventions and making them readily available to families and communities consistent with the recommendations put forth by Williams and Chang (2001). To accomplish this, large-scale evaluations of treatment models will need to be conducted following assessment strategies outlined by Morral et al. (2004) that seek to control and adjust for outcome differences based on assessed pretreatment characteristics that are known to affect outcome differentials.

The detailed case study assessing five outdoor behavioral healthcare programs showed that alternative treatment programs are being developed by the private sector to meet the demands of private-pay consumers looking for alternatives. Though some positive outcomes were identified, including a shift in motivation and a significant reduction in substance-use frequency posttreatment, the study had several limitations and generated several interesting questions that highlight the need for research into these types of innovative treatment options for adolescents. Several interesting conclusions were generated from the case study that would seem to warrant further investigation. First, OBH treatment showed a 93% completion rate of treatment for adolescents who were shown to be extremely unmotivated at admission but had shifted to a more pronounced desire to change depreciative behaviors at discharge. This completion percentage is significantly higher than other treatment options and may be appropriate for adolescents unwilling to commit to more structured treatment. Second, most adolescent clients were unmotivated and most had been coerced into treatment by parents or other adult figures in their lives. This is supported by the findings developed through analysis of the stages of change profiles that indicated that the majority of clients were in the reluctant and unmotivated profiles at admission. Third, many clients had shifted their willingness to change at the end of treatment and had begun actively working on their issues. Further supporting this finding is the data that show that 75% of all clients were engaged in some type of aftercare treatment after completion of the program. Fourth is the finding that adolescents seeking these alternative treatment options have significant substance-use issues evidenced by PEI scores; and, moreover, the majority of these adolescents had tried other forms of treatment that are reasoned not to have worked for them. They simply needed something different than traditional residential or outpatient talk therapy could provide. This finding is critical and one that should be looked into with further research. Finally, some positive outcomes were noted but should be treated with caution due to the limitations inherent in the study, namely, that there was no comparable control group used and that the only data available was self-reported by adolescents. Together, these findings suggest that alternative treatments for adolescents should continue to be evaluated, developed, and identified, making the suggestions put forth by Williams and Chang and other researchers in the area of substance-abuse treatment research a reality for parents and adolescents seeking these services.

REFERENCES

Amini, F., Zilberg, N. J., Burke, E. L., & Salasnek, S. (1982). A controlled study of inpatient versus outpatient drug abusing adolescents: One year results. *Comprehensive Psychiatry, 23*, 436–444.

Ashery, R., Robertson, E., & Kumpfer, K. (Eds.). (1998). Drug abuse prevention through family interventions. *NIDA Research Monograph 177*. Rockville, MD: United States Department of Health and Human Services.

Behrens, E., & Satterfield, K. (2006). *Report of findings from a multi-center study of youth outcomes in private residential treatment*. Presented at the 114th Annual Convention of the American Psychological Association at New Orleans, Louisiana, August, 2006.

Belding, M. A., & Iguchi, M. Y. (1996). Stages of change in methadone maintenance: Assessing the convergent validity of two measures. *Psychology of Addictive Behaviors, 10*(3), 157–66.

Burns, B. J., Costello, E. J., Angold, A., Tweed, D., Stangl, D., Farmer, E. M., et al. (1995). Children's mental health service use across service sectors. *Health Affairs, 14*, 147–59.

Catalano, R. F., Hawkins, J. D., Wells, E. A., Miller, J., & Brewer, D. (1990). Evaluation of the effectiveness of adolescent drug abuse treatment, assessment of risks for relapse, and promising approaches to relapse prevention. *The International Journal of Addictions, 25*, 1085–1140.

Cohen, J. (1988). *Statistical power analysis for the behavioral sciences* (2nd edition). Hillsdale, NJ: Erlbaum.

Cooley, R. (2000). How big is the risk in wilderness treatment of adolescents? *International Journal of Wilderness, 6*(1), 22–27.

De Leon, G., Melnick, G., & Kressel, D. (1997). Motivation and readiness for therapeutic community treatment among cocaine and other drug abusers. *American Journal of Drug and Alcohol Abuse, 23*(2), 169–89.

De Leon, G., Melnick, G., Kressel, D., & Jainchill, N. (1994). Circumstances, motivation, readiness and suitability (the CMRS scales): Predicting retention in therapeutic community treatment. *American Journal of Drug and Alcohol Abuse, 20*(4), 495–515.

Dennis, M., Godley, S. H., Diamond, G., Tims, F. M., Babor, T., Donaldson, et al. (2004). The Cannabis Youth Treatment (CYT) study: Main findings from two randomized trials. *Journal of Substance Abuse Treatment, 27*, 197–213.

Faggiano F., Vigna-Taglianti F. D., Versino E., Zambon A., Borraccino A., & Lemma P. (2006). School-based prevention for illicit drugs' use. Art. No.: CD003020. DOI: 10.1002/14651858.CD003020.pub2. Retrieved May 29, 2007, from http://www.thecochranelibrary.com

Foxcroft, D., Ireland, D., Lowe, G., & Breen, R. (2006). Primary prevention for alcohol misuse in young people. *Addiction, 101*(7), 1057–59.

Godley, M. D., Godley, S. H., Dennis, M. L., Funk, R. R., & Passetti, L. L. (2006). The effect of Assertive Continuing Care on continuing care linkage, adherence, and abstinence following residential treatment for adolescents with substance use disorders. *Addiction, 102*, 81–93.

Godley, M. D., Kahn, J. H., Dennis, M. L., Godley, S. H., & Funk, R. R. (2005). The stability and impact of environmental factors on substance use and environmental problems after adolescent outpatient treatment for cannabis abuse or dependence. *Psychology of Addictive Behaviors, 19*(1), 62–70.

Grella, C. E., Hser, Y. I., Joshi, V., & Rounds-Bryant, J. (2001). Drug treatment outcomes for adolescents with comorbid mental and substance use disorders: Findings from the DATOS-A. *Journal of Nervous and Mental Disease, 189*, 384–92.

Hesselbrock, M., Babor, T., Hesselbrock, V., Meyer, R., & Workman, K. (1983). Never believe an alcoholic? On the validity of self-report measures of alcohol dependence and related constructs. *International Journal of Addictions, 18*, 593–609.

Hser, Y., Grella, C. E., Hubbard, R. L., Hsieh, S. C., Fletcher, B. W., Brown, B. S., et al. (2001). An evaluation of drug treatment for adolescents in four U.S. cities. *Archives of General Psychiatry, 58*, 689–95.

Johnston, L. D., O'Malley, P. M., Bachman, J. G., & Schulenberg, J. E. (2006). *Monitoring the Future national survey results on drug use, 1975-2005*. Volume I: Secondary school students (NIH Publication No. 06-5883). Bethesda, MD: National Institute on Drug Abuse, 684 pp.

Kaminer, Y., Burleson, J. A., & Goldberger, R. (2001). Psychotherapies for adolescents with alcohol and other substance abuse: Three- and nine-month post treatment outcomes. *Alcoholism: Clinical and Experimental Research, 25S*, 90A.

Kaminer, Y., Burleson, J. A., & Goldberger, R. (2002). Cognitive-behavioral coping skills and psychoeducation therapies for adolescent substance abuse. *Journal of Nervous and Mental Disease, 190*, 737–45.

Kazdin, A. E., & Crowley, M. (1997). Family experience of barriers to treatment and premature termination from child therapy. *Journal of Consulting and Clinical Psychology, 65*, 453–463.

Lamb, S., Greenlick, M. R., & McCarty, D. (1998). *Bridging the gap between practice and research: Forging partnerships with community-based drug and alcohol treatment*. Washington, DC: National Academy Press.

Latessa, E. (2004). The challenge of change: Correctional programs and evidence-based practices. *Criminology and Public Policy, 3*(4), 547–60.

Leaf, P. J., Alegria, M. C., Goodman, S. H., Horwitz, S. M., Hoven, C. W., Narrow, W. E., et al. (1996). Mental health service use in the community and schools: Results from the four-community MECA study (methods for the epidemiology of child and adolescent mental disorders study). *Journal of the American Academy of Child and Adolescent Psychiatry, 35*, 889–97.

McConnaughy, E., & Prochaska, J. O. (1983). Stages of change in psychotherapy: Measurement and sample profiles. *Psychotherapy: Theory, Research, and Practice, 20*, 368–75.

McManus, M. A. (2003). *Is the health care system working for adolescents?* Washington, DC: Maternal and Child Health Policy Research Center.

Melnick, G., De Leon, G., Hawke, J., Jainchill, N., & Kressel, D. (1997). Motivation and readiness for therapeutic community treatment among adolescents and adult substance abusers. *American Journal of Drug and Alcohol Abuse, 23*(4), 485–506.

Miller, W. R., Brown, J. M., Simpson, T. L., Handmaker, N. S., Bien, T. H., Luckie, L. F. et al. (1995). What works? A methodological analysis of the alcohol treatment literature. In R. K. Hester & W. R. Miller (Eds.), *Handbook of alcoholism treatment approaches* (2nd ed., pp. 12–44). Needham Heights, MN: Allyn & Bacon.

Morral, A., McCaffrey, D., & Ridgeway, G. (2004). Effectiveness of community-based treatment for substance-abusing adolescents: 12-month outcomes of youths entering Phoenix Academy or alternate probation dispositions. *Psychology of Addictive Behaviors, 18*(3), 257–68.

Pantalon, M. V., & Nich, C. (2002). The URICA as a measure of motivation to change among treatment-seeking individuals with concurrent alcohol and cocaine problems. *Psychology of Addictive Behaviors, 16*(4), 299–307.

Pavuluri, M. N., Luk, S. L., & McGee, R. (1996). Help-seeking for behavior problems by parents of preschool children: A community study. *Journal of the American Academy of Child and Adolescent Psychiatry, 35*, 215–22.

Pompi, K. F. (1994). *Therapeutic communities: Advances in research and applications.* (Monograph No. 144). Washington, DC: National Institute of Drug Abuse.

Pompi, K. F., & Resnick, J. (1987). Retention in a therapeutic community for court-referred adolescents and young adults. *American Journal of Drug and Alcohol Abuse, 13*(3), 309–25.

Prochaska, J. O., & DiClemente, C. C. (1983). Stages and processes of self-change of smoking: Toward an integrative model of change *Journal of Consulting and Clinical Psychology 51*(3), 390–395.

Public Health Services Office. (1986). *Children's mental health: Problems and service—A background paper.* Office of the Surgeon General. Washington, DC: U.S. Government Printing Office.

Public Health Services Office. (2000). *Report of the surgeon general's conference on children's mental health: A national action agenda.* Washington, DC: Department of Health and Human Services.

Russell, K. C. (2000). Exploring how the wilderness therapy process relates to outcomes. *Journal of Experiential Education, 23*(3), 170–76.

Russell, K. C. (2003). An assessment of outcomes in outdoor behavioral healthcare treatment. *Child and Youth Care Forum, 32*(6), 355–81.

Russell, K. C. (2005). Two years later: A qualitative assessment of youth-well-being and the role of aftercare in outdoor behavioral healthcare treatment. *Child and Youth Care Forum, 34*(3), 209–39.

Russell, K. C. (2006). Evaluating the effects of the Wendigo Lake Expedition program for young offenders. *Journal of Youth Violence and Juvenile Justice, 4*(2), 185–203.

Russell, K. C. (2007). *A national survey of outdoor behavioral healthcare programs in the United States. Technical Report # 2,* Outdoor Behavioral Healthcare Research Cooperative, University of Minnesota, Minneapolis, MN, 62.

Shuffelt, J. L. & Cozza, J. J. (2006). Youth with mental health disorders in the juvenile justice system: Results from a multistate prevalence study. *Research and Program Brief*, June 2006. Delamar, NY: National Center for Mental Health and Juvenile Justice.

Stinchfield, R. D. (1997). Reliability of adolescent self-reported pretreatment alcohol and other drug use. *Substance Use and Misuse, 32,* 63–76.

Substance Abuse and Mental Health Services Administration. (2006). *Results from the 2005 national survey on drug use and health: National findings.* (No. DHS Publication No. SMA 06-4194). Rockville, MD.

Weisz, J. R., Weiss, B., & Donenburg, G. R. (1992). The lab versus the clinic: Effects of child and adolescent psychotherapy. *American Psychologist, 47,* 1578–85.

Williams, J. R., & Chang, S. Y. (2001). A comprehensive and comparative review of adolescent substance abuse treatment outcome. *Clinical Psychology: Science and Practice, 7,* 138–66.

Winters, K. C. (1999a). Treating adolescents with substance use disorders: An overview of practice issues and outcomes. *Substance Abuse, 20*(4), 203–25.

Winters, K. C., & Henley, G. A. (1989). *The personal experience inventory test and user's manual.* Los Angeles: Western Psychological Services.

Winters, K. C., Stinchfield, R., Oplans, E., Weller, C., & Latimer, W. W. (2000). The effectiveness of the Minnesota Model approach in the treatment of adolescent drug abusers. *Addiction, 95*(4), 601–12.

Winters, K. C., & Stinchfield, R. D. (1995). *Current issues and future needs in the assessment of adolescent drug abuse (No. 156)*. Rockville, MD: NIDA Research Monograph.

Winters, K. C., Stinchfield, R. D., Henley, G. A., & Schwartz, R. H. (1991). Validity of adolescent self-report of alcohol and other drug involvement. *The International Journal of the Addiction, 25*(11A), 1379–95.

Winters, K. C., & Stinchfield, R. D. (1999). Adolescent treatment. In R. E. Tarter, R. T. Ammerman, & P. Ott (Eds.), *Sourcebook on substance abuse: Etiology, epidemiology, assessment and treatment*, (pp. 350–361). New York: Allyn and Bacon.

Recovery Support Meetings for Youths: Considerations When Referring Young People to 12-Step and Alternative Groups

Lora L. Passetti, MS
William L. White, MA

ABSTRACT. Participation of young people in recovery support meetings is a promising yet largely understudied area. This article reviews the history of youth involvement in meetings, summarizes current research, and discusses issues to consider when making referrals. Professionals may want to research local meetings, help young people structure time before and after meetings, become familiar with group customs, investigate a variety of support groups, interact with support group service structures, develop a list

---

Lora L. Passetti, MS, is Research Projects Manager and William L. White, MA, is Senior Research Consultant, Chestnut Health Systems, Bloomington, IL 61701.

Preparation of this manuscript was supported by funding from the Center for Substance Abuse Treatment, Substance Abuse and Mental Health Services Administration, Department of Health and Human Services through the Strengthening Communities—Youth project (grant no. TI13356) and the National Institute on Drug Abuse, National Institutes of Health (grant no. 1 RO1 DA 018183 and fellowship no. 5 F31 DA17406 03). The content of this publication does not necessarily reflect the views or policies of the Department of Health and Human Services or the National Institutes of Health. The authors wish to acknowledge helpful feedback from Susan Godley on drafts of this manuscript.

of reliable group members to connect youths to the recovering community, and implement assertive referral strategies.

RECOVERY SUPPORT MEETINGS FOR YOUTHS: CONSIDERATIONS WHEN REFERRING YOUNG PEOPLE TO 12-STEP AND ALTERNATIVE GROUPS

Following addiction treatment, most adolescents struggle with recovery and relapse, and high relapse rates have been reported during the first 90 days after discharge (Brown et al., 1993). Participation in professionally directed continuing care groups can enhance substance use outcomes, but a substantial proportion of youths do not attend them unless assertive approaches that transfer responsibility of linkage and retention from the client to the clinician are employed (Godley, Godley, & Dennis, 2001; Godley, Godley, Dennis, Funk, & Passetti, 2002; Godley, Godley, Dennis, Funk, & Passetti, 2006). Peer-led community-based recovery groups are another potential source of support for youths that can complement acute care interventions (Humphreys et al., 2004). As free resources available in many communities, such groups can provide reminders of the negative consequences of substance use and the benefits of abstinence. Members offer experientially based advice, are available 24 hours a day, and provide encouragement and opportunities for substance-free social events and interactions (Kaskutas, Bond, & Humphreys, 2002; Kelly, Myers, & Rodolico, in press). Such potential benefits merit further attention for youths.

Participation of young people in recovery support meetings is a promising yet largely understudied area in the field of substance abuse research. The purposes of this article are to (1) review the history of youth involvement in recovery support meetings, (2) summarize current research on young people and recovery support groups, and (3) discuss issues professionals may want to consider when referring youths to 12-step and alternative groups, including strategies for linking young people to meetings. Much of this paper will focus on Alcoholics Anonymous (AA) and Narcotics Anonymous (NA) because of their longevity, membership size, geographical dispersion and availability, and the number of scientific studies of their relationship to long-term recovery outcomes.

HISTORY OF YOUTH INVOLVEMENT
IN RECOVERY SUPPORT MEETINGS

Professionally directed and peer-based support structures for young people seeking recovery from severe alcohol and other drug problems have evolved over the past two centuries in tandem with youthful substance use trends (White, 1999). Nineteenth-century recovery-support societies such as the Washingtonians and the Ribbon Reform Clubs sponsored "cadet" branches for young inebriates and launched "youth rescue" crusades (White, 1998). Many leaders of these efforts started their own downfalls as youth. One of them even became known on the temperance lecture circuit as the "saved drunkard boy" (Foltz, 1891). Young people were admitted to nineteenth-century inebriate homes, inebriate asylums and private addiction cure institutes; but there was no specialized adolescent treatment, or youth-focused branch of such institutional aftercare groups as the Keeley Leagues (White, 1998). Alcohol problems among young people waned in tandem with the growth of the American temperance movement.

The heroin epidemic of the early twentieth century spurred rising juvenile arrests, the rejection of thousands of World War I draftees, and the admission of adolescents to morphine maintenance clinics that operated in 44 communities between 1919 and 1924 (Terry & Pellens, 1928). Of the more than 7,500 addicts registered at the Worth Street Clinic in New York City, 743 were under the age of 19 (Hubbard, 1920), but there is no record of any peer-based recovery support structures linked to these clinics. This lack of specialized recovery support resources continued as admissions of persons under age 21 to the two federal "narcotics farms" rose from 22 in 1947 to 440 in 1950. The dramatic rise of juvenile narcotic addiction in New York City in the early 1950s led to increased admissions to local hospitals (New York Academy of Medicine, 1953) and the 1952 opening of America's first specialized addiction treatment facility for juveniles— Riverside Hospital. The eventual closure of Riverside in 1962 following studies confirming posttreatment relapse rates of more than 95% led some to speculate that the Achilles heel in the Riverside Hospital design was its inability to transfer institutional learning to the natural environment of those it treated (Gamso & Mason, 1958).

Peer-based recovery support structures for young people in the mid-twentieth century rose from three sources: AA, adaptations and alternatives to AA, and faith-based recovery ministries. Young People's Groups in AA ("young people" then defined as AA members under age 35) began in the

1940s in cities such as Cleveland (1944), Los Angeles (1945), Philadelphia (1946), New York City (1947), and San Diego (1948). The number of groups increased through the 1940s to the point they commanded a special section of the 1950 International Convention of AA. In 1958, the growing network of Young People's Groups formed the International Conference of Young People in Alcoholics Anonymous and hosted their first convention in Niagara Falls, New York. That annual event now draws more than 3,000 young AA members from all over the United States (Special Composition Groups in A.A., 2002).

Young People's Groups were started in AA to escape the status very young members had as curiosities at meetings. The first *AA Grapevine* articles on young people in AA were published in the late 1940s under such titles as "Young Men Solve Meeting Problems" and "A Plea for the Young in Years," and the number of such articles grew significantly in the 1960s and 1970s. Over that span, ages of "young AA members" dropped from the thirties into the early twenties and then into the teens. A review of articles on young people in AA published in the *AA Grapevine* between 1948 and 1978 reveals that the young people who entered AA in these years faced incredulity and suspicion ("You're too young to be an alcoholic!"), condescension and disdain ("I've spilled more booze than you've drunk."), criticism ("We don't want to hear about those other drugs."), or were fawned over ("You are so lucky to have come to AA so young!"). A review of similar articles over the past 25 years reveals that such attitudes weakened as the average age of AA members progressively declined. In 1994, a regular feature of the *Grapevine* ("Youth Enjoying Sobriety") was begun that focused on young people in AA. Between 1948 and 2006, more than 100 articles have appeared in the Grapevine that focused on young people recovering within AA (B. Weiner, personal communication, November 30, 2006). Alateen, founded in 1957, also served as a source of support for adolescents who struggled with the alcoholism of a parent and a pathway of entry into recovery for some of these young people who went on to develop similar problems in their teen years.

Several events contributed to the rise of young people and very young adolescents entering AA. Lowered age of onset of regular alcohol and other drug use in the United States and the trend toward use of multiple drugs have accelerated the development of severe alcohol and other drug problems and triggered help-seeking at ever younger ages. Increased public awareness of alcohol and other drug (AOD) problems and resources to resolve them along with reduced stigma may have increased the flow of young people into AA. The growing representation of youths may also signify a cumulative effect of young people in AA carrying a message of hope to others their age experiencing AOD problems and the growth of adolescent treatment programs that link their clients to AA for posttreatment recovery support. Additionally, AA has made an effort to reach out to young people through youth-oriented pamphlets (*Young People and AA*, *Too Young?*) and a film (*AA and Young People*).

Other adaptations of AA's 12-step recovery program have attempted to reach out to young people. NA has attracted young people since its founding in the late 1940s and early 1950s. In 2005, there were over 21,500 registered NA groups holding over 33,500 meetings weekly. The birth of Potsmokers Anonymous (1968), Pills Anonymous (1975), Chemically Dependent Anonymous (1980), Cocaine Anonymous (1982), Heroin Anonymous, and Crystal Meth Anonymous reflect the continued evolution of AOD problems in America and the 12-step adaptations that have risen in response to them. There has also been a growth in secular alternatives to 12-step programs. These include Women for Sobriety (1975), Secular Organization for Sobriety (1985), Rational Recovery (1986), Self Management and Recovery Training (SMART) (1994) and LifeRing Secular Recovery (1999). Explicitly religious approaches to addiction recovery include Alcoholics Victorious (1948), Alcoholics for Christ (1976), Overcomers Outreach (1977), Liontamers Anonymous (1980), and such recent groups as Ladies Victorious and Celebrate Recovery. Organizations such as Teen Challenge provide a religious alternative to secular treatment but have not generated autonomous, peer-based recovery support groups analogous to those linked to AA and NA.

The equivalent of AA's Young People's groups has not been created in these various recovery support programs, although such youth-oriented tracks could appear in the future. Queries to groups listed in the recovery mutual aid guide posted at the Faces and Voice of Recovery Web site (http://www.facesandvoicesofrecovery.org/resources/support_home.php) revealed only "a few" young people's NA meetings and one designated young people's meeting (Holland, Michigan) in Alcoholics Victorious. The first recovery support group organized specifically for adolescents in recovery is Teen-Anon (1999). Teen-Anon, affiliated with the California-based Streetcats Foundation for Youth and the National Children's Coalition, has variations of its program for Christian teens, Jewish teens, and lesbian, gay, and bisexual youth.

Current Research on Youth Involvement in Recovery Support Meetings

The vast majority of research related to recovery support meetings has been conducted with adults attending 12-step-oriented groups, and a substantial body of published work supports the clinical practice of referring adults to 12-step meetings, recommending regular attendance, and encouraging involvement (Bond, Kaskutas, & Weisner, 2003; Connors, Tonigan, & Miller, 2001; Humphreys et al., 2004; Kissin, McLeod, & McKay, 2003; McKellar, Stewart, & Humphreys, 2003; Moos & Moos, 2004). On the other hand, research aimed at examining the effects of support group involvement on treatment and recovery outcomes for youths is still in its beginning stages. Studies have focused on youth participation in 12-step meetings, and no published studies of involvement in alternative groups were identified for this review.

The handful of existing studies designed to explore the helpfulness of young people's involvement in 12-step groups shows promise in this approach, yet this body of work is far from conclusive. To date, it indicates that adolescents who attend AA and/or NA after residential substance abuse treatment are more likely to remain abstinent, engage in less frequent substance use, and have better posttreatment outcomes than those who do not (Alford, Koehler, & Leonard, 1991; Hsieh, Hoffman, & Hollister, 1998; Kelly & Myers, 1997; Kelly, Myers, & Brown, 2000; Kelly, Myers, & Brown, 2002; Kennedy & Minami, 1993). Two of these studies identified self-help meeting attendance as one of the most powerful discriminators of abstinence from substances up to 6 and 12 months after discharge (Hsieh, Hoffman, & Hollister, 1998; Kennedy & Minami, 1993). Table 1 provides further information about sample characteristics and outcomes of adolescent studies described throughout this section. More detailed descriptions can also be found in a review article by Kelly & Myers (2007).

In their review of the literature on adolescent participation in AA and NA, Kelly & Myers (2007) suggest that, while evidence is starting to accumulate that youths may benefit from participation in 12-step groups, conclusions on this subject are limited in four main ways: (1) only a small number of studies has been conducted; (2) all known published research has concentrated on adolescents discharged from residential or inpatient treatment, but no studies have yet examined 12-step involvement with adolescents treated in an outpatient setting; (3) research designs have been purely observational in nature, restricting the ability to make judgments about the effectiveness of youth participation in 12-step meetings; and

TABLE 1. Studies of Adolescents' Participation in Recovery Support Groups: Sample Characteristics, Settings, and Selected Outcomes

Authors (Year)	n	Mean Age	Female	Race/Ethnicity	Setting /a	Selected Outcomes
Alford, Koehler, & Leonard (1991)	157	16	38%	Not reported	Inpatient CD hospital unit	At 2 years post-discharge, youth who attended AA/NA at least weekly were significantly more likely to be abstinent or essentially abstinent than were those who attended less often or not at all.
Hohman & LeCroy (1996)	70	15	60%	Not reported	Residential CD treatment program	Adolescents who affiliated with AA post-discharge were more likely to have had prior treatment, friends who did not use drugs, less parental involvement in treatment, and more hopelessness.
Hsieh, Hoffman, & Hollister (1998)	2,317	Not reported	37%	2% African-American 90% Caucasian 2% Hispanic 4% Other	24 residential CD treatment programs	Post-treatment variables, especially attendance at AA/NA or other self-help support groups, were the most powerful discriminators of substance abuse status at 6 and 12 months post-discharge.

(Continued on next page)

TABLE 1. Studies of Adolescents' Participation in Recovery Support Groups: Sample Characteristics, Settings, and Selected Outcomes (Continued)

Authors (Year)	n	Mean Age	Female	Race/Ethnicity	Setting /a	Selected Outcomes
Kelly & Myers (1997)	43	15	61%	84% Caucasian 16% Other	Inpatient CD treatment program	More frequent AA/NA attendance was related to less frequent substance use at 3 months post-discharge. Those who attended groups with at least a substantial proportion of teens had significantly better substance use outcomes.
Kelly, Myers, & Brown (2000)	99	16	60%	4% African-American 78% Caucasian 16% Hispanic 2% Other	2 inpatient CD treatment programs	After controlling for factors such as aftercare attendance and intake substance use levels, 12-step meeting attendance during the first 3 months post -discharge contributed uniquely to substance use outcome variance at 3 and 6 months post-discharge.

| Kelly, Myers, & Brown (2002) | 74 | 16 | 62% | 8% African-American 70% Caucasian 18% Hispanic 4% Other | 2 inpatient CD treatment programs | Adolescents with greater substance use severity were more motivated for abstinence and more likely to attend and to affiliate with 12-step groups in the first 3 months post-discharge. Higher frequency of attendance and greater affiliation were associated with better post-treatment substance use outcome. Affiliation did not predict outcome over and above attendance. |
| Kelly, Myers, & Brown (2005) | 74 | 16 | 62% | 8% African-American 70% Caucasian 18% Hispanic 4% Other | 2 inpatient CD treatment programs | Greater age similarity to other meeting members was found to positively influence 12-step meeting attendance rates and the perceived importance of attendance. It was also marginally related to increased step-work and (at 6 months post-discharge) less substance use. Greater age similarity at meetings was not related to an increased likelihood of having a sponsor or engaging in social activities with 12-step members. |

(Continued on next page)

Table 1. Studies of Adolescents' Participation in Recovery Support Groups: Sample Characteristics, Settings, and Selected Outcomes (Continued)

Authors (Year)	n	Mean Age	Female	Race/Ethnicity	Setting /a	Selected Outcomes
Kelly, Myers, & Rodolico (in press)	Study 1:74; Study 2: 377	Study 1: 16; Study 2:17	Study 1: 62%; Study 2: 49%	Study 1: 8% African-American 70% Caucasian 18% Hispanic 4% Other Study 2: 2% African-American 81% Caucasian 5% Hispanic 12% Other	Inpatient CD treatment programs	Study 1: Aspects of AA/NA that youth liked best were general group dynamic processes related to universality, support, and instillation of hope; Study 2: The most common reason for discontinuing attendance was boredom/lack of fit, followed by relapse. Youths with prior AA/NA participation were significantly older and were more likely to have had prior CD treatment, prior psychiatric treatment, and a parent that attended AA/NA.
Kennedy & Minami (1993)	91	17	21%	92% Caucasian 8% Other	Inpatient/wilderness CD treatment program	Compared to adolescents who participated in AA/NA, those who did not had fourfold higher odds of relapse during the first 12-months post-discharge. AA/NA attendance and severity of drug use problems were the two best predictors of relapse.

/a: CD = chemical dependency.

(4) the 12-step construct has largely been measured in terms of attendance, pointing toward the need for additional information related to other dimensions of involvement, such as sponsor utilization, reading and comprehension of 12-step literature, and youths' understanding of the steps and how they are worked. Kelly & Myers (2007) advocate that future research studies include outpatient populations, focus on comparative efficacy and effectiveness studies of youth involvement in 12-step programs, better measure the 12-step construct, enhance understanding of developmentally specific barriers to participation, include process studies to inform practice guidelines for professionals, collect more data regarding the frequency, spacing, intensity, and duration of 12-step participation by youths, and test 12-step facilitation efforts for adolescents.

Complicating efforts to maximize the benefits of youth attendance at recovery support meetings is the fact that, as with adults (Galaif & Sussman, 1995; Kelly & Moos, 2003), a large number of adolescents who begin going to 12-step meetings eventually stop. One study revealed that the percentage of adolescents reporting attendance at one or more 12-step meetings dropped from 75% at 3 months postresidential discharge to 59% at 6 months (Kelly, Myers, & Brown, 2000). Another study discovered that 60% of adolescents in residential treatment attended 12-step meetings during the first 3 months after discharge, but only 38% did so at 12 months (Kennedy & Minami, 1993).

Adolescents who are more likely to attend 12-step meetings and/or to become involved with them tend to present for treatment with more severe substance abuse problems (Kelly, Myers, & Brown, 2002), have friends who use little to no substances, have been admitted to treatment more than once, experience more feelings of hopelessness, and receive less family participation in their treatment (Hohman & LeCroy, 1996). Further evidence suggests that professional inpatient programs with a 12-step orientation facilitate AA and/or NA participation immediately following treatment for a number of clients, at least in the short term (Kelly, Myers, & Rodolico, in press; Passetti & Godley, 2008).

Results from a recent study of adolescents discharged from residential substance-abuse treatment indicate that, in general, they perceived AA and/or NA to be important and helpful in their recovery; yet just over one in four perceived participation to be of little or no importance. On average, they felt connected to these recovery support groups; yet approximately one in five reported little or no feeling of connection to them. Aspects of AA and/or NA that youths reported liking the most were general group dynamic processes related to universality, support, and instillation of hope.

The most common reasons adolescents reported for dropping out of 12-step groups included boredom, lack of fit with the group, and relapse. To a lesser extent, lack of perceived need to continue, low motivation, and the removal of external pressures to attend were also mentioned. The authors concluded that general group therapeutic factors, rather than 12-step-specific ones, were most valued by adolescents during early stages of recovery and AA and/or NA exposure (Kelly, Myers, & Rodolico, in press).

Given the promise yet inconclusiveness of current research in the area of youth 12-step group involvement, providing clear recommendations for professionals working with youths experiencing substance abuse problems is challenging. Several issues, concerns, and barriers to the participation of young people have been raised in the literature or anecdotally by clinicians from adolescent treatment programs and are discussed below for further consideration.

Issues to Consider When Referring Youths to 12-Step and Alternative Support Groups

Potential iatrogenic effects of group interventions. One concern articulated in the literature on group interventions with youths is the potential of peers to contribute to the escalation of problem behaviors among young adolescents through "deviancy training." Data from some research conducted with at-risk youths suggested that certain peer-group interventions unintentionally increased adolescent problem behavior and negative life outcomes in adulthood under some circumstances (Dishion, McCord, & Poulin, 1999; Dishion, Poulin, & Barraston, 2002). These consequences may be impacted by the characteristics of group participants, the skill of group leaders, and the intervention context (Dishion & Dodge, 2005; Gifford-Smith, Dodge, Dishion, & McCord, 2005). Importantly, these studies focused on preventive interventions for at-risk youth who were in pre- or early adolescence and had not yet developed a substance use disorder (Burleson, Kaminer, & Dennis, 2006).

Research with adolescents who have already developed substance use disorders has failed to identify peer contagion effects of group interventions. For example, Waldron et al. (2001) did not find negative outcomes for the group intervention included in their randomized trial of four substance-abuse treatment models. Results from the Cannabis Youth Treatment (CYT) experiment (Dennis et al., 2004) indicated that all three group therapy conditions were associated with reduced substance use and problems during treatment and a follow-up period. Relative to individual and family interventions, there was no evidence of iatrogenic effects from group treatment in one of the largest randomized trials of adolescent substance abuse treatment. Additional examination of CYT data revealed that the composition of group members in terms of conduct disorder symptoms was not associated with worse substance use, psychological, environmental, or legal treatment outcomes. In fact, there was a slight advantage for youths with conduct disorder to be included in groups consisting of members with less severe symptoms. No results suggested that youths presenting with less severe conduct disorder failed to improve on outcome measures when exposed to youths with more severe symptoms, supporting the idea that group therapy for adolescents with substance use disorders is safe and effective (Burleson et al., 2006). Finally, a review of 66 studies by Weiss et al. (2005) did not discover any real evidence of systematic iatrogenic effects of group treatment of antisocial youths over the age of eleven.

These findings demonstrate that group interventions run by clinicians may not have negative effects on young people solely by virtue of the fact that they contain other youths with substance use disorders and behavioral problems. Recovery support meetings, however, are not traditionally run by treatment professionals and are frequently comprised of mostly adults. Anecdotally, some clinicians have expressed apprehension about adolescents' attendance at 12-step meetings dedicated to youths. One issue of concern was that youth groups tend to consist of a large gathering of newcomers (i.e., those without long-term sobriety) who lack the ability to offer recovery-related wisdom and, in some cases, who lack an investment in recovery. Another concern was that young people who tend to make poor relationship choices could form inappropriate relationships with other adults or adolescents in these meetings. Both sets of circumstances may test youths' ability to remain clean and sober (Passetti & Godley, 2008).

No detailed research investigating potential harmful effects of same-aged or older recovery support group members on youths has been identified; however, in response to these issues, professionals who refer youths to recovery support groups may want to consider working with parents and caregivers to structure and supervise youths' time before and after meetings to minimize the opportunity for negative interactions. Caregivers and professionals may also want to closely monitor attendance experiences and contacts made with other group members.

Age composition of recovery support group meetings. While 12-step-oriented treatment approaches and referrals of youths to recovery support meetings are prevalent (Drug Strategies, 2003; Jainchill, 2000), recent membership surveys of three common 12-step support groups reveal that less than 3% of their members are under the age of 21 (Alcoholics Anonymous, 2005; Cocaine Anonymous World Services, 2006; Narcotics Anonymous World Services, 2005). Rates of youth membership in 12-step alternative support groups are largely unknown, but a survey of LifeRing members indicated that less than 1% were under the age of 20 (LifeRing, 2005). Even though meetings dedicated to youths exist in some (but not all) communities, these statistics suggest that typical 12-step meetings consist largely of adults. Furthermore, Kelly and Myers (1997) found that 65% of the 12-step meetings attended by adolescents in that study were comprised mainly of older individuals. Such findings are meaningful because the substance-use patterns and related problems of adults often differ from those of youths. For example, adolescents in treatment tend to use multiple substances concurrently and experience fewer medical complications, fewer withdrawal symptoms, and significantly shorter histories of substance abuse than adults (Brown, 1993; Stewart & Brown, 1995). They also tend to have less substance-abuse problem recognition and motivation for abstinence (Tims et al., 2002). Adults may face difficulties related to loss of employment, loss of housing, and troubled relationships with spouses and children that youths cannot always identify with in their own lives.

Practice guidelines released by the American Psychiatric Association (1995) advise that young people generally function better in groups that consist of age-appropriate peers in addition to older members and that clients most likely benefit from groups containing individuals of similar age. Interviews with 28 clinicians employed in adolescent substance-abuse treatment programs across the country revealed that age composition of group members was one of the most common factors considered when referring adolescents to 12-step meetings (Passetti & Godley, 2008). Research conducted to date supports the belief that those youths who attend meetings with at least a substantial proportion of adolescents after inpatient treatment have significantly better substance-use outcomes (Kelly & Myers, 1997; Kelly, Myers, & Brown, 2005), higher frequency of attendance, and greater perceptions of the importance of meeting attendance. Greater age similarity, however, was not found to be related to the increased likelihood of having a sponsor or engaging in social activities with other 12-step group members (Kelly, Myers, & Brown, 2005). Additionally, while interviews with clinicians indicated that they perceived adolescents to have difficulty relating to adults, a few mentioned that some youths seemed to prefer adult meetings for the wisdom and praise provided by older individuals (Passetti & Godley, 2008).

Based on this information, professionals referring youths to recovery support meetings may want to locate groups that attract larger percentages of youths in an effort to maximize attendance, involvement, and substance use outcomes; however, close monitoring of experiences and contacts with other group members may be warranted given concerns described earlier. Some clinicians have noticed that young people tend to like NA more than AA because it attracts a younger and more diverse crowd (Passetti & Godley, 2008). Professionals may help youth by speaking with them about their comfort level at meetings consisting mainly of adults and by recognizing that some youths could opt to attend a mixture of meetings (i.e., some with more youths and some with mostly adults). Additionally, professionals may want to emphasize that other adolescents have benefited from support groups by feeling less lonely and more supported in their recovery efforts.

Ability of youths to understand and/or "buy into" program concepts. Related to the issue that young people may not relate well to adults is the concern that youths may have difficulty understanding and embracing ideas framed in adult language in recovery support groups, particularly ones grounded in the 12 steps. Concepts such as "acceptance," "surrender," and "spirituality" in 12-step programs are suspected to be too abstract for adolescents to grasp (Deas & Thomas, 2001; Passetti & Godley, 2008). Due to their relatively short substance use histories, youths may also find it problematic to admit powerlessness over alcohol or other drugs and commit to lifelong abstinence, especially if they do not meet criteria for substance dependence (Passetti & Godley, 2008).

Little systematic investigation has explored how young people perceive and interpret common concepts in recovery support groups. Preliminary results from qualitative interviews with adolescents in residential substance abuse treatment indicate that some young people acknowledge feelings of powerlessness over substances and recognize that their lives are unmanageable. For example, certain adolescents experienced loss of control over substance usage, school or work problems, strained relationships with other people, and substance-related legal involvement. The idea of "hitting bottom" was harder to identify with, and some youths interviewed struggled with spirituality and comprehending 12-step literature. Steps related to making a fearless moral inventory and direct amends to people harmed were sometimes perceived as confusing or frightening (Passetti, 2006). Interestingly, adolescents participating in the research conducted by Kelly et al. (in press) did not report that the spiritual content of 12-step meetings was one of the main reasons for stopping attendance. On the other hand, 12-step-specific content was not a major reason for attending meetings early in the recovery process. Both of these studies focused on youths admitted to residential treatment who tend to have more severe substance use histories than those admitted to less intensive treatment modalities; therefore, no conclusions can be drawn about the perceptions of young people with less severe substance use problems.

Since certain recovery support program concepts may be difficult to understand for some adolescents, professionals may want to review the language, concepts, and practices in those programs to prepare youths for what to expect during meetings (Forman, 2002) as well as to correct any misconceptions that may interfere with willingness to attend meetings. Youths can be encouraged to discuss any concerns, confusion, or anxiety with other group members or sponsors.

Severity of youths' substance use and related problems. In one study, clinicians working in adolescent substance abuse treatment programs were more likely to refer youths to 12-step meetings if they presented with a high severity of substance use or were diagnosed with substance dependence rather than abuse. If adolescents demonstrated problems with substance use over a period of time or experienced serious or numerous consequences from their use, they were referred more frequently. A history of prior substance abuse treatment admissions and a greater openness to admitting that substance use was problematic also helped some clinicians determine that referrals were appropriate (Passetti & Godley, 2008).

While a previously described study indicated that adolescents with more severe substance use problems were more likely to attend 12-step meetings (Kelly, Myers, & Brown, 2002), no research has confirmed or refuted the idea that youths with less severe substance use problems do not benefit from recovery support groups, and debate on this issue exists. Passetti and Godley (2008) reported differing views articulated by various clinicians. Some felt that many adolescents will not go on to have lifelong issues with substances and that stories heard during 12-step meetings would be sensationalized. Others believed that exposing youths to 12-step groups could help them to explore the ideas of powerlessness and acceptance and to feel more comfortable accessing recovery support groups in the future if needed. Furthermore, adolescents may hear other people's stories and realize that their substance use was more serious than they originally thought. Future research is needed in this area.

Differences in recovery support models. When making referrals to recovery support groups, professionals would benefit from becoming familiar with the models from which they operate (Laudet, 2003), the activities in which members engage (Chappel & DuPont, 1999), and the subcultures that might exist (Holleran & MacMaster, 2005). In the case of AA or NA, knowledge of the 12 steps and 12-step concepts would enable professionals to speak meaningfully with youths and to make the most informed referrals. Acquiring and reading group literature, visiting groups' internet sites, attending open meetings, and speaking with group members facilitate the process of learning group rules, concepts, language, and activities and the identification of group principles and guidelines, including membership requirements (White & Kurtz, 2006). For example, the only requirement for membership in AA is a desire to stop drinking (Alcoholics Anonymous World Services, 1972). If youths are not sure that they have a drinking problem or are reluctant to commit to abstinence, referrals to open meetings that welcome the general public rather than closed ones that are only for individuals who want to address a drinking problem may be more appropriate.

Familiarity with the variety of recovery support groups offered is important as well (Chappel & DuPont, 1999; Laudet & White, 2005; White & Kurtz, 2006). Not every youth will like 12-step meetings, and as established earlier, many stop attending over time. Some youths may find attending more than one type of group meeting helpful. By knowing about existing alternatives, professionals can provide youths with a menu of options for ongoing recovery support. Links to several mutual support groups can be found at the Faces and Voices of Recovery Web site mentioned above.

Differences in local recovery support group meetings. In addition to knowledge about different support groups, information about specific meetings of those groups can help guide referral practices. Significant variation exists among individual support group meetings within the same fellowship, network, or association, both across and inside geographic regions (Montgomery, Miller, & Tonigan, 1993). Differences in cohesiveness, independence, aggressiveness, and expressiveness have been found between AA meetings as well as differences in the perceived amount of focus on working the steps and the 12-step program (Tonigan, Ashcroft, & Miller, 1995). One meeting is not necessarily like another.

Since recovery support group meetings can differ greatly from one another, professionals may benefit youths by gathering information about particular meetings in youths' communities and then using this data to match an individual young person with particular meetings based on needs, preferences, and cultural background (Humphreys et al., 2004; Laudet, 2003; Passetti & Godley, 2008). Important considerations may include which ones have young participants, consist of members with long-term abstinence, or have adult members that welcome young people (Passetti & Godley, 2008). For certain youths, the number of people that normally attend, a smoking or nonsmoking designation, and/or substance of choice of group members may help determine which meeting to recommend. Other youths may be interested in meetings dedicated to certain groups of people based on gender or sexual orientation, speaker or discussion meetings, and/or meetings devoted to discussions of particular steps or traditions in 12-step- oriented groups (Forman, 2002; Passetti & Godley, 2008). In the case of AA, it may be relevant to know which meetings are more or less tolerant of individuals who are dependent on substances other than alcohol (Passetti & Godley, 2008). Youths may need to be encouraged to try a variety of meetings before finding ones that they feel the most comfortable attending (Caldwell, 1998; Passetti & Godley, 2008).

Professionals can learn about local recovery support group meetings in several ways. Colleagues and staff members of local substance-abuse treatment agencies, particularly those who have identified themselves as recovering, may be valuable sources of information (Chappel & DuPont, 1999; Passetti & Godley, 2008). Youths with prior meeting experience can provide insights from their perspectives (Passetti & Godley, 2008). Additionally, professionals not in recovery may want to attend open meetings in targeted communities to become familiar with the dynamics of those specific groups. Meeting lists can often be obtained by calling groups at contact numbers listed in the local telephone directory or from the Internet.

The ability to recommend certain meetings for youths depends on the availability and accessibility of meetings in a given area. Urban and sub-urban regions will more likely have a range of options than small towns and rural locations. If a youth lives in a small town with only one adult AA meeting and has no transportation, choices are limited without creative intervention. School and employment schedules and curfews may also impact which meetings youths are able to attend. A lack of available recovery support meetings in some geographical areas is triggering interest in telephone-based and internet-based recovery support services (Skinner et al., 2001; Kaminer & Napolitano, 2004). A helpful guide to such online recovery support groups can be found at the Faces and Voices of Recovery Web site.

Working with recovery support groups to connect youths to the recovering community. Most recovery support groups have service structures and procedures governing relationships with treatment organizations and other institutions. In AA, Hospitals and Institutions Committees or Treatment Facilities Committees work with organizations to bring meetings into facilities, encourage participation, coordinate temporary contact programs, and help arrange the purchase and distribution of literature (Alcoholics Anonymous, 2006). Other 12-step groups typically have similar structures in place (White & Kurtz, 2006). When working with youths, professionals may decide to contact such committees to facilitate involvement in the recovering community. Committee members may also be willing to help start meetings that might attract larger numbers of youths if they do not exist in a certain area.

Assertive linkage versus passive referral. In adult populations, assertively linking individuals to recovery support groups has proven to be a more successful strategy than passively recommending them to attend (White & Kurtz, 2006). Assertive linkage procedures may involve early referral to support groups, education about the potential benefits and risks of meeting attendance, ongoing monitoring of involvement and obstacles, and discussion of each person's prior experiences with, responses to, and perceptions of participation (Laudet, 2003; Ogborne, 1989; White & Kurtz, 2006). One study demonstrated that directly connecting someone to a 12-step group representative, rather than only providing meeting information and verbal encouragement, increased 12-step group attendance (Sisson & Mallams, 1981). While another study did not find greater attendance rates, referral procedures that proactively introduced adults to 12-step group volunteers, addressed concerns, set attendance goals, and encouraged finding a sponsor and a home group fostered greater involvement in 12-step activities, such as providing a service (e.g., setting up and taking down tables and chairs for meetings) and obtaining a sponsor. Those adults that received this intervention demonstrated significantly higher abstinence rates from substances other than alcohol than those who did not, and those with less previous meeting attendance were more likely to attend a greater number of meetings (Timko, DeBenedetti, & Billow, 2006).

There have been additional recommendations to incorporate motivational interviewing principles into efforts to link individuals with support groups. A focus on enhancing motivation to change and to abstain from substances, substance use problem acknowledgement, and recognition of the need for external support may promote attendance (Cloud et al., 2006; Laudet, 2003; White & Kurtz, 2006). In one study with adults admitted to an alcohol detoxification program, a 12-step motivational enhancement condition did not increase attendance at 12-step groups or improve drinking outcomes; however, the motivational approach was found to be more effective with individuals with little prior 12-step group experience (Kahler et al., 2004).

None of the above linkage strategies have been empirically tested with youths. Research in this area is needed to identify the most effective and appropriate referral strategies for young people. Motivational enhancement techniques may be especially appropriate for this population because of their tendency to have low substance use problem recognition and to have less experience with recovery support groups (Kelly, Myers, & Rodolico, in press). One study has provided preliminary information about the relationship between referral strategies of adolescent substance abuse treatment clinicians and rates of self-help meeting attendance. Analyses of interviews with clinicians from eight sites across the United States revealed that staff located at sites with the highest overall rates of adolescent self-help meeting attendance tended to engage in certain activities that the other sites did not or did to a lesser extent. They actively linked youths to the recovery community in the following ways: (1) by bringing them to sober social activities sponsored by support groups (e.g., young peoples' conferences and sober dances, picnics, and retreats); statewide activities of young people in AA can be identified on the state conferences of young people in AA Web sites (see http://www.e-aa.org/links/index.php?PID=9); (2) by working with service structures of support groups to host meetings and to locate good role models for youths; (3) by creating formal and informal networks of trusted people to accompany youths to meetings and/or to introduce them to the group; (4) by monitoring recovery support group attendance postdischarge through continuing care or case management; and (5) by helping youths identify and approach potential sponsors and then by interacting with and screening those sponsors for appropriateness. Appropriate sponsors possessed a good understanding of the 12-steps, worked the steps themselves, and had their own sponsor (Passetti & Godley, 2008).

Given these findings, professionals attempting to enhance youth attendance at recovery support groups may want to research support group-sponsored activities in youths' communities and assemble a list of reliable, trustworthy, and diverse individuals who can serve as temporary guides to a particular support group (Forman, 2002; Johnson & Chappel, 1994; White & Kurtz, 2006). Group members who have experience with or are willing to work with young people and are knowledgeable about local meetings may be identified through the committees of various support groups, consultation with colleagues, prior experience with youths who are connected into the recovering community, or communication with staff at substance-abuse treatment facilities. Ongoing monitoring of youths' interactions with group members, especially sponsors, and of their experiences at meetings may assist professionals in assessing the relationships that are formed, as well as reactions and obstacles to participation.

CONCLUSION

Further research is clearly needed into the effectiveness of youth involvement in recovery support groups and into the usefulness of various referral strategies. Referrals to such groups are a promising avenue for future investigation. To assist young people in this area, professionals may want to engage in the following activities: (1) help young people structure their time before and after meetings and monitor their interactions with group members to minimize situations that may lead to relapse; (2) become familiar with group customs and languages to prepare youths for meetings, make appropriate referrals, and clear any misunderstandings; (3) research the characteristics of local meetings, including age composition of members, so that referrals can be tailored based on youths' needs, preferences, and cultural backgrounds; (4) investigate the variety of recovery support groups offered in a given area to provide youths with a menu of options; (5) recognize that some youths may need to try a diversity of meetings before finding one (or a combination) that feels comfortable; (6) interact with recovery support group service structures and develop a list of reliable group members to connect youths to the recovering community; and (7) implement assertive rather than passive referral strategies, including connecting youths to sober social activities sponsored by support groups, helping youths identify and approach sponsors, screening sponsors for appropriateness, monitoring attendance, and monitoring reactions to experiences and program concepts.

REFERENCES

Alcoholics Anonymous. (2005). *Alcoholics Anonymous 2004 membership survey.* New York: AA World Services.

Alcoholics Anonymous. (2006). *AA guidelines: Treatment facilities committees.* Retrieved, March 15, 2007 from http://www.aa.org/en_pdfs/mg-14_treatfacilcomm.pdf

Alcoholics Anonymous World Services. (1972). *A brief guide to Alcoholics Anonymous.* New York: AA World Services.

Alford, G. S., Koehler, R. A., & Leonard, J. (1991). Alcoholics Anonymous—Narcotics Anonymous model inpatient treatment of chemically dependent adolescents: A 2-year outcome study. *Journal of Studies on Alcoholics, 52*, 118–26.

American Psychiatric Association. (1995). Practice guidelines for the treatment of patients with substance abuse disorders: Alcohol, cocaine, opioids. *American Journal of Psychiatry, 152* (Nov. suppl.), 1–59.

Bond, J., Kaskutas, L. A., & Weisner, C. (2003). The persistent influence of social networks and Alcoholics Anonymous on abstinence. *Journal of Studies on Alcohol, 64*, 579–88.

Brown, S. A. (1993). Recovery patterns in adolescent substance abuse. In J. S. Baer, G. A. Marlatt, & R. J. McMahon (Eds.), *Addictive behaviors across the life span: Prevention, treatment, and policy issues* (pp. 161–83). Newbury Park, CA: Sage.

Brown, S. A., Vik, P. W., & Creamer, V. A. (1989). Characteristics of relapse following adolescent substance abuse treatment. *Addictive Behaviors, 14*, 291–300.

Burleson, J. A., Kaminer, Y., & Dennis, M. L. (2006). Absence of iatrogenic or contagion effects in adolescent group therapy: Findings from the Cannabis Youth Treatment (CYT) study. *American Journal on Addictions, Supplement 1, 15*, 4–15.

Caldwell, P. E. (1998). Fostering client connections with Alcoholics Anonymous: A framework for social workers in various practice settings. *Social Work in Health Care, 28*, 45–61.

Chappel, J., & DuPont R. (1999). Twelve-step and mutual-help programs for addictive disorders. *Psychiatric Clinics of North America, 22*, 425–46.

Cloud, R. N., Besel, K., Bledsoe, L., Golder, S., McKiernan, P., Patterson, D., et al. (2006). Adapting motivational interviewing strategies to increase posttreatment 12-step meeting attendance. *Alcoholism Treatment Quarterly, 24*, 31–53.

Cocaine Anonymous World Services. (2006). *Membership Survey*. Retrieved, March 15, 2007 from http://www.ca.org/survey.html

Connors, G. J., Tonigan, J. S., & Miller, W. R. (2001). A longitudinal model of intake symptomatology, AA participation, and outcome: Retrospective study of the Project MATCH outpatient and aftercare samples. *Journal of Studies on Alcohol, 62*, 817–25.

Deas, D., & Thomas, S. E. (2001). An overview of controlled studies of adolescent substance abuse treatment. *American Journal of Addiction, 10*, 178–89.

Dennis, M., Godley, S. H., Diamond, G., Tims, F. M., Babor, T., Donaldson, J., et al. (2004). The Cannabis Youth Treatment (CYT) study: Main findings from two randomized trials. *Journal of Substance Abuse Treatment, 27*, 197–213.

Dishion, T. J., & Dodge, K. A. (2005). Peer contagion in interventions for children and adolescents: Moving toward an understanding of the ecology and dynamics of change. *Journal of Abnormal Child Psychology, 33*, 395–400.

Dishion, T. J., McCord, J., & Poulin, F. (1999). When interventions harm: Peer groups and problem behavior. *American Psychologist, 54*, 755–64.

Dishion, T. J., Poulin, F., & Barraston, B. (2002). Peer group dynamics associated with iatrogenic effects in group interventions with high-risk young adolescents. *New Directions in Child and Adolescent Development, 91*, 79–92.

Drug Strategies. (2003). *Treating teens: A guide to adolescent programs*. Washington, DC: Drug Strategies.

Foltz, A. (1891). *From hell to heaven and how I got there: Being the life history of a saved bar keeper, with stirring addresses on the temperance question.* Lincoln: Hunter Printing House.

Forman, R. F. (2002, October). One AA meeting doesn't fit all: 6 keys to prescribing 12-step programs. *Current Psychiatry, 1*, 16–24.

Galaif, D. R., & Sussman, S. (1995). For whom does Alcoholics Anonymous work? *International Journal of the Addictions, 30*, 161–84.

Gamso, R., & Mason, P. (1958). A hospital for adolescent drug addicts. *Psychiatric Quarterly, Supplement, 32*, 99–109.

Gifford-Smith, M., Dodge, K. A., Dishion, T. J., & McCord, J. (2005). Peer influences in children and adolescents crossing the bridge from developmental to intervention science. *Journal of Abnormal Child Psychology, 33*, 255–65.

Godley, S. H., Godley, M. D., & Dennis, M. L. (2001). The Assertive Aftercare Protocol for adolescent substance abusers. In E. Wagner & H. Waldron (Eds.), *Innovations in adolescent substance abuse interventions* (pp. 311–29). New York: Elsevier Science.

Godley, M. D., Godley, S. H., Dennis, M. L., Funk, R., & Passetti, L. L. (2002). Preliminary outcomes from the assertive continuing care experiment for adolescents discharged from residential treatment. *Journal of Substance Abuse Treatment, 23*, 21–32.

Godley, M. D., Godley, S. H., Dennis, M. L., Funk, R. R., & Passetti, L. L. (2006). The effect of assertive continuing care on continuing care linkage, adherence, and abstinence following residential treatment for adolescents with substance use disorders. *Addiction, 102*, 81–93.

Hohman, M., & LeCroy, C. W. (1996). Predictors of adolescent AA affiliation. *Adolescence, 31*, 339–52.

Holleran, L. K., & MacMaster, S. A. (2005). Applying a cultural competency framework to twelve step programs. *Alcoholism Treatment Quarterly, 23*, 107–20.

Hsieh, S., Hoffman, N. G., & Hollister, D. C. (1998). The relationship between pre-, during-, and post-treatment factors, and adolescent substance abuse behaviors. *Addictive Behaviors, 23*, 477–88.

Hubbard, S. (1920). The New York City Narcotic Clinic and different points of view on narcotic addiction. *Monthly Bulletin of the Department of Health of New York, 10*(2), 33–47.

Humphreys, K., Wing, S., McCarty, D., Chappel, J., Gallant, L., Haberle, B., et al. (2004). Self-help organizations for alcohol and drug problems: Toward evidence-based practice and policy. *Journal of Substance Abuse Treatment, 26*, 151–58.

Jainchill, N. (2000). Substance dependency treatment for adolescents: Practice and research. *Substance Use and Misuse, 35*, 2031–60.

Johnson, N. P., & Chappel, J. N. (1994). Using AA and other 12-step programs more effectively. *Journal of Substance Abuse Treatment, 11*, 137–42.

Kahler, C. W., Read, J. P., Ramsey, S. E., Stuart, G. L., McCrady, B. S., & Brown, R. A. (2004). Motivational enhancement for 12-step involvement among patients undergoing alcohol detoxification. *Journal of Consulting and Clinical Psychology, 72*, 736–41.

Kaminer, Y., & Napolitano, C. (2004). Dial for therapy: Aftercare for adolescent substance use disorders. *Journal of the American Academy of Child and Adolescent Psychiatry, 43*, 1171–74.

Kaskutas, L. A., Bond, J., & Humphreys, K. (2002). Social networks as mediators of the effect of Alcoholics Anonymous. *Addiction, 97*, 891–900.

Kelly, J. F., & Moos, R. (2003). Dropout from self-help groups: Prevalence, predictors, and counteracting treatment influences. *Journal of Substance Abuse Treatment, 24*, 241–50.

Kelly, J. F., & Myers, M. G. (1997). Adolescent treatment outcome in relation to 12-step group attendance. Abstracted in *Alcoholism: Clinical and Experimental Research, 21*, 27A.

Kelly, J. F., & Myers, M. G. (2007). Adolescents' participation in Alcoholics Anonymous and Narcotics Anonymous: Review, implications, and future directions. *Journal of Psychoactive Drugs, 39*, 259–269.

Kelly, J. F., Myers, M. G., & Brown, S. A. (2000). A multivariate process model of adolescent 12-step attendance and substance use outcome following inpatient treatment. *Psychology of Addictive Behavior, 14*, 376–89.

Kelly, J. F., Myers, M. G., & Brown, S. A. (2002). Do adolescents affiliate with 12-step groups? A multivariate process model of effects. *Journal of Studies on Alcohol, 63*, 293–304.

Kelly, J. F., Myers, M. G., & Brown, S. A. (2005). The effects of age composition of 12-step groups on adolescent 12-step participation and substance use outcome. *Journal of Child and Adolescent Substance Abuse, 15*, 63–72.

Kelly, J. F., Myers, M. G., & Rodolico, J. (in press). What do adolescents think about 12-step groups? Perceptions and experiences of two AA-exposed clinical samples. *Journal of Substance Abuse.*

Kennedy, B. P., & Minami, M. (1993). The Beech Hill Hospital/Outward Bound adolescent chemical dependency treatment program. *Journal of Substance Abuse Treatment, 10*, 395–406.

Kissin, W., McLeod, C., & McKay, J. (2003). The longitudinal relationship between self-help group attendance and course of recovery. *Evaluation and Program Planning, 26*, 311–23.

Laudet, A. (2003). Attitudes and beliefs about 12-step groups among addiction treatment clients and clinicians: Toward identifying obstacles to participation. *Substance Use and Misuse, 38*, 2017–47.

Laudet, A., & White, W. (2005). An exploratory investigation of the association between clinicians' attitudes toward twelve-step groups and referral rates. *Alcoholism Treatment Quarterly, 23*, 31–45.

LifeRing. (2005). *2005 LifeRing Participant Survey: Results.* Retrieved, March 15, 2007 from http://www.unhooked.com/survey/2005_lifering_participant_survey.htm

Margolis, R., Kilpatrick, A., & Mooney, B. (2000). A retrospective look at long-term adolescent recovery: Clinicians talk to researchers. *Journal of Psychoactive Drugs, 32*, 117–25.

McKellar, J., Stewart, E., & Humphreys, K. (2003). Alcoholics Anonymous involvement and positive alcohol-related outcomes: Cause, consequence, or just a correlate? A prospective 2-year study of 2,319 alcohol-dependent men. *Journal of Consulting and Clinical Psychology, 71*, 302–8.

Montgomery, H. A., Miller, W. R., & Tonigan, J. S. (1993). Differences among AA groups: Implications for research. *Journal of Studies on Alcohol, 54*, 502–4.

Moos, R. H., & Moos, B. S. (2004). Long-term influence of duration and frequency of participation in Alcoholics Anonymous on individuals with alcohol use disorders. *Journal of Consulting and Clinical Psychology, 72*, 81–90.

Narcotics Anonymous World Services. (2005, October). *Information about NA*. Retrieved, March 15, 2007 from http://na.org/basic.htm

New York Academy of Medicine. (1953). *Conferences on drug addiction among adolescents*. New York: The Blakiston Company.

Ogborne, A. C. (1989). Some limitations of Alcoholics Anonymous. *Recent Developments in Alcohol, 7*, 55–65.

Passetti, L. L. (2006, March). *Adolescents' perceptions of the 12 steps and 12-step philosophy*. Presentation at the Joint Meeting on Adolescent Treatment Effectiveness, Baltimore, MD.

Passetti, L. L., & Godley, S. H. (2008). Adolescent substance abuse treatment clinicians' self-help meeting referral practices and adolescent attendance rates. *Journal of Psychoactive Drugs, 40*, 29–40.

Sisson, R. W., & Mallams, J. H. (1981). The use of systematic encouragement and community access procedures to increase attendance at Alcoholics Anonymous and Al-Anon meetings. *American Journal of Drug and Alcohol Abuse, 8*, 371–76.

Skinner, H., Maley, O., Smith, L., Chirrey, S., & Morrison, M. (2001). New frontiers: Using the internet to engage teens in substance abuse prevention and treatment. In. P. M. Monti, S. M. Colby, & T. A. O'Leary (Eds.), *Adolescents, alcohol, and substance abuse: Reaching teens through brief interventions* (pp. 297–318). New York: Guilford. (2002, December). Retrieved December, 2002 from AAHistoryLovers@yahoo.groups.

Stewart, D. G., & Brown, S. A. (1995). Withdrawal and dependency symptoms among adolescent alcohol and drug abusers. *Addiction, 90*, 627–35.

Terry, C. E., & Pellens, M. (1928). *The opium problem*. Montclair, NJ: Patterson Smith.

Timko, C., DeBenedetti, A., & Billow, R. (2006). Intensive referral to 12-step self-help groups and 6-month substance use disorder outcomes. *Addiction, 101*, 678–88.

Tims, F. M., Dennis, M. L., Hamilton, N., Buchan, B. J., Diamond, G. S., Funk, R., et al. (2002). Characteristics and problems of 600 adolescent marijuana abusers in outpatient treatment. *Addiction, 97*, 46–57.

Tonigan, J. S., Ashcroft, F., & Miller, W. R. (1995). AA group dynamics and 12-step activity. *Journal of Studies on Alcohol, 56*, 616–21.

Waldron, H. B., Slesnick, N., Brody, J. L., Turner, C. W., & Peterson, T. R. (2001). Treatment outcomes for adolescent substance abuse at 4- and 7-month assessments. *Journal of Consulting and Clinical Psychology, 69*, 802–13.

Weiss, B., Caron, A., Ball, S., Tapp, J., Johnson, M., & Weisz, J. R. (2005). Iatrogenic effects of group treatment for antisocial youth. *Journal of Consulting and Clinical Psychology, 73*, 1036–44.

White, W. (1998). *Slaying the dragon: The history of addiction treatment and recovery in America*. Bloomington, IL: Chestnut Health Systems.

White, W. L. (1999). A history of adolescent alcohol, tobacco and other drug use in America. *Student Assistance Journal, 11*(5), 16–22.

White, W., & Kurtz, E. (2006). *Linking addiction treatment and communities of recovery: A primer for addiction counselors and recovery coaches*. Pittsburgh, PA: Institute for Research, Education, and Training in Addictions.

Twelve Step Meeting—Step Two

Recovery School Students

Jeffrey has entered the room "workingsobriety.com"

s_k_011 has entered the room "workingsobriety.com"

s_k_011: is anyone in here? just want to see if i made it in right?

Andrew has entered the room "workingsobriety.com"

austinm62 has entered the room "workingsobriety.com"

austinm62: Am I in the right place?

s_k_011: I think so I was not sure either

Andrew: yeah according to Jeffrey's email this is the right place

austinm62: k

s_k_011: ok

austinm62: whats up with noone showing up?

s_k_011: yeah it was just us three last time aren't there suppose to be a couple more people

Andrew: I don't know, almost noone replied to any of my emails when I was trying to set up the first meeting

Andrew: That's why it took so long to get going

Andrew: there are 6 or 8 people altogether

austinm62: yeah, i guess 3 is better than 0

Andrew: guess so

s_k_011: yeah

s_k_011: whats the step/topic tonight?

Andrew: We have yet to do Steps 2 and 12

During the course of arranging these on line meetings, the procedure for entering the chat room was changed due to technical difficulties. Note how the initial discussion moves immediately to the most important questions of the moment: first, whether this chat room is the right place to meet, and second, an examination of who is showing up. This sensitivity to process exemplifies one of the major changes that occurs in recovery from addiction. The "elephant in the living room" becomes the topic of conversation , rather than the source of denial.

Note also the rapid move towards acceptance, led by Austin, who not coincidentally is the chair of the meeting.

s_k_011: oh ok cool

Andrew: It's Austin's call as chair for this week

austinm62: oh I didn't realize I was chairing sorry

austinm62: just thought I was organizing, lol

Andrew: oh hah no prob, if you want to chair you can

Andrew: not too much to do

austinm62: Ok well lets get started.

s_k_011: do you think anyone else is coming

austinm62: If they come we'll fill them in when they get here

s_k_011: sounds good

austinm62: we all know the rules and formailities, so the

topic for this week is step 2 and 12. Would anyone like to start?

Andrew: should we do both or just one or the other? austinm62: well, we can do both but if we have to choose

just do 2nd step

s_k_011: we could do one and then the other if there is time

austinm62: sure lets do that

austinm62: Ok so step 2 we came to believe that a power greater than ourselves could restore us to sanity

austinm62: My name is austin and Im an addict

s_k_011: hi austin

Andrew: Hi Austin

austinm62: this is a wierd step for me being that I currently identify as an athiest

austinm62: So I guess i'll first go into my history with step 2

austinm62: I came into the program as an athiest

austinm62: I felt tremendous pressure to beleive in some form of higher power when I was in treatment

austinm62: the counselors and my sponsor kept telling me to fake until I make it

austinm62: So I did and with time my life got better

austinm62: at the time I attributed the positve phemonena occuring in my life to God

The position of authority that the meeting chair holds is supported by the members of the meeting. Unlike environments characterized by capricious exercise of authority, the environment of recovery supports authority that is mutually negotiated at all times. Andrew and Austin model this negotiation in exemplary fashion.
Lol=laugh out loud
The question of whether anyone else is coming may refer to the late entrance of Vijay at the last meeting.

Note again the negotiation around the meeting topic (Step 2 and/or 12); how each member voices their opinion and then authorizes the chair to make the decision. This process is consistent with the understanding of the group having its own Higher Power determined by the group conscience according to the second of the Twelve Traditions of AA.

Recognizing the absence of a benevolent Higher Power during the active phase of addiction may potentiate finding a Higher Power during recovery. The slogan "fake it until you make it" opens up the possibility of seeing evidence of a Higher Power. Austin articulately describes an operational definition of Higher Power: that to which he can attribute the positive phenomena in his life. Moving towards that Higher Power then leads to positive changes. However, even many people in recovery in Twelve Step programs confuse the spirituality of these programs with austinm62: This started a new phase in my recovery where I attempted to identify and re-negotiate my personality to fit with the conception of god

austinm62: It was a struggle from day one and i never really became comfortable being a "believer".

austinm62: I always felt more or less alienated by the spiritual aspects of the program austinm62: I eventually started to realize that no matter how hard I tried to believe, or even forced myself to believe, that I was just trying to shove a square peg in a round hole

austinm62: I am and probably will always be an atheist

austinm62: This realization really put my program into serious doubt

austinm62: "How can I remain a member of a 12-step group and be an atheist?"

austinm62: "How can I talk to my sponsor about this without him trying to convert me agian?"

austinm62: I eventually stopped going to the meetings I had been becausee I felt too much spiritual and religious pressure to believe as they did.

austinm62: I left AA and started going to a local NA meeting

austinm62: there I met a sponsor who also identified as an atheist

austinm62: This actually had nothing to do with NA in general, just a coincidence

austinm62: Anyways, he helped me to redefine what a higher power can be

austinm62: and made me feel as though it is ok to be an atheist and be in a 12-step program

austinm62: I started at that piont to identify principles and ultimately the power of the group as my higher power

austinm62: THis is where I more or less stand on my

higher power beliefs today

austinm62: An additional not on step 2...

austinm62: Restore to sanity is a crucial portion of step 2

a religion which demands belief in a specific God.

The process of "carrying the message of recovery" (see the Step Twelve meeting later in this book) is also frequently confused with religious evangelism or conversion. In fact, many alcoholics and addicts in recovery do not believe in a traditional god, and have established meetings for atheists and agnostics (AAAA-Atheists and Agnostics in AA).

Actually, the oral tradition in Twelve Step programs states that "my higher power may get you drunk."

Here Austin describes a common path to defining a higher power as the support of a loving group.

Interesting slip, "not" for "note"
Coming to believe in a higher power may facilitate the admission that one's addictive behavior is a form of insanity,

austinm62: If we use the 12-step pop-definition, insanity is trying the same thing over and over agina, expecting different results

austinm62: That definately categorized my life, in fact it still does from time to time today.

austinm62: I don't know if I give this definition the ultimate defintion of insanity but the idea behind the label is fitting

austinm62: When I work on my recovery, i am making conscious efforts to break negative cycles of behavior, both substance related behaviors and many other lifestyle behaviors that leave me in a negative place.

austinm62: Well, I've been sharing too long, so thanks.

Andrew: Thanks Austin

s_k_011: thanks austin

Andrew: !

austinm62: Hi andrew

s_k_011: Hi andrew

Andrew: I can definately relate to feeling some kind of pressure to get a higher power during treatment

Andrew: I was raised Catholic, and in fact I went to Easter mass today with my family, but I think that hindered my belief in a higher power

Andrew: I went to a Catholic high school and resented the strict religious point of view

Andrew: so when I started treatment and meetings, these steps were a little unnerving to see

Andrew: (2 and 3 and 11)

Andrew: but one of the huge reliefs I found was that not only can it be a higher power of my understanding, but I don't even have to put a definition or label on it

Andrew: I still held, and still hold, some beliefs from my christian upbringing, but it has evolved so much

Andrew: And since I was definately living an insane life and I saw so many people in the meetings were doing much better thanks to a higher power, I started praying and believing in some higher power, which I still can't and don't define or label

and that being restored to sanity is a process, not an event.

Ironically, after sharing these important thoughts on the second step, Austin reveals some possible shame about the length of his comments. He then recognizes Andrew, who volunteers to share next.

Andrew continues the theme of confusing the spiritual concept of a higher power with the religious concept of God, in his case, his understanding of a Catholic God.

Sometimes, the process of

Andrew: And one final point, "came to believe" is definatly true for me, it was certainly a process rather than a sudden experience or decision, and it's something I still have occasional doubts about, but my reliance on my higher power keeps growing

Andrew: Thanks for listening, I'll pass

austinm62: thanks andrew

s_k_011: thanks andrew

s_k_011: !

Andrew: Hi Stef

austinm62: hi stef s_k_011: My name is stef i am an alcoholic an addict

s_k_011: I was raised believing in the christian god and going to a non denominational church

s_k_011: as i started to use drugs and alcohol i didn't really care about "god" I blamed a lot of my problems s_k_011: on god

s_k_011: Once I came into the program and saw the steps that had god in them, I also saw as we understood

s_k_011: I had mentioned in meetings that I was unsure of what god was, some people kind of pressured the religious god and others shared that it was as you understand and came to believe

s_k_011: I do not have a label on my god either. I do believe in god. And since I have been praying it has made a difference in my life

s_k_011: Though as andrew mentioned my understanding of god is always growing. I do not put a label cause I am alway open to other peoples believes and opinons

s_k_011: I do not know exactly who my god or higher power is but i know that there is something out there and when i pray it helps

s_k_011: and like you said andrew "came to" it is a process for me not a instant decision

s_k_011: but the other part of step 2 "restore us to sanity" I am definatly alot more sane then i was when i was using and even more then when i was first getting sober

s_k_011: I do not think i will ever be completely sane but i do know that the program and god has helped restore me to some sanity.

recovery results in a changed attitude about religion. Prayer comes to mean a process of asking for help rather than complying with a formula.

Here we find an illustration of group conscience at work. No one member of the group makes a decision on behalf of the group to end the discussion. Austin notes that the group has the option of continuing discussion on Step Twelve or ending. Another group conscience is sought and accomplished. Further decisions are discussed and negotiated about contacting other members and setting up leadership and schedule for the next meeting.

s_k_011: Though I can still have many insane moments in my life

s_k_011: well thank you for listening and sharing. I will pass with that

Andrew: Thanks Stef

austinm62: thanks stef

austinm62: Does anyone want to add anything else on step 2? I personally am done with this topic

s_k_011: nope i am done thanks

Andrew: No, I'm done too, thanks

austinm62: Well, we only have 15 mins left for step 12 if we're going to talk about that topic. Do you think we should end now or have a very short discussion of step 12?

s_k_011: doesn't matter to me whatever you guys think

Andrew: I think we should wait because we might be able to get a better turnout, what do you think?

austinm62: Yeah that sounds good

s_k_011: yeah i agree

austinm62: Stef you want to email everyone this week?

austinm62: Maybe chair next time?

s_k_011: sure but i do not have anyones email adress

s_k_011: would you want to email them to me by any chance?

austinm62: Did you save any of the emails?

Andrew: I can email them to you

s_k_011: um possibly

Andrew: I have one more to add anyway

s_k_011: ok that would be really cool if you could andrew?

austinm62: ok cool

s_k_011: so next sunday this time good??

austinm62: Next sunday same time

Andrew: sounds good

austinm62: good for me

s_k_011: alright then i will start emailing once i get the list of adresses =)

austinm62: Ok, well thanks for coming andrew and stef, see you both next week

s_k_011: So see you guys next week then?

Andrew: You too, good night all.

austinm62: good night\

s_k_011: thanks! good night and have a good week

austinm62 has left the room (logged out)

s_k_011: see ya on sunday

Andrew has left the room (logged out)

s_k_011: how do you log out

s_k_011: nevermind stupid question

s_k_011 has left the room (logged out)

Recovering addicts often use other people to speak on behalf of a power greater than themselves, usually being careful not to make one person into a Higher Power, but relying on a group conscience.

Recovery High Schools: A Descriptive Study of School Programs and Students

D. Paul Moberg, PhD

School of Medicine and Public Health, University of Wisconsin

Andrew J. Finch, PhD

Vanderbilt University

ABSTRACT. High schools specifically designed for students recovering from a substance use disorder (substance abuse or dependence) have been emerging as a continuing care resource since 1987. This study of

D. Paul Moberg, PhD, is in the Population Health Institute, University of Wisconsin School of Medicine and Public Health, Madison, WI 53726-2397.

Andrew J. Finch, PhD, is in the Department of Human & Organizational Development, Vanderbilt University, Nashville, TN 37203.

Funding for this research was provided by the National Institute on Drug Abuse, Grant # R21-DA-019045. We are indebted to Barbara Hill for managing many of the details of this research and participating in most of the site visits. We particularly wish to thank the staff and students of the following schools for their enthusiastic participation in this research: Aateshing–Cass Lake, MN; Archway Academy–Houston, TX; Clean & Sober–Santa Rosa, CA; Clean & Sober–Petaluma, CA; Community High–Nashville, TN, Gateway Program–St. Paul, MN, Horizon High–Madison, WI, INSIGHT–White Bear Lake, MN; Phoenix Academy–San Rafael, CA; Safe Harbor–Spring Lake Park, MN; Serenity High–McKinney, TX; Sobriety High–Burnsville, MN; Sobriety High–Maplewood, MN; Sobriety High–Edina, MN; SOAR–Broomfield, CO; Solace Academy–Chaska, MN; Transitions High–Harrisburg, PA; and Winfree Academy–Dallas, TX.

17 schools provides the first systematic description of recovery school programs and their students. The most common school model is that of a program or affiliated school, embedded organizationally and physically with another school or set of alternative school programs. Although embedded, there are serious efforts to maintain physical separation of recovery school students from other students, using scheduling and physical barriers. Affiliation with public school systems is the case for most recovery schools and seems to be a major factor in assuring fiscal and organizational feasibility.

The students in the recovery high schools studied were predominantly White (78%), with about one-half from two parent homes. Overall parent educational levels suggest a higher mean socio-economic status (SES) than in the general population. Most students (78%) had prior formal treatment for substance use disorders, often concomitantly with treatment for mental health concerns, and were often referred by treatment providers. Students came with a broad and complex range of mental health issues, traumatic experiences, drug use patterns, criminal justice involvement, and educational backgrounds. The complexity of these problems clearly limits the enrollment capacity of the schools.

Retrospective pretest-to-posttest analysis suggests significant reduction in substance use as well as in mental health symptoms among the students. Students were very positive in their assessment of the therapeutic value of the schools but less enthusiastic regarding the educational programs. The school programs appear to function successfully as continuing care to reinforce and sustain the therapeutic benefits students gained from their treatment experiences.

INTRODUCTION

High schools specifically designed for students recovering from a substance use disorder[1] (substance abuse or dependence) began opening in the United States in 1987, with the opening of Sobriety High in Minnesota. According to the Association of Recovery Schools (ARS), this continuing care model has slowly grown since that time to include 31 high schools in 10 states. With some exceptions (Godley, Godley, Dennis, Funk, & Passetti, 2002; McKay, 2001; Spear & Skala, 1995; Winters, Stinchfield, Opland, Weller, & Latimer, 2000), overall research about posttreatment continuing care is sparse. Even more sparse is research conducted on recovery schools, which has been limited to theses and dissertations (e.g., Finch, 2003; Rubin, 2002; Teas, 1998) and unpublished reports (Moberg, 1999; Moberg & Thaler, 1995). Despite a lack of cross-school research and no published model for replication, growth has been impressive. Most of the schools have opened in the last 7 years. Recovery high schools received federal recognition in summer 2002 when the Center for Substance Abuse Treatment (CSAT) funded a 3-day conference for existing recovery school administrators. Hazelden Press recently published a manual by Dr. Finch, "Starting a Recovery School: A How-To Manual" (Finch, 2005).

As recovery schools generate awareness and more states and foundations consider funding such schools, exploratory research is needed to describe and explicate school models to inform replication and prepare for rigorous evaluation of the effectiveness of recovery schools. This paper provides initial results from an ongoing descriptive research project designed to begin evaluating this promising model for providing continuing care for adolescents with substance use disorders. Specifically, we describe the characteristics of the existing recovery high schools and their students, addressing the following questions:

- What services are provided in recovery schools?
- What educational and therapeutic models are being implemented?
- How are these schools funded to assure institutional viability?
- What goals exist for the schools and their students?
- What are the characteristics of the students in terms of substance use disorder, treatment history, comorbidity, and socioeconomic status?
- How do students gain access to the programs?

Further work with these data will attempt to develop a descriptive typology of recovery school programs and assess the feasibility of conducting more rigorous research. The data will also be examined to enhance our understanding of issues affecting the long-term institutionalization and viability of recovery school programs, which has been problematic to date. Thus we are laying the groundwork for future studies to prospectively evaluate the cost effectiveness of these programs of continuing care for adolescents with substance use disorders.

The methodology for this study was built upon prior single-site research on recovery schools conducted independently by the authors. Site visits were scheduled for each participating school and included document review, observation, staff interviews and surveys, student surveys, and interviews with key external constituents.

TERMINOLOGY

The concepts of "treatment" and "recovery" are evolving. Indeed, until recently, much less focus was placed in the United States on adolescent treatment than on prevention of adolescent substance abuse. As in any growing field, terminology, though often elusive, is important in attaining a common level of understanding. Some terms used frequently in this paper are "substance abuse," "dependence," "treatment," and "recovery." They are defined here.

Substance Abuse and Dependence

This paper uses the term "substance use disorder" to encompass both substance dependence and substance abuse, each of which is considered a substance use disorder in the Diagnostic and Statistical Manual of Mental Disorders, 4th edition (DSM-IV) (American Psychiatric Association, 1994). According to the DSM-IV, "The essential feature of Substance Abuse is a maladaptive pattern of substance use manifested by recurrent and significant adverse consequences related to repeated use of substances" (American Psychiatric Association, 1994, p. 182). The DSM-IV preempts a diagnosis of substance abuse with one of substance dependence if a person's pattern of substance use has ever met the criteria for substance dependence. Dependence is defined as, "a cluster of cognitive, behavioral, and physiological symptoms indicating that the individual continues use of the substance despite significant substance-related problems" (American Psychiatric Association, 1994, p. 176). These problems can be categorized as tolerance, withdrawal, or compulsive use behaviors. Thus substance use without "recurrent and significant adverse consequences" is not sufficient to warrant a substance use disorder diagnosis, nor does it qualify students for participation in a recovery school.

The Substance Abuse and Mental Health Administration (SAMHSA) provides this clarification:

> Dependence is considered to be a more severe substance use problem than abuse because it involves the psychological and physiological effects of tolerance and withdrawal. Although individuals may meet the criteria specified for both dependence and abuse, persons meeting the criteria for both are classified as having dependence, but not abuse. Persons defined with abuse do not meet the criteria for dependence.

(Substance Abuse and Mental Health Services Administration, 2006, p. 67)

Much of the national data referenced in this study were collected from the National Survey on Drug Use and Health (NSDUH), conducted annually by SAMHSA. Substances monitored by the NSDUH include alcohol and illicit drugs, such as marijuana, cocaine, heroin, hallucinogens, and inhalants, and the nonmedical use of prescription-type psychotherapeutic drugs (Substance Abuse and Mental Health Services Administration, 2006).

Treatment

"Treatment" is an evolving concept, especially for adolescents. The NSDUH creates a distinction between "specialty treatment" for a substance use disorder and more generalized treatment. The NSDUH defines specialty treatment as

> treatment received at any of the following types of facilities: hospitals (inpatient only), drug or alcohol rehabilitation facilities (inpatient or outpatient), or mental health centers. It does not include treatment at an emergency room, private doctor's office, self-help group, prison or jail, or hospital as an outpatient. An individual is defined as needing treatment for an alcohol or drug use problem if he or she met the DSM-IV (APA, 1994) diagnostic criteria for dependence on or abuse of alcohol or illicit drugs in the past 12 months, or if he or she received specialty treatment for alcohol use or illicit drug use in the past 12 months. (Substance Abuse and Mental Health Services Administration, 2006, p. 73)

These distinctions helped guide our understanding of the students in the schools, and they represent the meaning of our terminology in the paper. As the term "specialty treatment" can be cumbersome, we use the term "treatment" synonymously. Note that we do not consider 12-step meetings to be "treatment" in the context of this paper.

Recovery and the Continuum of Care

"Recovery" may be the most ambiguous of the terms discussed here. While recovery has often been considered to begin once treatment ends (i.e., "aftercare"), this understanding has proven insufficient. Since many people who meet the criteria for a substance use disorder do not ever receive treatment, recovery cannot be contingent upon the receipt of specialty treatment. Indeed, the field has embraced a "continuum of care" paradigm to replace the traditional, linear intervention-treatment-aftercare mindset. In his plenary presentation at the 2007 Joint Meeting on Adolescent Treatment Effectiveness (JMATE), Dr. Jack Stein, an administrator in SAMHSA's Center for Substance Abuse Treatment (CSAT), suggested that the field has started to view recovery as beginning with the decision to get treatment rather than after treatment ends (Stein, 2007). This corresponds well with Bill White's definition of "recovery" in his addiction recovery glossary as

> the process of resolving, or the status of having resolved, alcohol and other drug problems. . . . While recovering conveys the dynamic, developmental process of addiction recovery, recovered provides a means of designating those who have achieved stable sobriety and better conveys the real hope for a permanent resolution of alcohol and other drug problems. The period used to designate people recovered from other chronic disorders is usually 5 years without active symptoms. (White, 2002, p. 29)

This view of recovery is consistent with that of the schools selected for this study. Recovery schools typically limit enrollment to students with a "substance use disorder," as defined above. While few schools require treatment, most of the students in these schools have received some form of specialty treatment prior to and/or during their enrollment. Furthermore, using White's distinction between "recovering" or "recovered," none of the students in this study had attained 5 years of sobriety. Presumably, as high schools are typically 4 years of school, no recovery school student would achieve the "recovered" status unless he or she stopped using in seventh grade.

BACKGROUND

Post-treatment continuing care or "aftercare" services for persons recovering from a substance use disorder have been described by researchers to be a "logical," "essential," and "important" component of the treatment continuum (Brown & Ashery, 1979; Hawkins & Catalano, 1985; McKay, 2001). According to the National Survey on Drug Use and Health

(NSDUH) (Substance Abuse and Mental Health Services Administration, 2006), 2.1 million youths aged 12 to 17 needed treatment for an illicit drug or alcohol use problem in the United States in 2005, and of this group, 181,000 youths received treatment at a specialty facility (8.6% of youths who needed treatment). This left an additional 1.9 million youths in the United States who "needed" treatment for a substance use disorder but did not receive it at a specialty facility.

Rates of substance use disorders are associated with age. In 2005, 8.0% of youths aged 12 to 17 had a substance use disorder, and this increased to 21.8% for young adults aged 18 to 25 (Substance Abuse and Mental Health Services Administration, 2006).

The lives underlying these statistics show youths suffering from a variety of adverse consequences, including fatal and nonfatal injuries from motor-vehicle accidents, suicides, homicides, violence, delinquency, psychiatric disorders, and risky sexual practices (Winters, 1999). Additionally, the rate of physical, sexual, and emotional traumatization is high among adolescents in substance treatment (Dennis, 2004). Thus, the risk of posttraumatic stress is high for students in recovery.

Adolescents often initiate drug use due to experimentation and social conformity. Compared to adults with a substance use disorder, teens exhibit shorter use histories, more involvement with alcohol and cannabis, and greater binge drinking and poly-drug abuse (Titus et al., 2002; Winters, Stinchfield, Opland, Weller, & Latimer, 2000). It is widely agreed that, while adolescents have many of the same issues as adults, the unique challenges of adolescence require treatment and continuing post-treatment interventions designed specifically for youth. Research conducted on aftercare programs has linked continuing care with positive treatment outcomes (Donovan, 1998; Godley, Godley, Dennis, Funk, & Passetti, 2002; Kelly, Myers, & Brown, 2000; Marlatt, 1985). Research on posttreatment continuing care in general, let alone on adolescent aftercare, is lacking.

Recovery and Schooling

For teenagers, school often sits at the heart of the relapse threat. Because they are minors, the majority of adolescents must return to their pretreatment neighborhoods and schools (in the case of residential treatment). Students treated as outpatients may never have a respite from drug-using peers in their school and neighborhood. One study found that virtually all adolescents returning to their old school reported being offered drugs on their first day back in school (Spear & Skala, 1995). Students who attend schools with high overall use levels are particularly susceptible to use (Cleveland & Wiebe, 2003; Piper, Moberg, & King, 2000). For many adolescents, schools not only represent the environment of previous use and contact with pretreatment drug-using friends but the emotional turmoil involved with life transitions (Isakson & Jarvis, 1999). When young people leave residential treatment or while receiving outpatient treatment, if a private school is not financially possible, their options usually are limited to their former school or dropping out.

Hawkins, Catalano, and Miller (1992) use the terms "risk factors" and "protective factors" in their study reviewing elements that contribute to adolescent substance use disorders (the former) as well as substance use avoidance (the latter). While their review is focused upon "the factors that have been shown to precede drug abuse," the concepts are salient for continuing care programs that have a goal of preventing relapse. Among the risk factors noted by Hawkins and colleagues are association with drug-using peers, alcohol or drug availability, physiological and genetic factors, and academic challenges. Svensson (2000) also situates time spent with friends and peer deviance among the most important risk factors. In addition to peer pressure, difficulty coping with negative feelings and interpersonal conflict can endanger a teen's newly established sobriety (Winters, 1999). Spear and Skala (1995) paint a picture of adolescent recidivism that includes the following:

- lack of involvement in productive activities;
- return to the environment of previous use;
- failure to establish social contact with nonusers;
- lack of family involvement;
- less likelihood of 12-step meeting attendance or leisure activities without drugs; and
- increased likelihood of engaging in activities with pretreatment friends.

Additionally, adolescent relapsers are less likely to stay in school and more likely to skip school. Succeeding academically can help students stay sober, which in turn can help them graduate. Poor academic performance is the "single strongest predictor of dropping out" (Gibson, 1997, p. 5), and adolescents who drop out of school have a higher risk of relapsing than those who finish school (Casemore, 1990). Among adults aged 18 or older, those who graduated from high school but did not attend any college and those who graduated from college had lower rates of substance use disorders (9.0 and 8.0%, respectively) than those who were not high school graduates and those with some college (10.2 and 10.3%, respectively) (Substance Abuse and Mental Health Services Administration, 2006). This implies that educational attainment is a factor in a person's ability to avoid abusing substances.

Vaillant (1988) finds that prosocial activities such as school assist the recovering person, and Resnick et al. (1997) believe "connectedness with school" is a general protective factor for adolescents. Under these premises, the first schools designed specifically to aid the newly sober teen opened in the late 1980s. According to White and Finch (2006), the first wave of recovery high schools opened between 1987 and 1998. These schools were truly experimental in nature, with the goal of "sober schooling" but no existing blueprints to guide them. Ecole Nouvelle (now Sobriety High) in Minnesota was established in 1986 and opened in a community center with four students and one teacher in 1987. Other early recovery high schools included several Minnesota schools: PEASE (Peers Enjoying a Sober Education) Academy (1989), the Gateway Program (1992), the Arona Campus (now Arona Academy) (1995), YES (Youth Education Sobriety) (1997, now closed), ExCEL Sober School (1998, now closed), and the Aateshing Program (1998). Early programs outside Minnesota included Unity High School in Phoenix, AZ (1992, now closed), Recovery High School in Albuquerque, NM (1992, now closed), Phoenix Academy in San Mateo, CA (1992), Thoreau High School in Woodland Hills, CA (1996), Oasis Academy (now Community High School) in Nashville, TN (1997), Santa Rosa (CA) Clean & Sober High School (1998), and the Summit School in Spokane, WA (1998, now closed).

Recovery High Schools and the Continuum of Treatment Care

The first recovery schools were designed to fit into the established treatment continuum of care. Winters (1999, p. 24) suggest that for adolescents, "the period right after completion of a treatment program, when the youth returns to family, peers, and the neighborhood, is often the time of greatest risk of relapse." Spear and Skala (1995, p. 346) concur that the first 60 days are "the greatest time of risk for each level of relapse," suggesting "the need for intense posttreatment services during this time." Students often transition into recovery high schools immediately upon leaving residential treatment or completing intensive outpatient programs. The schools thus are designed to reduce the relapse risk factors in a student's experience by incorporating a "social bonding" perspective similar to the one advocated by Hawkins and colleagues (1992).

Moving to a life without drugs represents a major life change for the students of recovery schools. Since alcohol and other illicit drugs are considered mind- or mood-altering, the removal of them affects how students experience the world. For drug dependent adolescents, alcohol and other drugs provide, among other things, support systems, coping mechanisms, recreational activities, and access to a peer group. A life without chemicals necessitates the replacement of each of these components or a decision to live without them. The support they receive in their first school experience after "getting clean and sober" can be a crucial factor in their ability to sustain their recovery. Most recovery high schools expect students to participate in mutual-aid programs to support their recovery from substance use disorders. Additionally, alternative-learning environments can provide peer support vital to a young person's attempts to avoid alcohol and drugs (Harrison & Hoffmann, 1987). With this goal in mind, recovery schools provide services to a specialized population with the intent of developing a strong internal community around a shared issue.

These schools fit the paradigm of continuing care within a "recovery management" system. Reviewing a number of recommended approaches to continuing care, Godley and colleagues (2002) summarize key components of posttreatment programs, suggesting they

(a) "offer sufficient intensity and duration of contact;
(b) target multiple life-health domains (e.g., educational, emotional, physical health, vocational, legal, psychiatric);
(c) be sensitive to the cultural and socioeconomic realities of the client;
(d) encourage family involvement;
(e) increase prosocial leisure habits;
(f) encourage compliance with a wide range of social services to provide additional support;
(g) focus on relapse prevention; and
(h) provide cognitive behavior and problem solving skill training to help reduce cravings and to cope with anger, depression and anxiety."

Recovery high schools focus on each of these domains during the school day, while providing an education and creating a nonusing social network. Hawkins and Catalano (1985) cite the "correlates of relapse" (p. 918) as absence of a strong prosocial network (including family, peer, and isolative factors), lack of involvement in productive roles or active recreational activities, negative emotional states, and physical symptoms.

PAST RESEARCH

Spear and Skala (1995, p. 356) state, "Post-treatment intervention research must focus on modalities or combinations of modalities that have a significant impact on recovery rates and behavior associated with establishing a drug-free lifestyle." They further elaborate, "At this point, the discussion is not about fine tuning interventions but rather identifying which post-treatment modalities have a significant impact on relapse rates for which adolescents." The call for literature on sound continuing care resources is still valid, and especially so for educational services. As an emergent form of recovery management for adolescents, these programs' structure, institutionalization, and effectiveness need to be better understood. By systemically describing and examining recovery high schools, this project aims to establish their place in the continuum of care and to understand practices across schools.

No multisite studies have been conducted on this model of schooling and continuing care before this study. Both the authors, however, have independently conducted previous single site case studies of recovery high schools.

Evaluation of Recovery High School, Albuquerque, New Mexico

Recovery High School (ARHS), located in Albuquerque, New Mexico, was an innovative alternative public high school for youth in recovery from substance use disorders. The development of the initial plan for the school, its implementation, and evaluation were funded through grants from the Robert Wood Johnson Foundation (see Diehl, 2002). Moberg and Thaler (1995) conducted an evaluation of this program, focusing on the feasibility and replicability of the program model and its institutionalization into the Albuquerque Public Schools (APS) and the Albuquerque community. This study provided a model for the data collection and analysis methods used in this paper.

Moberg and Thaler (1995) concluded that the ARHS model—as modified over the life of the project—is feasible programmatically, with impressive evidence of therapeutic effectiveness but limited educational success. The programmatic feasibility was limited by the high per pupil costs encountered due to the severity of the presenting problems among the students who were attracted to the program. The nature of the students also led to an emphasis on therapy over traditional educational experiences. Thus the model the emerged is that of a day-treatment program for students with substance use and co-occurring disorders, provided in an alternative educational setting. Structural and governance issues that plagued the program from its inception were never overcome. Criteria for assessing institutionalization—a commitment by the school district to continue the program, success in developing other funding sources, the development of routine ongoing relationships with other schools, and the maintenance of stable referral relationships in the community—were in general not accomplished.

Evaluation of Chicago Preparatory Charter High School

The Robert Wood Johnson Foundation subsequently funded the evaluation of another attempt to develop a recovery high school benefiting from the lessons learned in the Albuquerque program. The evaluation was funded to provide an external evaluation of the implementation, feasibility, and preliminary effectiveness of the Chicago Preparatory Charter High School (CPCHS) program, partially funded by the Foundation. CPCHS was established as a charter school within the Chicago Public Schools to support students in their recovery from substance use disorders, while providing a rigorous educational program leading to a high school diploma. Due to premature closure of the school, resulting from a failure to implement the very well conceived plan, the evaluation was not implemented (Moberg, 1999).

Boundaries and a Sense of Place at "Recovery High School"

Finch's (2003) study centered on the dynamics of recovery within one recovery high school. His study utilized ethnographic data to examine Recovery High School (RHS), a private school with 25 students who had entered voluntarily and agreed to work "programs of recovery" for a substance use disorder. A key finding concerned the effect of boundaries upon the sense of place within the school experienced by staff and students at RHS. The research focused on naturally occurring events, which were the usual events of the classrooms and the school being studied. RHS attempted to support the recovery of its students, and boundaries existed to define the sense of place in the community. Findings showed that supports and threats did not align neatly with permeable or firm boundaries. Some students found rigid structures helpful, while others preferred the freedom of permeability. Ultimately, the individual personalities and mental health of the collective staff and students involved with the school determined the appropriate levels of structure and flexibility necessary to provide a healthy learning environment.

Thus, past research has examined single schools, emphasizing initial implementation, feasibility and institutionalization, as well as microlevel interaction patterns within a school. The current study builds on this work to provide a multisite examination of recovery schools.

Association of Recovery Schools (ARS)—Definition of Recovery Schools

The Association of Recovery Schools (ARS) is a network of recovery high schools developed in 2002. ARS has developed membership criteria for schools that wish to join the association. These criteria guided (but did not completely limit) the selection of schools for this study. Officially recognized recovery high schools are expected to fit each of the following criteria:

- "Recovery schools at the secondary level meet state requirements for awarding a secondary school diploma. Such schools are designed specifically for students recovering from substance abuse or dependency. . . .
- Recovery Schools provide academic services and assistance with recovery (including post-treatment support) and continuing care. However, they do not generally operate as treatment centers or mental health agencies.
- Recovery Schools require that all students enrolled in the program be in recovery and working a program of recovery determined by the student and the School. Consequences of relapse are addressed by the individual School.
- Recovery Schools offer academic courses for which students receive credit toward a high school or college degree. At the secondary level, schools assist students in making the transition into another high school, college, or a career.
- Recovery Schools are prepared through policies and protocols to address the needs of students in crisis, therapeutic or other. These procedures can involve
  - full or part-time licensed counselors on staff, or

- out-sourced counseling contracts through which a specific outside agency consults with staff in the event of a student crisis or relapse" (Association of Recovery Schools, 2007).

Because there is a remunerative obligation for membership and because these criteria have no evidence base, membership in ARS was not a requirement for participation in this study. By providing a frame that was deliberatively conceived by professionals and recovering students, however, the ARS membership criteria did serve as a guide for defining schools that were invited to participate.

METHODS

The study was conducted as an exploratory, descriptive analysis with the goal of yielding a typology of the schools and their operative program theories/models. Survey data provided information on the staff and on the students attending these schools. While an outcome study is needed, it was determined that a rigorous experimental or quasi-experimental trial would be premature before (a) understanding the nature of programs in operation and (b) assessing the feasibility of an outcome study.

The prior projects described above and the ARS guidelines for membership set the stage for the project. A general design and approach for studying the characteristics of recovery schools and their students was established and demonstrated to be useful in the Albuquerque and Chicago studies. Student data collection tools and mechanisms were piloted in these two schools. Additionally, a new small school was used as a pilot site for the current study before scheduling the official site visits.

The complete project included startup, protocol and survey development, and contracting with recovery schools to assure their participation; a one-day site visit to each of the participating schools during which survey and interview data were collected; and data analysis, interpretation, and presentation of reports and publications. Data collection occurred over three school semesters. As the study of the Albuquerque Recovery High School discovered, the program evolved considerably over its first year of operation. With this in mind, our sample of schools was limited to 18 high schools (17 research sites and one pilot) that fit the ARS defining criteria (above) and that had been operating for at least 2 years. Data collected included observational field notes, interviews, documents (school charters, policy manuals, student handbooks, and accountability reports), anonymous surveys of students, staff and administrators, and various secondary data such as school administrative data, attendance reports, graduation rates, and other reports available from the schools. This paper provides an initial analysis of student survey and site visit data.

Site Visits

A central component of the methodology was the use of in-person site visits of at least one full day on site. Site visits facilitated collection of survey data but also complemented and extended that data by allowing for exploration of the school and community, direct observation of settings and activities, and access to key individuals for interviewing. Site visits were conducted by teams of two to three researchers (though in two cases, only one researcher visited due to the extremely small size of the schools), in order to allow for multiple insights, differential expertise, cross-validation of findings, and enhanced scope. Increased validity of results was facilitated by this team approach. Due to IRB concerns regarding protection of human subjects, students were not interviewed.

As the purpose of the site visits was to gather descriptive information about the programs and students rather than to carry out a complete natural-istic inquiry or case study, we conducted scheduled, relatively standardized oral interviews (LeCompte, Preissle, & Tesch, 1993) with administrators, teachers, counselors, and other key personnel, such as volunteers or Board Members. We also attempted to interview at least one external constituent from each school's interorganizational network (such as school district ad-ministrators and referring treatment providers.) Interviewees were chosen based on discussions with school leaders and accessibility on the day of the site visit.

The interviews used detailed interview guides (tailored to the type of respondent) to assure that all the conceptual areas of interest were covered at each site. While the interview guide provided structure, relevant probes and exploration of relevant divergent topics were also incorporated to maximize the learning from these interviews.

Observations were conducted during academic classes, staff meetings, and therapeutic programs (such as community meetings and "check-in" groups) and other routine activities. Interview data was collected on the nature, structure, and general goals of confidential therapy sessions, both individual and group, from staff perspectives (since these could not be directly observed). Also, facility tours were conducted during each visit, along with observation of the surrounding neighborhoods. Similar to the limitations placed on the interviews, observational data focused upon specific details of the events rather than an attempt to glean the representational nature, frequency, or participants' sense of the events. With written permission of the participants, interviews were recorded and subsequently transcribed and erased.

Surveys

Administrators: In each school the responsible administrator was asked to complete a survey that summarized information about the school program itself. This included items about the organizational and physical structure of the school, number and characteristics of students, number and characteristics of staff, testing and employment policies, and other related items. A number of these items were adapted from the National Center for Education Statistics' annual Schools and Staffing Survey (U.S. Department of Education, 2004).

School staff: All staff were invited to complete anonymous surveys that included information specifically about their own demographic background, training, credentials and attitudes regarding education and recovery. Included in the survey were a series of attitude questions regarding operational aspects of the recovery school. (Staff survey data are not included in the present article.)

Students: An anonymous survey was developed for students to complete during the site visit. Since the limitations of our funding and the purpose of the project limited us to one survey opportunity with no follow-up data, a "retrospective pretest posttest" design was incorporated into the survey (Pratt, McGuigan, & Katzev, 2000; Hill & Betz, 2005). The content of the survey adapted the Global Appraisal of Individual Needs-Quick (GAIN-Q) (Dennis, Titus, White, & Unsicker, 2005) as the basic instrument. The GAIN-Q contains a brief subset of items from the comprehensive GAIN-I, which is being used extensively in adolescent treatment programs and provides us with ready comparisons of the students-in-recovery schools to youth receiving treatment in other settings. GAIN-Q items, which form scales on substance use disorders, emotional health, and behavioral health, were included. In addition, we included standard items and/or our own constructed measures on educational, juvenile justice and treatment history; opinions and satisfaction with the recovery school; self perception/self esteem (Rosenberg & Rosenberg, 1978); and basic demographics.

Protection of Participants: To assure anonymity for the survey respondents and to obtain an IRB waiver of written parental consent, the student survey was designed so that all demographic items were on a separate page, which was removed from and stored separately from the remaining items at the end of each survey administration. The schools sent IRB-approved informational letters (prepared by our research staff) to all parents and students prior to site visit days, with instructions on who to contact on the school staff if they wished to withhold consent from student involvement—which none did. Thus by not requiring written consent, and separating demographics from other data, no record of student identity or means of inferentially linking substantive responses to individual students is possible. All student surveys were conducted by our research team with no involvement of local school staff, were held by our staff and were removed from the schools immediately at the conclusion of the site visit. Students were not interviewed. Staff interviewed and recorded at site visits signed informed consent forms.

FINDINGS

In this section, we summarize what we have learned to date about the programmatic, organizational, and physical characteristics of recovery schools themselves. We then provide descriptive information on the students, their history and background, their self-reported behaviors, and their perceptions of the schools. Future articles will provide diagnostic estimates, compare these students to other adolescent treatment samples, and conduct further analysis of co-occurrence of the various complex concerns the students are struggling with. Survey and depth interview data from staff will be analyzed in future reports.

As described earlier, our study included 18 schools—the first school in Wisconsin was included as a pilot to test our data-collection tools and methods, and the subsequent 17 were included in the final data. Those 17 were in the following states (number of schools in parentheses):

- California (3)
- Colorado (1)
- Minnesota (8)
- Pennsylvania (1)
- Tennessee (1)
- Texas (3)

The sample approximated the national distribution of schools, with Minnesota, California, and Texas being the only states with more than one school in operation more than 2 years, and Minnesota being the only state with more than 10 recovery high schools.

Self-Referential Language

While for heuristic purposes this study uses the term "recovery high schools"—in line with the language of the Association of Recovery Schools—programs use a number of titles. In keeping with frequent embedding of recovery schools in larger organizations, some participants referred to the schools as "programs" rather than "schools," even though the school had its own staff and student base. In many cases, staff, students, literature, and stakeholders of the same school might each refer to it differently. Some of the referential terms other than recovery school—which was most common in discussions with the researchers—included: "sober school," "alternative school," "community school," "charter school," and "area learning center." The original schools in Minnesota were commonly known as "sober schools," and this term was used most often by people associated with schools in that state. School representatives universally embraced their designation as "schools" or "school programs" rather than "treatment."

Area Learning Centers (ALC) are an organizational form that is unique to Minnesota. These programs were authorized by the Minnesota State Legislature in 1987 as part of the so-called "second chance law" for secondary and postsecondary students (Boyd, Hare, & Nathan, 2002). ALCs are an educational program modality serving students with certain emotional and behavioral needs, including substance use disorders. Interestingly, participants often referred to this incorrectly as "Alternative Learning Center."

Characteristics of Schools and Models

Most of the schools were embedded organizationally and physically, with students separated from other programs. While facilities and staff might be shared with another program or school, students were not. In every case, students spent the entire day in a homogeneous recovery school setting. Students were referred primarily from treatment programs and parents, and in some cases juvenile justice. It was rare that a student's prior school was the referral source.

The schools had small enrollments, usually ranging from 12 to 25 students. Staff and administrators stated a preference to remain small, even though official and budgeted enrollments were usually larger than

FIGURE 1. Recovery High School Facilities (n = 17)

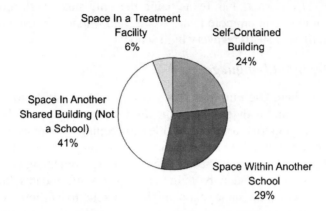

attendance observed during site visits (which on average was about 65% of the official number). This could be accounted for by the variance of school population over the course of a school year. Many schools see enrollment changes daily and most at least weekly to semiweekly. Based on the administrators' surveys, turnover is such that the total number of students enrolled at the fall official enrollment count is estimated to be 45% of the total students who enroll over the course of a school year. The median stated capacity was 35 students, but median enrollments on the days of researcher visits were 75% of that stated capacity.

School Facilities

As can be seen in Figure 1, facilities varied widely, with most schools sharing space with another school or program.

The seven schools that shared space with another building usually did so with a business or nonprofit organization. In one case, the school was one of multiple nonprofit programs located in a church facility. Only one school was located in an alcohol and drug treatment facility, and this was an outpatient treatment center.

In the five schools that shared space with another school, there was usually some division, such as a wall, doorway, or floor between the recovery school and the other school. Classrooms were distinct and were not shared at the same time. While students might take classes in the "other" part of the building, this was due to the teachers' location, and the nonrecovery school students would not be present. In several cases, schools altered start times so that the recovery school students would start, eat lunch, and leave at times different from the nonrecovery school students to minimize the opportunity for interaction. The total stated enrollment capacity of the 17 school facilities was 648.

School Funding

Funding was usually tied to enrollment, as schools were allotted funds on a per pupil basis by the local districts. To have some income certainty, most schools combined public funding with other fees, donations, and in two cases an actual "tuition" was charged.

Two of the schools received no public funding. Of the 15 that did receive public funding, the ratios provided were as follows:

- 75–100%: 8
- 50–75%: 4
- 25–50%: 1
- Data not provided: 2

The median amount of public or tax-based funding was 80%. The two most common public school funding categories were alternative schools/area learning centers (9) and charter schools (5).

Admission Requirements

Schools were selected for this study based on their assertion that their school was designed for students in recovery from a substance use disorder. We found that admission criteria around this description varied. No school required an official diagnosis for admission, and the usual criteria corresponded more with Alcoholics/Narcotics Anonymous's requirement of "a desire to quit drinking/using." Sobriety duration prior to enrollment ranged from no official number of days stated up to 30 days of sobriety prior to admission.

Corresponding to the "stages of change" model (DiClemente, Schlundt, & Gemmell, 2004; Prochaska, DiClemente, & Norcross, 1992), students were admitted who described their stage of recovery anywhere from contemplation through active recovery maintenance, though schools stated a desire to enroll students only in active recovery maintenance. Three schools had arrangements with the juvenile justice system to admit students on probation for alcohol and drug or other violations. Most schools stated an openness to accept students who exhibited symptoms of a substance use disorder who had a "willingness" to stop drinking/using, even if the student had no official diagnosis and did not exhibit all the symptoms of dependence or abuse. This appeared often to be driven by budgetary needs and responsiveness to community needs.

Most schools required some type of prior treatment for substance use, though this was undefined. Usually, this meant outpatient treatment. The three schools with juvenile justice agreements did not require prior treatment, and many students in these schools were coerced to attend by judges and parole officers. In the other schools, however, enrollment was almost completely voluntary on the part of students and their families. Recovery schools were seen as a school choice to support an alcohol- and drug-abstinent lifestyle.

Frameworks of Recovery and Therapeutic Support

All schools included support groups during the academic day, many holding these groups once (or more) per day. All schools utilized some variant of the 12-step or Minnesota Model (Winters et al., 2000; Room, 1998), with an expectation of ongoing abstinence while attending the school.

One-on-one counseling was readily available across the schools as well. All schools involved a counselor or therapist, though some contracted with treatment centers to provide this service rather than having someone on staff. Counseling credentials for staff members varied. Most common were licensed alcohol and drug counselors, licensed professional counselors, and licensed professional social workers. Therapeutic approaches ranged from the confrontational style of traditional alcoholism counseling to various forms of client-centered motivational approaches.

Academic Programs

Most schools shared academic staff with other schools or programs. The schools sharing facilities with other schools usually shared the parent organization's administration and teachers. Most schools, however, had at least one or two dedicated staff members.

Teaching and learning was individualized and self-paced, often tutorial in nature. Class sizes were small, ranging from 2 or 3 students up to 10–15, depending on the enrollment of the school. Schools usually blended grade levels into one class or subject, and sometimes blended multiple subjects into one class period. A few schools only had one or two teachers available for the entire school. These schools used an externally created modular curriculum aligned with state standards. Schools employed licensed or license-eligible teachers.

The academic programs were designed to either transition students from drug treatment to their regular schools (n = 3) or to graduate them from the recovery high school (n = 9). The remaining schools indicated flexibility on this goal depending on the student's needs and choices. Typically, there was no set limit on length of stay, and some schools regularly had students enrolled for three or all 4 years of high school.

Summary Observations

While more precise exploration remains to be done, some general conclusions can be made about the schools. Schools tend to

- be more publicly than privately funded;
- have more voluntary than involuntary enrollment;
- emphasize recovery maintenance and support more than primary treatment;
- balance their emphasis between academics and therapeutics;
- offer an eclectic recovery-support model that incorporates 12-step philosophy more than a 12-step exclusive model;
- be integrated with another school/program rather than be freestanding;
- share facilities with another school/program rather than stand alone;
- share staff with another program rather than employ dedicated staff;
- have slightly more intent to graduate their own students rather than transition them to another school; and
- have funding based on enrollment rather than sum-certain funding.

As these data are examined in more detail, we will be able to quantify these distinctions more accurately. Part of the complexity of that process is that school descriptions often varied across a school's staff both in interviews and surveys. In some cases, it is difficult, if not impossible, to place a school completely in one category or another on these continua due to conflicting staff reports. This is due in part to the evolving nature of these schools as well as the lack of an explicit model for most recovery schools to follow.

STUDENTS IN RECOVERY HIGH SCHOOLS

The demographic characteristics of the 321 students who completed surveys in the 17 schools we studied are summarized in Table 1. Here

TABLE 1. Demographic Characteristics of 321
Students in 17 Recovery High Schools

	Percent
Grade Level	
Eighth	<1%
Ninth	12
Tenth	25
Eleventh	35
Twelfth	27
Sex	
Female	46
Male	54
Ethnicity	
American Indian	4
Asian or Pacific islander	3
African American/Black	3
Hispanic/Latino	7
White/Caucasian	78
Other/Mixed	4
Family Structure	
Two Parent Home	54
Mother only	22
Father only	10
Other relatives	5
Other	4
Father Education: (64 missing)	
LT High School	10
High School Graduate	28
Some College or Technical School	19
College Degree	22
Advanced Degree	21
Mother Education: (53 missing)	
LT High School	8
High School Graduate	30
Some College or Technical School	16
College Degree	30
Advanced Degree	16

we see that most of the students are classified as being in 10th, 11th or 12th grades, with 11th being the grade level with the largest enrollment. There is a slight overrepresentation of male students (54%). Most students (78%) are White, followed by 7% Hispanic/Latino and 4% American Indian. African American students are underrepresented at 3% of enrolled

TABLE 2. Treatment History for 321 Students in 17
Recovery High Schools

	Percent
Past treatment for Substance Abuse or Dependency	78
Inpatient or residential	54
Outpatient	55
Past treatment for mental health problem	49
Inpatient or residential	23
Outpatient	25
Currently receiving treatment outside the school	48
For substance use	18
For mental health	16
For both	22

students. For comparison, White non-Hispanics made up 69.1% of the total US population in 2000; African Americans made up 12.9%, Hispanic or Latinos 12.5%; and American Indians 0.9% (2000 U.S. Census, Table DP-1).

Family structure reported by the students included 54% in two-parent homes (compared to 65.3% of all households with children in the US in 2000) and 22% living with mother only (close to the 19% nationally). Parental educational attainment, our only indicator of socioeconomic status, shows that 43% of fathers and 46% of mothers had a college degree or more; 55% reported at least one parent had a college degree or higher. Twenty-four percent of the US population aged 25 years and over in 2000 had a college degree (US Census Table DP-2), suggesting that recovery schools are serving a population at higher than average SES.

Students had fairly extensive treatment histories for substance use disorders as well as various mental health issues (Table 2). Seventy-eight percent reported past substance treatment, including 54% with at least one episode of inpatient or residential service and 55% with outpatient treatment. Sixty percent reported an arrest history, and 20% were currently on probation or parole. Mental health-specific treatment had been received by 49%, and nearly half were currently receiving outside treatment services. Currently, 80% report participating at least weekly in AA, NA, or some other form of 12-step group (often a requirement for continued enrollment in a recovery school).

In keeping with the extensive treatment histories, the primary reported referral source (Table 3) to the recovery school was a substance treatment

TABLE 3. Referral Source for 321 Students in 17 Recovery High Schools

	Percent
Referred by:	
Substance treatment facility	50
Self	25
Friends/family	20
Therapist	15
Previous school	12
Probation/parole	11
Immediately Prior Setting:	
Treatment setting	42
Another school	33
Regular school	21
Alternative, charter, etc.	12
Out of school/ not attending	22
Incarcerated	5

TABLE 4. Student Substance Use Behaviors and Symptoms—Before and Now (n = 291)

	Pct Before*	Pct Now	p
Weekly use of alcohol, marijuana or other drugs	90	7	<.001
Use caused to feel depressed, nervous, suspicious, uninterested, other psychological problems	77	12	<.001
Used in dangerous or unsafe situation	82	10	<.001
Use caused repeated problems with the law	57	8	<.001
Reports tolerance	81	7	<.001
Reports withdrawal problems	71	18	<.001
Used larger amounts, more often or longer time than meant to	84	11	<.001
Continued in spite of medical, psychological or emotional problems	78	10	<.001

*"Before" is based on retrospective report at the time of survey regarding "the 12 months before your started this school."

facility (50%). This was followed by self referral (25%) and friends or family (20%). Immediately prior to entering the recovery school, 42% reported they had been in a treatment setting, 33% in another school, and 22% out of school and/or not attending.

Self-reported student substance use patterns are summarized in Tables 4–6. A sampling of symptoms used for diagnosis of substance use disorders is

TABLE 5. Student Drug Use Patterns 90 Days Before Entered School and Past 90 Days (n = 174 students who have been in school at least 90 days)

	Mean (s.d) Before	Mean (s.d.) Now*	p
Days abstinent	28.5 (36.8)	266.1 (258.8)	<.001
Days used alcohol	33.6 (35.4)	3.5 (11.2)	<.001
Days drank 5 or more drinks at one time	31.3 (34.2)	3.0 (11.1)	<.001
Days used cannabis	47.2 (40.0)	3.1 (12.3)	<.001
Days used other drugs	30.9 (37.3)	2.8 (10.5)	<.001
Smoked cigarettes in last 30 days	NA	91% (67% daily)	NA

*Total days since entered school; not limited to 90 days.

TABLE 6. Student Drug Use Abstinence 90 Days Before Entered School and Since Entered School (n = 174 students who have been in school at least 90 days)

	Pct Before	Pct Now*	p
Percent abstinent from all alcohol and other drugs	20	56	<.001
Percent abstinent alcohol	24	62	<.001
Percent abstinent cannabis	30	71	<.001
Percent abstinent other drugs	40	74	<.001
Percent *of days* abstinent	32	82	<.001

*Since started school, not limited to 90 days.

shown in Table 4. Here we see that, using the retrospective pretest approach, all symptoms were reported to be very significantly (p < 0.001) reduced when students were asked to report what their use was like during the 12 months before entering the school (while in the community) compared to currently while attending a recovery school. For example, reports of at least weekly use of alcohol, cannabis or other illicit drugs were reduced from 90% to 7% at the time of the survey. Nearly one in five students (18%) reported continued withdrawal symptoms, however.

Table 5 provides student reports of their current drug use patterns, for those students who have been enrolled 90 or more days in the school. Students report a mean of 28.5 days abstinent in the prior 90 days before they entered the school. They reported an average of 266 days abstinent since entering the schools. These numbers translate to 32% of all days abstinent before entering the school, compared to 82% of all days since

TABLE 7. Selected Student Mental Health Symptoms—Before* and Now (n = 291)

	Pct Before	Pct Now	p
Feel very trapped, lonely, sad, blue, depressed or hopeless about the future	73	31	<.001
Have no energy, losing interest in work, school, friends, sex or other things you cared about?	60	20	<.001
Thought about ending your life or committing suicide	53	16	<.001
Felt very anxious, nervous, tense, fearful, scared, panicked....	68	44	<.001
Trembling, heart racing, restless...	60	40	<.001
Very distressed, upset when reminded of the past	65	55	.003
Had a hard time expressing feelings, even to people you cared about.	83	49	<.001
Had a hard time paying attention at school, work or home.	86	63	<.001
Been unable to stay in a seat or where you were supposed to be	71	41	<.001
Bothered by any nervous, mental or psychological problems?	69	33	<.001
Disturbed by memories of things from the past that you did, saw or happened to you?	76	55	<.001

*"Before" is based on retrospective report at the time of survey regarding "the 12 months before your started this school."

they entered the school. Similarly, we see large, significant reductions in days using alcohol, "binge" drinking, days using cannabis, and days using other drugs. Current cigarette use was nearly universal (91%) among the students in recovery schools, however.

Reported rates of complete abstinence from drug use were also calculated (Table 6). Continuous abstinence from all alcohol or other drugs increased from 20% during the 90 days before entering the school to 56% at the time of the survey. Complete abstinence since entering the school was reported by 62% for alcohol, 71% for cannabis, and 74% for other drugs.

To report meaningful contrasts to the 90 days before entering the school, these data are reported for the 174 students with at least 90 days in the school (54% of our sample). When we look at abstinence for all students completing our survey, we find a slightly higher rate of reported complete abstinence since entering the school (59% versus 56%), perhaps due to shorter time at risk.

TABLE 8. Student Opinions about their Progress (n = 290–315)

How do you feel you *are* doing NOW compared to before coming to this school...	Better	Same—Good	Same—Not Good	Worse
Academically (school work and grades)	71%	18%	6%	5%
Emotionally	59	28	8	5
With your alcohol/drug issues	80	14	6	1
With family issues	57	28	11	4
With peer/friendship/social issues	56	33	7	4

TABLE 9. Student Opinions about their Recovery Schools (n = 290–315)

	Strongly Agree	Agree	Disagree	Strongly Disagree
I came to this school completely voluntarily	42%	33%	17%	8%
I get more attention here than I did at my other high schools	55	31	10	4
I think classes are easier here than at other schools	26	45	24	5
I spend a lot of time doing homework after school	2	13	45	40
This school has a high quality academic program	14	55	23	8
I think this school offers a good clinical/therapeutic program	42	43	9	5
I think the clinical program here is better than at other treatment programs I have been to	18	35	35	12
Overall, I am satisfied with this school	47	40	9	4

Concomitant with the reported reductions in substance use are significant reductions in mental health symptoms (Table 7). Symptoms of depression, suicidal ideation, anxiety, and ADHD all decreased significantly at the time of the survey, relative to the year prior to entering the school. The percentage reporting they are bothered by any nervous, mental or psychological problem dropped from 69% to 33%. While also dropping significantly, symptoms of posttraumatic stress disorder remain high at 55%.

Students were asked to provide their opinions about their progress, comparing how they felt at the present compared to before coming to this school (Table 8). Here we see the most improvement is reported regarding improvement in alcohol/drug issues (80% better than before, 14% the same-good), followed by academic progress (71% better, 18% same-good). Emotional, family and peer issues are also reported to be improved.

Finally, students were asked a number of opinion items regarding their recovery school (Table 9). Highlights of these data are that about 75% report they came to the school completely voluntarily; 86% report they get more attention than they did at other high schools, 85% agree the school offers a good clinical/therapeutic program, and 87% report overall satisfaction (47% strongly). Indicators of perceived academic rigor are less strong. Most (71%) agree that classes are easier than at other schools; only 15% agree they "spend a lot of time doing homework after school"; and, while 69% agree that the school has a "high quality academic program," only 14% "strongly agree" with this statement.

DISCUSSION

The data collected for this study provide the first systematic description of recovery-school programs and their students. Based on selection process and knowledge of the range of recovery schools, we believe the 17 schools studied are representative of the 34-some schools in existence at this time. As a new phenomenon, recovery schools are dynamic in nature and vary in student population size and stability, financial and governance arrangements, and staffing, organizational and physical arrangements. The most common school model is that of a program or affiliated school embedded organizationally and physically with another school or set of alternative school programs. Although embedded, recovery-school students are physically separated from other students through serious efforts to maintain physical separation, using scheduling and physical barriers in most cases studied. Affiliation with public school systems is the case for most recovery schools and seems to be a major factor in assuring fiscal and organizational feasibility.

The students in the recovery high schools studied slightly overrepresented male students (54%), were predominantly White (78%), with about one half from two-parent homes. Overall, parent educational levels suggest a higher mean SES than in the general population. Most students (78%) had prior formal treatment for substance use disorders, often concomitantly with treatment for mental health concerns, and were often referred by treatment providers. Students came with a broad and complex range of mental health issues, traumatic experiences, drug-use patterns, criminal justice involvement, and educational backgrounds. The complexity of these problems clearly limits the enrollment capacity of the schools.

Retrospective pretest-to-posttest analysis suggests significant reduction in substance use as well as in mental health symptoms among the students in recovery schools. Students were very positive in their assessment of the therapeutic value of the schools but with less enthusiastic but positive ratings of the educational programs. The school programs do appear to successfully function as continuing care to reinforce and sustain the benefits students gained from their treatment experiences.

LIMITATIONS

The limitations of this descriptive study are consistent with our intent to conduct pilot or feasibility research. We expect that our results will further elucidate models for recovery schools and begin to describe the students and programs. We do not intend to draw any more than general impressions about effectiveness at this time. The limitations that prohibit drawing firm conclusions include the sample selected for the study, which we believe is representative but which was not randomly selected from all known recovery schools. The site visits were short (1 day) and capture only a brief snapshot of what we have learned are very dynamic environments in terms of resources, staffing, student enrollment, and organizational characteristics. By selecting schools with at least a 2-year history, we assured some level of stability, but nonetheless our results must be seen to represent only a snapshot in time for these schools.

The student survey data also have a number of serious limitations. Since this is a preliminary report, we have not completed the programming needed to score all the diagnostic scales tapped by our survey, so we have instead reported on a sampling of representative items in this paper. Future articles will include analysis of a number of scales and will compare to data on other adolescent populations in treatment. The retrospective pretest-posttest design, while having some evidence of validity (e.g., Pratt et al., 2000), is not an adequate substitute for a longitudinal design with multiple data-collection points. Respondents to these surveys can be expected to slightly heighten or reduce the contrasts between the before and after items, depending on demand characteristics of the situation and their personal circumstances. However, this design remains superior to a purely single point-in-time measurement, which was our only alternative in this study.

Since we used a self-completed paper and pencil survey, there are a number of data quality problems that would be reduced in an interview situation or a computer-aided self-interview (CASI) system. These data quality and missing data problems have been resolved by careful data cleaning and, where data are missing, using the general assumption of "missing at random" in our analysis. Thus we have reported results assuming that the distribution would be the same if every student had completed every item in this paper.

As the data collected were descriptive in nature, this study did not address effectiveness of recovery schools, although such an assessment is needed and is a planned next step in our research. Furthermore, both time and cost limitations did not allow for a deep naturalistic inquiry. Such case studies will be needed to complement future evaluative research.

Finally, while there is extensive literature on self-report of adolescent behaviors, it is commonly acknowledged that biological validation of self-reported drug use is desirable in rigorous treatment research situations. In our case, the situations of survey reporting were structured to elicit honest responses with no repercussions, so our estimates of use rates are likely relatively close to reality. However, any future rigorous studies we conduct of this population would incorporate urinalysis into the design.

FUTURE RESEARCH

We anticipate that this descriptive study will set the stage for a multi-site service effectiveness study. A lack of understanding currently exists about what tools recovery schools utilize to serve their students, who the students are, whether they show effects for students significantly different from those attained by recovering students attending nonrecovery schools, and how student and programmatic differences affect outcomes. There are two critical endpoints in future research. On the program level, institutionalization with a stable flow of appropriate students and funding is critical. On the student level, relapse avoidance (or, at minimum, significantly reduced substance use and reduction of problems in other life areas) is the most critical outcome, with successful educational attainment a highly related and important secondary outcome. Our future research will address these issues, informed by the results of this preliminary work.

NOTE

1. The term "substance use disorder" is used in this paper to refer to either substance abuse or dependence, as defined by the DSM-IV (American Psychiatric Association, 1994).

REFERENCES

American Psychiatric Association. (1994). *Diagnostic and statistical manual of mental disorders: DSM-IV* (4th ed.). Washington, DC: American Psychiatric Association.

Association of Recovery Schools. (2007). *Membership criteria.* Retrieved June 19, 2007, from http://www.recoveryschools.org/applicants_info.html#criteria

Boyd, W. L., Hare, D., & Nathan, J. (2002). *What really happened? Minnesota's experience with statewide public school choice programs.* Center for School Change, Hubert H. Humphrey Institute of Public Affairs, Minneapolis: University of Minnesota.

Brown, B. S., & Ashery, R. S. (1979). Aftercare in drug abuse programming. In R. L. DuPont, A. Goldstein & J. A. O'Donnell (Eds.), *Handbook on drug abuse* (pp. 165–73). Rockville, MD: Department of Health Education and Welfare, Public Health Service, Alcohol, Drug Abuse, and Mental Health Administration, National Institute on Drug Abuse.

Casemore, B. P. (1990). *Teen drug use: Impacts and outcomes.* Washington, DC: U.S. Department of Education Office of Educational Research and Improvement.

Cleveland, H. H., & Wiebe, R. P. (2003). The moderation of adolescent-to-peer similarity in tobacco and alcohol use by school levels of substance use. *Child Development, 74*(1), 279–91.

Dennis, M. L. (2004). Traumatic victimization among adolescents in substance abuse treatment: Time to stop ignoring the elephant in our counseling rooms. *Counselor*, April, 36–40.

Dennis, M. L., Titus, J. C., White, M., & Unsicker, J. (2005). *Global Appraisal of Individual Needs—Quick.* Bloomington, IL: Chestnut Health Systems.

Diehl, D. (2002). Recovery high school. In S. L. Isaacs & J. R. Knickman (Eds.), *To improve health and health care, Vol. V: The Robert Wood Johnson anthology* (pp. 143–175). San Francisco, CA: Jossey-Bass.

DiClemente, C. C., Schlundt, D., & Gemmell, L. (2004). Readiness and stages of change in addiction treatment. *American Journal on Addictions, 13*(2), 103–19.

Donovan, D. M. (1998). Continuing care: Promoting the maintenance of change. In W. R. Miller & N. Heather (Eds.), *Treating addictive behaviors* (2nd ed., pp. 317–336). New York: Plenum.

Finch, A. J. (2003). A sense of place at Recovery High School: Boundary permeability and student recovery support. Unpublished PhD dissertation, Vanderbilt University, Nashville, TN.

Finch, A. J. (2005). *Starting a recovery school: A how-to manual.* Center City, MN: Hazelden Publishing and Educational Services.

Gibson, J. T. (1997). Rekindling the spirits of throw-away children. *New Directions for School Leadership, 6,* 1–9.

Godley, M. D., Godley, S. H., Dennis, M. L., Funk, R., & Passetti, L. L. (2002). Preliminary outcomes from the assertive continuing care experiment for adolescents discharged from residential treatment. *Journal of Substance Abuse Treatment, 23*(1), 21–32.

Harrison, P. A., & Hoffmann, N. G. (1987). *CATOR Report: Adolescent residential treatment, intake and follow-up findings.* St. Paul: Ramsey Clinic.

Hawkins, J. D., & Catalano, R. F. (1985). Aftercare in drug abuse treatment. *The International Journal of the Addictions, 20*(6 & 7), 917–45.

Hawkins, J. D., Catalano, R. F., & Miller, J. Y. (1992). Risk and protective factors for alcohol and other drug problems in adolescence and early adulthood: Implications for substance abuse prevention. *Psychological Bulletin, 112*(1), 64–105.

Hill, L. G., & Betz, D. L. (2005). Revisiting the retrospective pretest. *American Journal of Evaluation, 26*(4), 501–17.

Isakson, K., & Jarvis, P. (1999). The adjustment of adolescents during the transition into high school: A short-term longitudinal study. *Journal of Youth and Adolescence, 28*(1), 1–26.

Kelly, J. F., Myers, M. G., & Brown, S. A. (2000). A multivariate process model of adolescent 12-Step attendance and substance use outcome following inpatient treatment. *Psychology of Addictive Behaviors, 14*(4), 376–89.

LeCompte, M. D., Preissle, J., & Tesch, R. (1993). *Ethnography and qualitative design in educational research* (2nd ed.). San Diego: Academic Press.

Marlatt, G. A. (1985). Relapse prevention: Theoretical rationale and overview of the model. In G. A. Marlatt & J. R. Gordon (Eds.), *Relapse prevention: Maintenance strategies in the treatment of addictive behaviors* (pp. 3–70). New York: Guilford.

McKay, J. R. (2001). Effectiveness of continuing care interventions for substance abusers. *Evaluation Review, 25*(2), 211–32.

Moberg, D. P. (1999). *Evaluation of Chicago Preparatory Charter High School. Final Grant Report to the Robert Wood Johnson Foundation.* Madison: University of Wisconsin Center for Health Policy and Program Evaluation.

Moberg, D. P., & Thaler, S. L. (1995). *An evaluation of Recovery High School: An alternative high school for adolescents in recovery from chemical dependence.* Madison, WI: University of Wisconsin Center for Health Policy and Program Evaluation.

Piper, D. L., Moberg, D. P., & King, M. J. (2000). The Healthy for Life Project: Behavioral outcomes. *Journal of Primary Prevention, 21*(1), 47–73.

Pratt, C. C., McGuigan, W. M., & Katzev, A. R. (2000). Measuring program outcomes: Using retrospective pretest methodology. *American Journal of Evaluation 21*(3), 341–49.

Prochaska, J. O., DiClemente, C. C., & Norcross, J. C. (1992). In search of how people change: Applications to addictive behaviors. *American Psychologist, 47,* 1102–13.

Resnick, M., Bearman, P., Blum, R., Bauman, K., Harris, K., Jones, J., et al. (1997). Protecting adolescents from harm: Findings from the National Longitudinal Study on Adolescent Health. *Journal of the American Medical Association, 278*(10), 823–32.

Room, R. (1998). Mutual help movements for alcohol problems in an international perspective. *Addiction Research 6,* 131–45.

Rosenberg, F. R., & Rosenberg, M. (1978). Self esteem and delinquency. *Journal of Youth and Adolescence, 7,* 279–94.

Rubin, B. T. (2002). *Changing lives through changing stories: A phenomenological study of adolescents in recovery from addiction.* Unpublished PhD dissertation, Vanderbilt University, Nashville, TN.

Spear, S. F., & Skala, S. Y. (1995). Posttreatment services of chemically dependent adolescents. In E. Rahdert & D. Czechowicz (Eds.), *Adolescent drug abuse: Clinical assessment and therapeutic interventions (NIDA Research Monograph 156)* (pp. 341–64). Rockville, MD: U.S. Department of Health and Human Services, National Institute on Drug Abuse.

Stein, J. (2007). *Adolescent treatment—The road forward: A CSAT perspective.* Paper presented at the Joint Meeting on Adolescent Treatment Effectiveness, Washington, DC.

Substance Abuse and Mental Health Services Administration. (2006). *Results from the 2005 National Survey on Drug Use and Health: National Findings.* Rockville, MD: Office of Applied Studies.

Svensson, R. (2000). Risk factors for different dimensions of adolescent drug use. *Journal of Child and Adolescent Substance Abuse, 9*(3), 67–90.

Teas, T. G. (1998). *Chemically dependent teens with special needs: Educational considerations for after treatment.* St. Paul, MN: Bethel College.

Titus, J. C., Dennis, M. L., White, M. K., Godley, S. H., Tims, F., & Diamond, G. (2002). An examination of adolescents' reasons for starting, quitting, and continuing to use drugs and alcohol following treatment (abstract). *Drug and Alcohol Dependence, 66(supplement 1),* s183.

U.S. Department of Education. (2004). *Schools and staffing survey: 2003–2004 school year, OMB No. 1850–0598.* Washington, DC: National Center for Education Statistics.

Vaillant, G. E. (1988). What can long-term follow-up teach us about relapse and prevention of relapse in addiction? *British Journal of Addiction, 83,* 1147–57.

White, W. L. (2002). An addiction recovery glossary: The languages of American communities of recovery [Electronic Version]. Retrieved June 11, 2007, from http://www.bhrm.org

White, W. L., & Finch, A. J. (2006). The recovery school movement: Its history and future. *Counselor, 7*(2), 54–57.

Winters, K. C. (Ed.). (1999). *Treatment of adolescents with substance use disorders (TIP 32).* Rockville, MD: U.S. Department of Health and Human Services, Public Health Service, Substance Abuse and Mental Health Services Administration, Center for Substance Abuse Treatment.

Winters, K. C., Stinchfield, R. D., Opland, E., Weller, C., & Latimer, W. W. (2000). The effectiveness of the Minnesota Model approach in the treatment of adolescent drug abusers. *Addiction, 95*(4), 601–12.

Restorative Justice

Angela Wilcox, MA

ABSTRACT. This article provides a first person narrative of one teacher's experience in three different recovery schools over more than a decade of teaching. The author discusses some of the recurring challenges and successes encountered by many recovery high schools and discusses key concepts such as the importance of a clear school mission, the role of restorative practices in recovery education, successful classroom methods, and the importance of communication and support between recovery schools.

If you don't know the trees you may be lost in the forest, but if you don't know the stories you may be lost in life. —Siberian Elder

There is emerging research about recovery schools that provides stakeholders with the data necessary to demonstrate their effectiveness. At the same time, there are stories flowing from these schools; they are the stories of students who say their lives were saved, of tearful parents who are grateful that their children are alive, of teachers and administrators gratified by

Angela Wilcox is lead teacher and an English teacher at Sobriety High School's North Summit Academy Campus, Maplewood, Minnesota.

student successes and healthy workplaces. This is the story of one teacher's decade in recovery schools. It is a story of schools and classrooms, politics and disappointments, and difficult lessons learned. It is a story of revelation and transcendence. Mostly, it is a story about young people in recovery, for it was hearing their stories that drew me to this work and helping them tell their stories that has been the heart of it. Sometimes, working in recovery schools has felt like being lost in the forest, without guide or landmark, but with each story shared, each mistake admitted and success celebrated, we learn to recognize the trees, and eventually, someday, create field guides that will allow future travelers to make their own way.

THE BEGINNING

My story begins, as many do, with a happy accident. A friend who worked at a "sober" school asked, offhand, if I knew any English teachers looking for a part-time teaching job. As it happened, I was, and her phone call secured me an interview. When I was shown to my English classroom after accepting the job, I looked around curiously and asked where they stored the books. Imagine how my wheels started spinning when I found out there weren't any. No materials, no library, thirty-five students in grades 9–12, and one English teacher. I had recently come from a position teaching in a large, wealthy public high school where I was part of a department of more than a dozen teachers. The curriculum was pre-approved by a committee and my course work was handed to me in nicely color-coordinated stacks of paper. I was terrified and exhilarated by the challenge before me. I haunted libraries and used bookstores, and bought armfuls of notebooks and pens. I drew on past experiences and created lesson plans from patchworks of other people's ideas that I thought might work in this setting. I wrote our daily classroom agenda on the blackboard, and I waited to see what would happen.

Initially, students were in shock; in this school, they hadn't had a teacher who required them to come to class every day, or to write things down, or to turn in homework. In years past, they had earned English credit for talking in group counseling sessions, under the heading of Interpersonal Communication. My first year was riddled with conflict and resistance. "This ain't no public school" was the frequent refrain as students demanded a return to their right to exercise self-care by leaving the classroom, playing computer solitaire, or ping-pong in the student lounge rather than attending classes. But there were also moments that transcended the battle: there were stories. I heard stories that students told in their writing and poetry, stories they told in response to reading assignments, and even fascinating stories they told to explain why they hadn't done their homework at all. Students came to me before and after school, bubbling over with stories that demanded being told and being heard. I discovered that my most important resource wasn't a new curriculum library but a willingness to listen, take these stories, and build my classroom around them.

As a young teacher, I was fortunate to attend several SEED workshops (Seeking Educational Equity and Diversity) and through them was introduced to an article by Emily Style called "Curriculum as Window and Mirror" (Style, 1988). This simple essay spoke deep truth to my experiences in the classroom. Style asserts that students need to be exposed to worlds outside of their own, the windows that schools can provide into things beyond their daily lives. But, she says, they also need mirrors that reflect their own life experiences back to them. Students learn best when the curriculum shows them something of themselves, as well as showing them places they might one day go. I began to realize, in my first year teaching at a recovery school, that there was a special set of mirrors that I would need to create to help my students find their place in my classroom. I needed to understand addiction, sobriety, and recovery so that I could find ways to reflect this back to them, and how those windows and mirrors could best help them grow into the people they wanted to become. It wasn't easy, and I often felt conflicted about how little I seemed to be accomplishing, but I loved working with these young people and was determined to find some way through.

In addition to the struggles over the shift in the academic culture, there were also battles about sobriety. How did we define it, why did we enforce it, and whose business was it, anyway? Why wasn't it okay, they wondered, to have a glass of wine with a parent on their birthday? Why did that have to count as a "relapse" if an adult gave permission and they didn't get drunk? Wasn't it enough, some wondered, that they didn't "wake and bake" every day? They wanted harm reduction. We wanted them to want recovery.

Our school had no template, no model, no Association of Recovery Schools, no chemical dependency counselor, no known peers in the field to call on for advice. We were building something that we knew was essential, but we didn't have the resources, the time, or the knowledge to do it the way it needed to be done—not yet. There were others doing the work we were doing, but we didn't know who or where they were and didn't understand the profound implications that making those connections would eventually have on our work.

One staff person, a woman who started teaching the same fall that I did, was in recovery herself. She started an AA meeting for students after school one day a week, and from this seed a small culture of recovery started to grow in our school. Students started to talk openly about the 12 steps. Phrases like "practice these principles in all our affairs" and "progress, not perfection" made their way into our community. Over time, it no longer felt like all my energy went into the song and dance of getting them to show up; more often now they were present, ready, and willing to figure out where this journey was going to take them. They wanted to write. And write they did.

Creative writing became one of the centerpieces of my English curriculum. It didn't require textbooks, and it was flexible. Students working at the third-grade or thirteenth-grade level could work together, learn from each other, and accomplish something meaningful. Most importantly, they loved it. They loved writing about themselves. They loved discovering the texture and variety of emotion that was part of a sober life. Rather than covering up all of their feelings by drinking or drugging, they were naming emotions. They were turning them over, personifying them, facing them down, and running after them. Things in the classroom were starting to hum. I had found one of the mirrors I needed to help my classroom make sense.

The changes that were taking place in the school community became clearer to the director, and he supported what I was trying to accomplish in my classroom in material ways. He ordered books: textbooks, workbooks, writing curriculum, and anything else he could find that he thought would be helpful. He allowed teachers to create policies that required students to maintain classroom attendance in order to earn credit. He cut out smoke breaks for students between classes. He added an hour to the school day in order to enrich class offerings to students. He refused to operate under a "poverty mentality," insisting that we bring in and use every resource we thought we needed in order to make the school a quality institution, both academically and culturally. He lead without ego, asking for advice and help, and then using his power to enact what he saw as best for students and teachers.

The range of ability levels in my classroom ran from barely literate to college level, and I talked to the director about how to meet the varying needs in an authentic way. One student in particular was a constant behavior problem in my classroom and refused to write *anything*. He was incredibly bright, verbally articulate, and read voraciously above his grade level, but he would not pick up a pen to save his life (or his grade). Eventually, I gave him the assignment of making a list of everything he had in his beloved and ever-present backpack, and when he did it, I realized that the reason he didn't write was because he couldn't write—the scrawl on the page looked like a kindergartener's work. He was unable to complete even that most basic task when it came to writing, and the coping mechanism he'd developed, which had helped him make it through grade school and junior high, was to act out until he got kicked out rather than admit his problem to his teachers. This felt beyond my ability to address in a classroom full of other struggling learners. We had no special education department, no liaison from the school district, and no services to address those with learning disabilities. Parents who enrolled their children were informed of this and had to make the decision about which was more important to them: special education or a sober school. I strongly advocated for bringing in a specialist who could work a few hours a week with students who needed to learn very basic reading and math skills. Immediately, our director put out a search and contracted with a woman who worked a few hours a week with our lowest-skilled students. Within months, the brilliant young man who could not write was writing. He was still far below grade level, but he was now openly discussing his struggles and being provided tools that helped him overcome something that had plagued him his entire school career. Eventually, his writing progressed and he was able to function with other students in my English classroom, turning in written work that I could read and respond to. The consultant was able to work with a small pull-out group of students in both English and math, and this addition to our school program made an enormous difference in how we were able to serve students. Over the years, that position evolved from a four-hours-a-week contract to a full-time special education teacher, serving up to 20 students with individualized education plans and working in conjunction with teams from their home schools to provide services, sometimes even transportation to and from our school.

The culture was taking shape in wonderful ways. Our students were learning and talking openly about enjoying school for the first time in their memories. They talked to us about it, they talked to their parents, and they talked to their friends—a lot of their friends. We were faced with a decision to start a waiting list, or to consider increasing the number of students we served. When I started teaching at the school in the fall of 1996, there were about 35 students. That number increased each year, until we had to consider renting additional space from the church and adding staff in order to keep class sizes small and continue to offer the model we'd created. We felt committed to serving as many students as we could, feeling that no one who wanted a safe, sober education should be turned away. However, when we increased to 75 students, it became quickly and painfully apparent that we had grown too large to feel the sense of community that had defined us. Our classrooms were no longer connected by one hallway, leaving some teachers and classrooms isolated from the main body of the school. We had grown too large to gather in one room in a way that allowed everyone to be seen and heard easily. After one year of operation with 75 students, we agreed that 60 to 65 students was the magic number for us, given our space and our staff; it provided us sufficient funding to maintain our current staff but kept the school small enough that we still felt like a community. We knew from this experience that it was better to ask a student to wait to be admitted than to compromise the integrity of our program.

A YEAR OF TRANSITION

After my third year at the school and many positive changes, the original and much-loved director made the decision to move on and was hired as the principal of a public school. We faced a new set of challenges but felt optimistic that with all we had accomplished, we could carry on the mission of the school under new leadership. The staff had played such an active and integral role in crafting the culture and vision, and we looked forward to what new energy and ideas this transition might bring.

Our new director came on board at the start of the next school year, armed with experience and a set of philosophies honed in to the alternative school world. This could have been a real asset to our community, as many of the elements that are successful in alternative schools work marvelously in recovery schools; but in the end, the conflict in understanding about the mission of our school deepened to a real crisis. The director insisted that the large public school we contracted with required us to admit any student who met the seven "alternative school" criteria, including being behind in credits, pregnant, or in legal trouble. It is significant that "committed to recovery" and "sober" are not on that list of criteria. Those of us who believed in a recovery school fought hard to maintain the expectation that students live a sober lifestyle, in or out of school. The director admitted many students to the program who had never been through treatment and thus didn't understand the basic principles of addiction and recovery. At the same time, we retained a core group of students who were committed to recovery and their 12-step program. The lack of clarity about the mission of the school within the staff had a profound impact on the culture. When one student came forward saying that she had been harassed by peers for being in recovery and didn't feel safe at the school, the director assured her we'd help her find a different school. When a student was accused of selling drugs in the boy's bathroom, the director argued that students didn't have to buy if they didn't want to and that they'd have to toughen up a bit if they were going to survive in the "real" world. Students, undoubtedly feeling the tension and responding as they must, acted out. There were physical fights, weapons threats, failing grades, and a general sense of malaise. Staff meetings, formerly one of our most cherished times to reflect and support each other in our work, became unbearably tense, to the point of open conflict and hostility. With a new baby and a toddler at home, my energy was already stretched thin, and the stress at work was taking a toll. I was ready to walk away from the whole thing, convinced that it had been a noble but ultimately unworkable dream. I was devastated.

Several of us on staff who had already seen the school through some difficult transitions had, over the course of the year, been trying to find a way to save the school we loved. My trusted colleagues encouraged me to hang on for a little while longer. We told our stories to the board in letters, in meetings, and in phone calls. Eventually, the accumulated power of our words made them realize what was at stake, and they asked us to work with them. Together, we crafted a written statement that would make our central mission concrete. The board was able to convince most of the core teaching staff to return for another year, assuring us that our voices would be honored and that the mission of the school protected. They found another director, making certain that he would support the recovery mission of the school. Skeptical but unable to let go of the glimpses I had seen of what could be, I stuck it out.

This transition year was a year of invaluable lessons. We learned that it is vital for the school to have a clear central mission and philosophy in writing, and that anyone hired in a position of power be committed to that mission. It sounds so obvious in retrospect, yet at the time the board was hiring a new director, the school's mission was understood and practiced by the founding director and the staff but not made explicit in any written form to facilitate the major transition that hiring a new director implied. The board, a group of dedicated community volunteers with little understanding of either addiction or recovery or of the education world, was not equipped to fill in these gaps on its own. In addition, there was no pool of experienced recovery school directors to draw from, so we had to hope that qualified candidates from the education world would be willing to learn about addiction and recovery as part of their new role. The first time, it didn't work. The second time, we got lucky.

SERVANT LEADERSHIP IN ACTION

Soon after the start of the next school year, it was clear that this new director had a heart of gold and a commitment to the sober mission of our school. He worked hard to earn our trust and to understand what had caused rifts between staff. Listening to our needs, he set aside staff time and searched out people who could foster healing and help us move forward together. As our staff rebuilt trust, the students responded again, this time in positive ways.

The issues that we faced became clearer as we were able to move past the basic struggle to protect the recovery mission of our school. We didn't have anyone on staff with professional training or experience working in a recovery community. The director approached the board of directors to convince them that having a chemical dependency counselor was vital to building a healthy recovery community in our school. There were some concerns that had to be addressed. Some wondered whether having a chemical dependency counselor on staff would confuse the mission, making it seem more like treatment than an educational program. I was one of those people. I felt we had worked so hard to create a solid program based around academics, and I worried that bringing in someone from the treatment world might dilute our mission to educate our students. We had tried being an "alternative" school and it had almost destroyed us. I was worried about what might happen if we became a treatment center/school and what kind of students it might attract. Our concerns and opinions were weighed, and the process felt open and respectful, but in the end the director felt strongly that to serve our students well, we needed someone who understood this central aspect of their lives.

He convinced the board to hire a licensed chemical dependency counselor on a part-time basis. Her job would be to work with individual students to support them in their recovery and to help the staff understand new ways we could work effectively with this population of students. Once the decision was made, I willingly dropped my skepticism and waited to see what this person could teach us that we hadn't already figured out on our own.

Quickly, I came to see the new chemical dependency counselor as an invaluable resource for both students and staff. In four years, I had learned that my instincts were often right, but now I had someone with many years experience who was eager to talk about how what I saw and taught in the classroom could support students in their recovery. Some of our policies and procedures, she pointed out, enabled students or undermined our goal of creating a healthy recovery community. She created a contract that challenged students to become totally honest without consequences; we needed to know who was really sober, for how long, and whether or not they really wanted to be in recovery. Students amazed us by rising to the challenge. We gathered the entire community—65 students—in a large circle and asked each one to state out loud what their sobriety date was and what their level of commitment to sobriety, and thus our school, would be. A few students admitted that they were using and were only attending this school to stave off the consequences that they would face if adults in their lives suspected. They were asked to consider, and then commit to, a lifestyle and to honor what we were trying to build by their choice. Others proudly stated their sobriety date and their firm commitment to living a life of recovery. It wasn't perfect, but it was a start, and most importantly, it was honest. We had given students a clear message: this is a program built around honesty. We will respect your choices, but we will also ask you to respect what we're trying to build.

Students and staff were taught new ways of understanding recovery in communities. We knew the term "relapse," but our new chemical dependency counselor taught us about "prolapse," as well. Not every incident of use, she showed us, necessarily means that someone has returned to active addiction. The chemical dependency counselor explained that when people use and immediately understand that this not what they want—they are honest about it with all the important people in their lives, and they show a renewed commitment to their recovery—that it is a prolapse. She asked us to set a policy at our school that would reflect the difference between the two kinds of "lapses." If students were immediately honest about their use and were able to articulate what changes they were going to make to remain sober, they would be welcome to stay in the community. If a student's use was discovered, or a confession was coerced by police, a parent, or a friend after the fact, the student would be asked to leave the community until he or she could gain a stable recovery.

The chemical dependency counselor also asked that we modify our policy about students revealing use by others in the community. As it was, we assured students that their concerns would be held in confidence if they came forward about another student. An honesty program included being willing to admit your concerns, she said, and told us she wouldn't act on "anonymous" information. We were very worried that this would have a negative impact on our community; if students didn't feel safe coming forward anonymously, one of our most important sources of information about what was really going on in the community would dry up. She assured us that this was common practice in recovery communities and that it would work. Once again, she was right, and it proved to be vital in helping build more authenticity into our community. Students felt safe. They felt trusted, and they felt a stake in this school. They proved they were willing to stand up and protect both the school and their own recovery by being honest about what was going on, even with their close friends. Students learned to talk directly to each other. They would offer their friend a chance to go confess to the chemical dependency counselor on their own, and if they chose not to, the person with concerns would go forward. Contrary to our fears, the number of students coming forward actually increased.

RESTORATIVE JUSTICE

The policy about asking students who relapsed to leave the school, though clearer now, was still very complicated. In a small community, one student's departure could have a major impact. Students always wanted to know exactly what happened and why this person had been asked to leave the school, but rules about confidentiality prevented us from sharing any of that information with students. Gossip in the hallways or classrooms would fill in the gaps, usually inaccurately, and often, it would create further drama and chaos. Students struggled to find ways to understand and have a voice in who remained in the community and who was asked to leave. They accused us of racism, favoritism, and bias, grieving the loss of each of their friends in ways that constantly disrupted our small community. They appealed to the staff to include a select group of students in the process of making decisions about discharges.

That winter, at an alternative education conference, the chemical dependency counselor and I attended a workshop on restorative justice. Immediately, it was clear that the tools that restorative justice would offer our school, especially talking circles, could be the missing piece in the puzzle of how to maintain a healthy recovery community that felt safe for everyone. The workshop was offered by the Minnesota Department of Education, which was providing grants to schools who would volunteer to serve as pilot sites for restorative justice in schools. I took an application, and with the backing of the board and school director, we became one of those pilot sites. This meant that our entire staff could go through a multiple-day training, with periodic follow-up training, for free. We also collected data at our site, documenting how often we used restorative practices instead of traditional disciplinary measures, like detention or suspension, and how our rates of student misbehavior changed as a result.

Restorative justice is a philosophy that is built on the idea that when there is harm done to someone in a community, it affects everyone. Each member of a community needs to find ways to heal, to have his or her voice heard, and to discern what his or her role should be in making things better. We had seen how much each student was affected when someone relapsed, when there was stealing, gossip, or drama, but usually those types of behaviors were dealt with in the office, behind closed doors with the perpetrators. Even the victim was often shut out of the process of responding to the transgression, with the assurance that it was being dealt with by the people in power. Restorative justice, through a variety of methods, offers everyone in the community a chance to say what happened, how they were impacted, what they need, and what they are willing to do to help make things better. Even people who seem to be peripherally involved in an incident can have important insight into how it has impacted the community. Often, the perpetrators have a story to tell about what led up to their actions that can give vital perspective to a community that hopes these people will change their harmful behavior. The stories shared and insight gained can be profoundly important in transforming and healing for everyone, not just those directly involved in the harm.

The most important change in the community after incorporating restorative circles was that we now had a tool to communicate with students if someone had relapsed and was going to have to leave the community. Students who were in the position of leaving the school were offered and encouraged to hold a circle with the community in order to tell them what they were planning to do to next, and to receive support and feedback. Remarkably, almost every student took advantage of this opportunity. They wanted the chance to say goodbye, make amends, and get support from the community. We quickly saw the benefits of this new model for our community; drama, gossip, and blame evaporated as students gained a voice in the processes that a healthy community required.

Circles gave our community a crucial tool that assured that every voice was heard and every story had a chance to be told. Each relapse or prolapse circle offered lessons that we could not teach in other ways. Students told, for example, the familiar story of what happened when they started spending time with their friends who still used drugs and alcohol. Many of these stories shared the common themes of teens who didn't believe a friend would put their recovery at risk, or who thought they could handle it or that they could walk away; they believed that they could control their desire to return to using. We all learned lessons about powerlessness from these stories, and soon students talked openly about incorporating the lessons learned from these circles into their own program of recovery.

One particularly powerful circle was called for a student who had made a conscious decision that he wanted to start using drugs again. He wanted to honor the community by leaving before he used, and to thank and say goodbye to each person who had touched him while he was a student there. It was a heartbreaking circle, with many tears shed and many who struggled to find the right words to help this young man see how frightened everyone was for him. A teacher stood, removed his shirt, and standing in his undershirt, tearfully told the story of the tattoo on his biceps—praying hands, which he had put there after the death of his younger brother from an overdose. He fiercely told this young man that he wasn't willing to watch him walk away, possibly to die, without telling him this story of the pain his brother's death had caused in the lives of everyone who loved him. Days later, the student returned to us, saying that he had been so moved by this circle, and especially by the story told by his teacher, that he had decided he had to find the strength to get sober again and remain with us. He graduated with almost a year of sobriety. I cannot think of any other appropriate way that this teacher could have shared this story in such a moving and powerful way but in the context of the circle, where every person is there not as his or her title but as another human being in the community; it was perfect.

Restorative practices shaped many elements of our school. We offered a circle to a parent who was struggling to feel heard and had been trying to play staff off of each other, even talking about mounting a law suit, in order to feel her child's needs were being addressed. The staff gathered in a circle and offered her a chance to tell her story to all of us and then to hear our stories about working with her child. The tension and anger was immediately replaced by a sense of calmness and respect, and all parties gained important perspective on what the problems were and agreed to move forward together for the student's benefit. The circle transformed the way we were able to work with the parent, and thus the student.

As the English teacher, I saw an opportunity to use circles to teach writing. For several years, I had attempted to incorporate the writer's workshop into my classroom, a model that puts student writing at the center of the curriculum and allows them opportunities to present their work to other writers and get feedback from them. The variety of learning disabilities and social difficulties in the student population prevented this model from working the way I wanted it to, but the idea of gathering in the now-familiar circle with a talking piece presented a new possibility. Using the work of teachers like Nanci Atwell (Atwell, 1998) and Linda Christensen (Christensen, 2000), who have successfully developed writing workshop models with a variety of students of all levels, and Roseanne Bane (Bane, 2005), who offers a brilliant concept about how to structure the process of giving feedback, I added the talking piece and came up with a highly successful model for my English classroom. Because the circle was already a place of trust, and the talking piece is a tangible symbol of permission to speak and assurance of being heard, students were able to take the enormous leap of presenting their work to peers and accepting concrete feedback on their writing. Students strove to create pieces they felt proud to present to their fellow writers, pushing the quality of writing to new levels. They wrote during lunch hours. Some snuck into the bathrooms of their group homes to share poetry after hours. A handful started reading at open-mike poetry readings, and one student even became a member of the Minnesota Poetry Slam team. Students who had long-refused to write, let alone share their writing with others, began to fill notebooks. The "read-around" (a phrase borrowed from Christensen and perfect to describe our circle gatherings) became so popular that I offered a read-around class as an after school elective. We had visitors from all over the world, including a U.S. Representative and a restorative justice expert from Australia, come to our classroom and leave with tears in their eyes, moved by the risks these young people took and the stories they told.

In the math classroom, similar leaps and bounds were occurring. Our new director had hired a math teacher with experience teaching College Prep Math (CPM),[1] a program developed by math teachers in conjunction with the University of California at Davis. The program focuses on taking abstract mathematical concepts, from pre-algebra to calculus, and making them visual and concrete for students. Classroom work is done in small groups; students ask questions and find answers together, rather than by individuals in desks watching the teacher at the board. These elements of the program, unusual in math classrooms, were highly successful with our students. Students were overcoming one of the most prevalent and powerful phobias in their academic history: fear of math. As they found success with the hands-on curriculum, and the support and engagement a group-centered classroom offered them, they began to believe in a new way that they could actually succeed as students. We were seeing gains in confidence and academic success that we had only dreamed about that first year I had started teaching.

MIX IT UP

Like all urban schools, we faced the challenge of understanding how our classrooms were impacted by the many differences between our students. There were differences of race and culture, of age and developmental level, of academic successes or failures, of family situation, socioeconomics, and the many other dividers that polarize students and make it challenging to create and sustain authentic communities and effective learning environments. Here again, the read-around and circles both played a vital role in helping us grow and learn. We were discovering, especially as deeper and more authentic stories emerged and the level of trust increased between members of the community, that all of those differences could melt away in the face of the disease of addiction and the power of recovery. With every read-around, with each pass of the talking piece around a circle, they would express surprise, amazement, and relief at hearing the experiences and feelings they had imagined too strange or shameful to admit come out of others' mouths. Often, these discovered connections would appear between the most unlikely pairs. Out of these unexpected connections, friendships emerged. Students marveled aloud at the experience of becoming close to someone who looked so different from themselves. I would smile in wonder myself as the preppy cheerleader from the suburbs bent her blonde head close to the girl with a pierced lip and a green Mohawk, sharing secrets between classes. With the common ground of their battle against addiction and the rewards of recovery, they were learning what this community had to offer them.

Now, when we asked students why they came to our school, or what kept them coming back every day, they said it was because this school was their family. They felt a deep connection that went far beyond what any traditional academic institution had ever offered them. Even when they were ill, tired, furious, jittery, or frustrated, when they drove each other (and us) crazy, when they disagreed with the rules or chafed against the ever-higher standards we tried to push them to achieve, they returned day after day, surpassing attendance requirements and the patterns of their own histories. Like family, we were the people who had to take them in when no one else would. Unlike many of their families, we actually did.

ASSOCIATION OF RECOVERY SCHOOLS

It was during this period of deep joy in our healthy community that the director and chemical dependency counselor were contacted about a new organization, an association of those working in schools dedicated to serving adolescents and young adults in recovery. A dozen or so representatives of those schools would gather in Washington, DC, in July of 2002 to make connections, talk about what worked, what didn't, and the possibility of building an organization that could support existing schools and promote the establishment of new schools around the country. When we returned to school that fall, the chemical dependency counselor was buzzing with excitement about the connections she had made and the possibilities she saw growing out of this fledgling group of counselors, administrators, and educators. Much of what we had learned, other schools had also discovered. We were not alone in this. Positive connections were forged with schools we had previously only heard about as competitors for our students. We began to feel that we were all colleagues in a growing field, rather than a few crazy people in a church basement. We started calling our school a "recovery" school, rather than a sober school, in order to accurately describe the intention of our program and to be consistent with other programs around the country doing similar work.

The formation of the Association of Recovery Schools (ARS) was a very important moment for all of us. Suddenly, the work we were doing took on new dimensions, as we realized we could take what we were learning and share it with others. Even more profound, we could turn to others to see what else was working and ask for advice, support, and perspective. In 5 years, the ARS has grown to include more than two dozen schools; and the summer conference, from that original 12 people, has grown 10 times. For me, the ARS has been the touchstone; as I have now worked at three different recovery schools, I can see the importance of building bridges between schools, and of reaching out to each other as colleagues rather than as competitors. The ARS provides a way for educators, administrators, and counselors to unite behind our common mission.

BEHIND THE CURTAIN

As all of us who had worked so hard to create a healthy recovery community enjoyed the fruits of our work and dug in to learn with our students, our director was facing struggles of his own. We were only able to fund about 70% of the operating budget of the school with the money we got from the state, so fundraising was crucial. Yet the demands of being the school administrator and the sole fundraiser for the school were much more than a full-time job. He shielded the staff from these struggles but talked openly and often with the board about the need for support in fundraising. After two years of strong, capable leadership, he chose to take a job in another district. He was clear with the board that he was leaving because, without committed fundraisers working in conjunction with the director, the school could not be sustained. He was no longer willing to live with the stress of trying to wear so many different hats, knowing that he couldn't succeed and that the school would suffer as a result. He respected the school and its mission, and hoped, he said, that his departure would spur the board to rethink the role of director and the vital question of who would work to raise funds to sustain the school.

He left us hoping that another lesson had been learned. Good leadership, devoted and experienced teaching staff, students who are actually in recovery, and solid programming can come together to create an excellent, safe, sober school; but without wise leadership and support from the agencies charged with sustaining the long-term health of the school, it will founder. A director in a school of our size, even one who is highly competent and committed, could not be expected to oversee the day-to-day operations of the school and also be charged with its long-term financial survival through fundraising and other related activities.

A PATTERN EMERGES

The departure of this wise leader ushered in a new series of challenges and successes. Subsequent directors faced the same difficulties of wearing too many hats, and the board continued to struggle to find the right leaders for a nearly impossible job. Through it all, dedicated people continued striving to offer the very best in recovery education they could, graduating increasing numbers of students and sending more and more of them on to post-secondary education. In my 11 years of work in recovery schools, I have taught at three different schools under seven different directors. At each school, I have seen the same elements succeed: small classes; innovative teaching staff, who are flexible and understand the basic concepts of working with young people in recovery; restorative practices to build and sustain a sense of community; and a clear and intentional dedication to the mission of the school to help students in recovery learn in a supportive environment. In a school like this, even students in very early recovery can thrive and succeed, both academically and interpersonally.

By the same token, the same challenges emerge at each school. Again and again, finding the right person to act as the director, and finding the right board of directors to support and guide that person through the running of the school, has proved crucial. The school cannot survive without a board that is willing to acquire an understanding of the complexity of the director's job, a commitment to supporting that role, and thus the school, through active ongoing fundraising. Whatever the funding source, whether it be tuition or public dollars, schools will be hard pressed to support the small classrooms and provide the necessary materials and support without additional funding in the form of grants, scholarships, and private donations.

Vision, energy, compassion, and experience are vital to the creation and sustenance of a school that can truly support students in recovery. And yet, as I have experienced both firsthand and through hearing the stories of others in the field, these are not enough. Creating a truly functional organizational structure for recovery schools is a constant challenge. There is no preexisting template for schools to follow. People trained in school administration aren't always able to understand the dynamics of working in a recovery school culture, and those from the recovery world are often at a loss when it comes to the complex politics of school administration. To function well, our classrooms need to have a low student–teacher ratio, and yet with smaller classrooms comes less funding from the state. How, then, can recovery schools hire and maintain adequate staffing with very limited funding? All of these challenges trickle down and have a profound impact on the day-to-day functioning of the school and the classroom culture. Many people with good intentions and a wide range of skills can still struggle to maintain sustainable schools.

And yet many schools continue, day by day and year by year, to overcome these obstacles, graduate increasing numbers of well-educated students, and turn the statistics about young people in recovery on their heads. All of the schools I have worked in are still thriving, though some in very different forms than they began. In a field where questions are still far more prevalent than answers, one thing is certain: it is through telling our stories, being honest about our struggles and failures, and celebrating our successes that we will continue to move closer to the day when every student who needs a recovery school can find one and that every student in a recovery school has the opportunity to thrive, both academically and in their recovery. That would be the happiest ending I could imagine.

NOTE

1. College Preparatory Mathematics (CPM). 1233 Noonan Drive, Sacramento, CA 95822, http://www.cpm.org

REFERENCES

Amstutz, L. S., & Mullet, J. H. (2005). *The little book of restorative discipline for schools: Teaching responsibility; creating caring climates.* Intercourse: Good Books.

Atwell, N. (1998). *In the middle: New understanding about writing, reading, and learning.* Portsmouth: Boynton/Cook.

Bane, R. (2005). *If you don't get what you want: Tips for getting the feedback you need.* http://www.rosannebane.com/main/art-feedback.htm, March 16.

Christensen, L. (2000). *Reading, writing, and rising up: Teaching about social justice and the power of the written word.* Milwaukee: Rethinking Schools.

Gruwell, E. (1999). *The freedom writer's diary: How a teacher and 150 teens used writing to change themselves and the world around them.* New York: Main Street Books.

Meiers, D. (2008). http://www.deborahmeier.com/.

Pranis, K. (2003). *Peacemaking circles: From crime to community.* St. Paul: Living Justice Press.

Pranis, K. (2005). *The little book of circle processes: A new/old approach to peacemaking.* Intercourse: Good Books.

Rethinking Schools. (2002). Milwaukee, WI. http://rethinkingschools.org/.

Style, E. (1988). "SEED Curriculum as Window and Mirror" (http://www.wcwonline.org/joomla/index.php?option=com_content&task=view&id=652&Itemid=127&Itemid=54) Wellesley Centers for Women website. First published in Listening for All Voices, Oak Knoll School monograph, Summit, NJ.

Zehr, H. (2002). *The little book of restorative justice.* Intercourse: Good Books.

A Secondary School Cooperative: Recovery at Solace Academy, Chaska, Minnesota

Monique Bourgeois, BS, LADC

ABSTRACT. The recovery school movement exploded across the nation in the late nineties and early part of the twenty-first century. Secondary and postsecondary recovery schools have become a vital part of the chemical dependency continuum of care and our nation's educational system. Solace Academy is a restorative practices high school designed for recovering chemically dependent students. Through the collaboration of professionals in Carver and Scott Counties, the Carver-Scott Educational Cooperative's Solace Academy recovery high school opened its' doors in the fall of 2001. Appropriately colocated with other programs provided by the Carver-Scott Educational Cooperative, Solace Academy provides a high school education, life skills and support for its recovering chemically dependent students. Co-location has insulated the existence of Solace Academy by shared staff, increased academic opportunities and financial stability. A typical day at Solace Academy is like and unlike many high schools across the nation. These similarities and differences have provided many lessons during Solace Academy's tenure.

Monique Bourgeois, BS, LADC, currently works for the Carver-Scott Educational Cooperative's (CSEC) Solace Academy recovery high school program. She is also the Department Head of Chemical Health with Carver-Scott Educational Cooperative school district. She has been involved with the Association of Recovery Schools (ARS) since its inception in 2003 as a committee member, Vice-Chair, Chair and Past Chair of the ARS Operating Committee.

INTRODUCTION

Recovery high schools are a relatively new concept in the educational and chemical dependency systems, but they have become a vital part of the chemical dependency continuum of care and our nation's educational system. In this article, I will share a personal perspective of a recovery high school, how we began, what a typical day is like, and what I have learned through my experiences at Solace Academy.

SOLACE ACADEMY

Solace Academy is a high school designed for students in recovery from chemical dependency. Located in Chaska, a Minneapolis suburb and open since the fall of 2001, Solace Academy is a part of District 930, the Carver-Scott Educational Cooperative, or "Co-Op." The Carver-Scott Educational Cooperative is a "joint-power" school district within Carver and Scott Counties in Minnesota. The cooperative serves a diverse range of people who need individualized or customized education and support and includes a broad range of alternative and special education offerings from early childhood though adulthood. Programs include Area Learning Centers, career and technical education, and special education programs.

Solace Academy is considered part of an Area Learning Center, and it is colocated with other Carver-Scott Educational Cooperative programs, primarily a secondary school alternative program called LINK. The mission of Solace Academy is to provide a safe, sober environment for chemically dependent students to meet their educational goals while encouraging healthy life choices. Solace provides a supportive, educational environment for up to 40 students in grades 9–12, who have successfully completed a chemical dependency treatment program. Consideration is given to students who have not had any treatment experience but are working on a program of recovery. Solace Academy requires adherence to continuing care plans, attendance of a minimum of two 12-step meetings weekly, ongoing contact with a sponsor, participation in random urinalysis and compliance with an enrollment contract.

Solace Academy adheres to the philosophy that

recovering students have a desire to maintain sobriety;

they need time in a chemically free environment to strengthen healthy living skills;

they need a safe group to practice coping skills;

they need a specialized learning environment to improve academic performance as well as academic credits; and

they need to experience positive, sober peer and community interaction to build success and create a vision for their future.

PROGRAM ORIGINS

A few years prior to the opening of Solace Academy, professionals in Carver and Scott Counties were struggling with how to address the recovery needs of high school aged students. Returning to the community after completing treatment, adolescent clients in Carver and Scott Counties had little or no support beyond a once-a-week aftercare program at the local treatment centers. According to Mike Coyne (personal communication, January 16, 2007), a former county social worker, "There were limited resources for students coming out of treatment." He adds that the professionals working with these students were seeing high rates of relapse and a return to active addiction. This gap in service spawned hopelessness for all involved: the client, the family, professionals, the community and the school systems.

Educational settings are designed to be safe, sober environments. Unfortunately, many students returning from chemical dependency treatment find that their educational settings are not safe, sober environments for them. Consider that for many students their school was the location of their heaviest substance access, use, and peer influence. The experience for a recovering teenage student, thus, has been described as being similar to asking an alcoholic adult to sit in a bar 7 hours a day, 7 days a week and not to drink. This is obviously a set-up for relapse; yet, this is what students were facing in Carver and Scott Counties when they would return from treatment to their schools. Sara Sones (personal communication, February 6, 2007), a Solace Academy alumnus, stated that after 3 days of returning to her home high school she "wanted to drink. I didn't want to stay at the home school and not be with those people." According to Sara, those "people" to whom she refers were her "using friends."

Over a two-year period, collaborative efforts began between Carver and Scott County's key stakeholders. The key stakeholders included human services, corrections, schools districts, and community members. A needs assessment and data from Drug and Alcohol Abuse Normative Evaluation System were utilized to support this exploration and to verify the gap in services for adolescents addressing their recovery. It was determined that the Carver-Scott Educational Cooperative would be the best vehicle to launch the new recovery school program, because it already provided multiple alternative high school programs within the two counties. Approval was sought from and given by the Carver-Scott Educational Cooperative member school districts to go ahead with the recovery high school, and professionals from those counties continued collaborating to create programming.

With other recovery high schools located within the Twin Cities, the recovery high school wheel did not need to be reinvented. Ideas from the other recovery high schools were utilized and adjusted to fit with the vision of the collaborative efforts. On September 10, 2001, "Dry High" was born. The name was later changed to Solace Academy.

INSTITUTIONAL STRUCTURE: THE VALUE OF A COOPERATIVE

If starting a recovery high school was as simple as collaboration between two counties' professionals and key stakeholders, more recovery high schools and college programs likely would exist throughout the United States today. Many recovery high school programs, however, have come and gone. Jeff Theis, Director of Development for the Carver Scott Educational Cooperative, attributes Solace Academy's survival to its being part of a cooperative. As previously noted, the Carver-Scott Educational Cooperative is a joint-powers school district. This means it has nine member districts throughout Carver and Scott Counties, and these member districts play an important role in determining what programs are needed, created, and maintained.

Cooperative Advantage #1—Ability to Share Staff and Resources

A main advantage of being part of a cooperative is the colocation with other programming that serves secondary school students. This allows staff to be shared between the programs, which enhances Solace's financial viability. Co-location has also resulted in availability of daily special education services and broader curricular offerings, such as physical education, art, music, a leadership class, T'ai Chi, senior seminar, service learning, and mentoring. These subject areas would be limited, at best, if Solace Academy were in a solitary location. The approximate student-to-professional ratio is 15 to 1, which is allowed to decrease based on the number of certified special education students in the program.

During the first 3 years of its existence, Solace Academy was colocated in the same building as a secondary alternative school called "LINK," an adult English Language Learners (ELL) program, an adult developmentally disabled program called "Living Skills," and an independent study program for students of all ages who were finishing their high school diplomas or working toward a GED. Unlike a typical school, these programs were all housed under the one roof of a single-story office building located in a business park.

Initially those involved in the planning of Solace Academy were concerned about its colocation with the alternative program called LINK. Because the purpose of having a recovery high school was to provide a safe, sober environment for students in recovery, planners wondered about the ability to support abstinence from alcohol and drugs if Solace Academy was located in the same building as another alternative program educating at-risk students. For this reason, boundaries were clearly laid with each student population to maintain the safest environment. As LINK, like Solace Academy, is an alternative program based in restorative practices, the staff who teach in Solace Academy also teach in the LINK program. The students, however, do not intermingle. When, for example, a subject is being taught in Solace Academy, it only contains Solace Academy students. Staff noticed, interestingly, that the students in the Solace Academy and LINK programs were not very interested in one another. On occasion, students in either program have known students in the opposite program, but rarely has this caused any concerns. When issues have risen, they have been handled in a restorative manner (to be addressed in more detail later).

Expansion and growth at the start of the fourth year of operation created an opportunity for Solace Academy to move to an adjoining building. The new, larger facility, created room for a gym, larger classrooms, and more office space. Solace Academy still utilizes the former building for art, the computer lab, and a conference room, but now there is more distinction between Solace and other programs.

Cooperative Advantage #2—Continuum of Care

Another advantage to being part of an educational cooperative is the connection to a continuum of care with Carver and Scott Counties to address substance use issues in Carver and Scott Counties. At approximately the same time Solace Academy came into existence in 2001, the educational cooperative along with Carver and Scott Counties began developing a model for a continuum of care to address substance use, abuse, and dependence within the two counties. The Carver-Scott Educational Cooperative identified gaps in service delivery, including a lack of chemical health services within the mainstream and alternative high school programs. With the increased accountability of school districts due to No Child Left Behind, there was an increased need to address issues that impeded students from graduating. Student substance use was identified as one of those issues. The cooperative felt that if students with chemical health issues could be reached and provided appropriate services, their chances of graduation would also increase, therefore helping their home school district to be more accountable.

The cooperative sought and obtained grant funding to add Chemical Health Specialists to the mainstream and alternative high schools within Carver and Scott Counties to provide prevention, intervention, and referrals related to substance use issues. Along with the placement of Chemical Health Specialists in the schools, the local chemical dependency treatment providers, and Solace Academy, the counties are slowly closing the gaps in chemical health services for adolescents. For Solace Academy students, this allows for a more seamless flow from intervention through treatment and then continuing care. Future expansion of this continuum of care will include the development of community coalitions to further address substance use in Carver and Scott Counties.

INSTITUTIONAL PHILOSOPHY: RESTORATIVE PRACTICES

During Solace Academy's development, current program manager Heather Bantle introduced the idea of implementing the philosophy of restorative practices as a basis within the school. Ms. Bantle was certified as a Family Group Conferencing Facilitator and Trainer through the International Institute for Restorative Practices. The institute's Web site (International Institute for Restorative Practices, 2007) describes restorative practices as being rooted "in 'restorative justice,' a new way of looking at criminal justice that focuses on repairing the harm done to people and relationships rather than on punishing offenders (although restorative justice does not preclude incarceration of offenders or other sanctions)."

The philosophy of restorative practices was born from the family group conferencing process that has been utilized by New Zealand's indigenous people, the Maori, for centuries. In the Maori ritual, the extended network of family and friends share the responsibility for a young person's behavior while involving the victims of that behavior in the process of resolution. Many other native tribes around the world use "circles," similar to the family group conferencing process of the Maori tribe, as a way to heal the community when harm has been done. The formalized ideas of family group conferencing or restorative justice and practices were introduced in the United States around 1994. According to the International Institute:

> The most critical function of restorative practices is restoring and building relationships. Because informal and formal restorative processes foster the expression of affect or emotion, they also foster emotional bonds. The late Silvan S. Tomkins's writings about psychology of affect (Tomkins, 1962, 1963, 1991) assert that human relationships are best and healthiest when there is free expression of affect—or emotion—minimizing the negative, maximizing the positive, but allowing for free expression. Donald Nathanson, director of the Silvan S. Tomkins Institute, adds that it is through the mutual exchange of expressed affect that we build community, creating the emotional bonds that tie us all together (Nathanson, 1998). Restorative practices such as conferences and circles provide a safe environment for people to express and exchange intense emotion. . . . Restorative practices are the science of building social capital and achieving social discipline through participatory learning and decision-making." (International Institute for Restorative Practices, 2007)

At Solace Academy, the use of restorative practices develops a sense of community. As stated by Ted Wachtel (1997) in *Real Justice*, "Community is not a place. Rather, it is a feeling, a perception. When people see themselves as belonging to a community, they feel connected. They have a sense of ownership and responsibility. They feel that they have a say in how things are run and a stake in the outcome."

Restorative practices, furthermore, align well with the 12-step model's focus on admitting, accepting, and taking responsibility for the care of one's disease and encouraging the development of bonds with other recovering addicts to improve and maintain a healthier, chemical-free lifestyle. As Solace Academy emphasizes the 12-step model of recovery and restorative practices readily fit that model, the two have fit together well in the school. All staff have been trained in restorative practices. It is integrated through everything we do. Solace Academy was the first recovery high school based on the principles of restorative practices. At least one other recovery high school, PEASE Academy in Minneapolis (described in this volume by Angela Wilcox), has integrated the principles into its program as well.

The social discipline window (Figure 1) is a simple but useful framework for understanding the implementation of restorative practices at Solace Academy. The window describes four basic approaches to maintaining *social norms* and *behavioral boundaries*. The four are represented as different combinations of high or low control and high or low support. The restorative domain combines both high control and high support and is characterized by doing things *with* people rather than *to* them or *for* them.

Figure 2 shows how restorative measures are utilized within in a continuum from informal to formal activities. Restorative practices can be

FIGURE 1. Social Discipline Window.

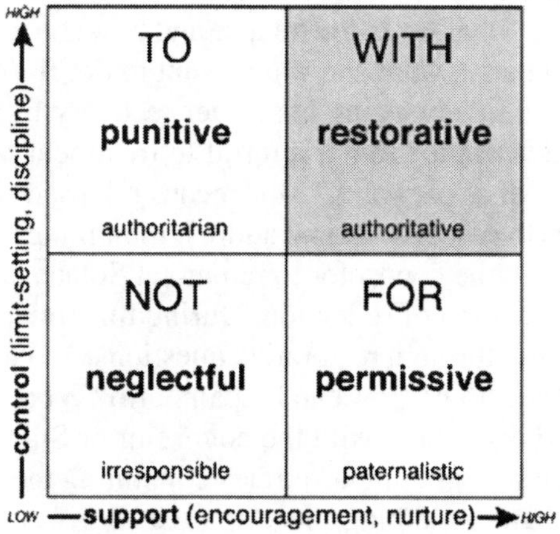

SOURCE: (International Institute for Restorative Practices, 2007)

FIGURE 2. Restorative Practices Continuum.

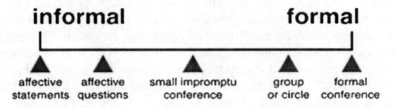

SOURCE: (International Institute for Restorative Practices, 2007)

as simple as addressing a disruptive student in class by using affective statements and questions to addressing a more serious issue such as relapse. We have found the best thing about the use of restorative practices at Solace Academy is how it allows for problems to be addressed in a respectful, solution-oriented manner, with a large emphasis on the student *owning* his or her problem and then finding solutions to resolve it.

Restorative Practices at Solace Academy: A Case Involving Relapse

This example of a relapse will demonstrate the utilization of restorative practices. For this example, the term "relapse" means the use of a nonprescribed mood-altering chemical after a period of sobriety. "Cindy," a student, has come forward and stated that she has relapsed. An individual session is held between Cindy and Solace's licensed alcohol and drug counselor to discuss what led to the relapse and how she would like to move forward, if indeed that is what she wants want to do. If a Solace Academy student is interested in advancing his or her recovery by remaining at the school, and it is determined that a referral to treatment is not needed, the student is placed "out of program." This means relapsed students take time out of their classes to reflect upon and address their relapse/recovery issues.

Cindy agrees with the counselor to remain at Solace, and thus is placed out of program for a time of reflection. During this time, she restoratively addresses her relapse through restorative questions: What happened? Who has been affected and how? How can I repair harm? What is my plan? After careful review and discussion with the counselor or Solace program manager, Cindy is then brought into a "circle" containing the Solace Academy community members. A talking piece is used to symbolize who has the floor to speak, and it always moves to the left in the circle. Cindy shares her restorative assignment with the community. As the talking piece moves left through the circle, the community has the opportunity to share how they have been affected and what they would like to see result from this experience. The talking piece continues to move around the circle until everyone has said what he or she needs to say regarding the relapse. By coming to the circle, sharing, and receiving feedback, Cindy is "restored" back into the community. This process also provides the community the opportunity to share how *they* have been affected by the student's relapse.

In using restorative practices at Solace Academy, our goal is to give the problem back to the person responsible for it in the first place. As Figure 1 identifies, giving the problem back does not imply neglecting of the issue, solving the issue for the person, or punishing someone for his or her issue. Restorative is about *resolving* issues with the student. At Solace Academy, we see these as valuable life skills that students can take with them for the rest of their lives.

OPERATIONAL STRUCTURE

Finances and Budgeting

Similar to any recovery school, Solace Academy has its challenges when it comes to its operating budget. Original start-up funding for Solace Academy was granted for 2 years by Carver and Scott Counties' Family and Children's Mental Health Collaboratives. These collaboratives consisted of county agencies and school districts. This funding allowed Solace Academy to begin with a budget that accommodated eight students the first year of operation and 15 students the second year. While the initial stated enrollments were small—and thus more costly—those collaborating on the development of Solace Academy wanted to ensure its success and sustainability over time. It was agreed that having a smaller student population the first 2 years would allow for the newly hired staff to familiarize themselves with students in recovery and the school's practical philosophy. The small size also provided staff the ability to adapt program needs with fewer variables.

The Carver-Scott Educational Cooperative develops its program budgets for the upcoming school year months before the actual school year starts. Budgeting is based on the number of students currently in the program and the anticipated return of students from one year to the next. Unfortunately, these estimates are not guarantees and can complicate the budgeting process. In reality, students may not return as expected for a variety of reasons, including graduation, a return to active using, or a transition back to their home schools or other programs. During its first 6 years, Solace Academy operated in the red and the black. Should Solace Academy student numbers fall below budget projections, the Solace Academy program budget can be supported by other, more financially stable programs within the educational cooperative.

Funding for Solace Academy comes from a variety of resources, including the following:

General Education revenue or Minnesota state "tuition" dollars;
Special Education funds;
Scott Family Net, the Family Services and Children's Mental Health Collaborative in Scott County; and
Grant funding from the Mdewakanton Sioux Community, the Park Nicollet Foundation, and the Minnesota Department of Health.

Additionally, the school has the flexibility to add or subtract staff based on the number of students currently in the program.

Admissions Process

Referrals to Solace Academy come from a variety of avenues such as treatment centers, social services, corrections, school personnel, and word of mouth. To enroll at Solace Academy, a prospective student needs to complete an application and interview. The application paperwork includes agreeing to the enrollment contract, signing of releases of information, completing a referral form, and writing a brief essay on the student's history, educational goals, and why he or she wants to be at Solace Academy. Once the application is received by Solace Academy, it is reviewed and an interview is scheduled.

The interview is held with the prospective student and parent(s), along with the licensed alcohol and drug counselor, the Program Manager, and an outside professional. A typical interview lasts 45–60 minutes and consists of (a) reviewing the application and (b) the potential student answering questions pertaining to his or her current state. The interview team then determines if the student is accepted or not. A large part of determining acceptance is a student's willingness to be at Solace Academy. That does not mean the student has to be overjoyed about attending Solace Academy, but he or she needs to convey a willingness to follow the enrollment contract and program expectations.

Potential students usually are not accepted to Solace Academy (1) if they are currently using or (2) they demonstrate an unwillingness to enroll at Solace Academy. The latter of the two is typically seen when students feel forced to apply by parents, probation officers, social workers, or treatment center staff.

If a student is accepted, the student, family, and home school district determine a start date. Solace always tries to have a student start as soon as possible, thus the school accepts students at any time throughout the quarter or semester. The process of completing an application and interviewing often indicates a student's willingness to be at Solace Academy. Virtually all students that apply and interview, therefore, are accepted. The school believes a student's desire to attend Solace is a key to success for the school and the student.

Academic Class and Therapeutic Group Schedule

Students at Solace Academy attend school Monday through Friday from 8 a.m. to 2:30 p.m. Class periods are approximately 50 minutes long. The school has a closed lunch, meaning students do not leave to get lunch elsewhere. There are the obvious reasons for having a closed campus, including that fact that our location makes it difficult for students to leave, get lunch, and return to school within the 25 minutes allotted. The school does offer a hot lunch program available for purchase. The Carver-Scott Educational Cooperative's main campus—located only five miles away—prepares and delivers the hot lunches, which is another advantage of being a part of a cooperative. Students also run a store with "nonnutritional" foods, and there are a refrigerator, a toaster, and microwaves available for students to use. Proceeds from the school store go back into the program for activities such as field trips, prom, and graduation.

Solace Academy has seven class periods. Typically, the school has at least two classes offered each period. As the counselor, I facilitate a therapeutic group with the students on an every-third-day rotation. Students receive academic credit for their group participation. While one third of the students are in group with me, other students are in a class such as current events or physical education. I determine the group composition, which lasts one quarter of the school year. Students, thus, change groups four times per year. This has not always been the case. In the school's first year, groups occurred twice daily with a longer, more therapeutic group in the morning and a short check-out group at the end of the day. As we have evolved, the current group schedule has worked well. The groups at Solace Academy have always been focused on supporting students' recovery. We do not do 12-step work or present assignments related to recovery but we do talk about all aspects of recovery and life.

Parental Involvement

Parental involvement and communication is highly encouraged while students are attending Solace Academy. There are two main ways this occurs. First, there are bimonthly parent support and educational groups that are just for parents. These groups provide an opportunity for parents not only to receive education and support but also to connect with the parents of the other recovering students at Solace Academy. Parents making this connection strengthen the supportive nature of the school. Second, quarterly conferences are held with the parent(s), student, and staff. Attendance is required for both parents and students. Additionally, communication takes place through midquarter and final quarter report cards, e-mail, and phone conversations.

Academic Goals

Solace Academy wants to work with students to best meet their academic goals. Students may choose to stay with us until they graduate, or they may choose to transition to another academic setting. Transitional possibilities include returning to their home school, other programming within the educational cooperative, or postsecondary educational options. The Carver-Scott Educational Cooperative, which is Solace Academy's school district, is *not* a diploma-granting school district. All students attending the cooperative's programs, therefore, follow their home school district's requirements for graduation. This does not lessen the academic rigor, but it does require strong collaboration between the Carver-Scott Educational Cooperative and a student's home school district to ensure requirements are being met.

If a student finishes his or her graduation requirements while attending a Carver-Scott Educational Cooperative program, the diploma is granted by the home school district, and it states the home school district's name on the diploma. Solace Academy does, however, hold its own graduation ceremony. On average, five students graduate each year. For students graduating from Solace Academy, or any recovery high school, it is about more than just getting a diploma. By the time students and families get to graduation day, most have endured an incredible amount of heartache. Graduation represents what recovery is all about: healing, serenity and gratitude. As Solace graduate, Sara Sones, stated, "The graduation ceremony was designed by us, and it was about us."

PERSONAL REFLECTIONS: LESSONS LEARNED

Education and Advocacy

Solace Academy has faced a constant need to educate and advocate. In Solace Academy's first years, education centered on helping school administrators understand the disease of chemical dependency and recovery and educating professionals, treatment centers, and the general public about what Solace Academy is and what it is not. Solace is not a treatment center and cannot be substituted for one. First and foremost, Solace Academy is a school that supports students in recovery, and it serves a niche in the education world. To legitimize our continued existence, we must continue to address the need to educate and advocate beyond our own system.

Importance of Connection with Other Schools

Initially, a board consisting of chemical dependency professionals from both Carver and Scott Counties provided advisory support. As the program developed and gained experience, the need for advisory support diminished. With Solace Academy located so close to several recovery high school programs in Minnesota, though, we began to connect with other recovery high school professionals. We have relied on this connection to share experiences and receive guidance and support. Because of our relationship with other recovery school professionals, the school did not have to "reinvent the wheel" each time a new situation was encountered. At the same time, we felt a sense of excitement to be on the cutting edge of an emerging concept in the world of education.

Enrollment and Fiscal Uncertainty

A huge lesson learned throughout our tenure is that there is an ebb and flow to the student population. The number of adolescent clients currently being served at local chemical dependency treatment programs directly impacts the enrollment at Solace Academy. When the treatment centers are busy, our demand increases, and when they are not busy, our demand decreases. We have noticed a tendency for the local adolescent treatment center population to be lower at the start of the school year, even though the progression of a person's chemical dependency will continue regardless of the school calendar. As a result, we begin to see an increase in referrals around November 1, as students begin completing treatment and start looking for other schooling options.

Another factor impacting our enrollment is relapse. Depending on the circumstances, some students *are asked to leave* the school after relapsing, some students *choose to leave,* and some return to treatment. This instability in student population translates into uncertain operating budgets relative to the rest the educational system. Such enrollment and fiscal uncertainty contributes to financial difficulties for recovery high schools.

The impact of enrollment variability is felt in school operations as well. The number students enrolled at Solace Academy can range from 15 to 30; and, like any group's dynamics, when group members are added or taken away, the group can struggle to adjust and return to homeostasis. One way Solace Academy has tried to handle this is by controlling the number of new students who can enroll during any given week. Once this limit was placed, we found that new students and current students both adjusted better, therefore creating a more stable, welcoming environment.

Countless times I have joked with potential and current students about the following statement: "The great thing about Solace Academy is that we are a small school; the bad thing about Solace Academy is that we are a small school." In truth, the small size has proven to be much more of an asset than a liability. A small school community fosters compassion and it creates opportunities for students to develop sober relationships in a safe, nurturing environment. The small size allows a student to develop a sense of responsibility and accountability to others that can get lost in a large school setting. At Solace Academy, everyone knows you, whether you like it or not; but ultimately, this is one of the school's strengths.

Relapse: Honesty, Integrity, and Boundaries

Two primary goals of Solace Academy are (a) to keep the program safe and (b) to maintain a high level of integrity. We feel these goals require both a staff committed to maintaining firm, consistent boundaries and a community based on honesty. Solace Academy recognizes that for some people, relapse is part of the recovery process. Thus, with integrity being an integral part of our community, it is expected that a student who has relapsed will be honest about it immediately. Such honesty ensures that the student can remain enrolled at Solace Academy. If a student needs further treatment services to address his or her relapse, appropriate referrals are made.

When a student hides his or her use or another student's use, we have seen that this secrecy begins deterioration in multiple life areas and negatively impacts the community at Solace Academy. These can be difficult situations to handle, because there is a fine line between what is best for the community and what is best for the individual student. Chemical dependency can lead to death, but recovery school staff can neither "fix" students nor guarantee sobriety. Sometimes, students relapse and never come back without explanation. This proves to be difficult for the community of staff and students because of the lack of closure. Solace Academy has let students go for dishonesty about their substance use or for enabling another student's use. There is always an underlying question, though, of what a staff person could have done differently to help this student. In hindsight, most of the time we have made the right decision, but it remains one of the most difficult things about my job.

On occasion, students will reapply for enrollment after they have left or been asked to leave. There have been some students who have left and come back a few times. When previous students return, however, they are not the same. Prior notions about these students can be thrown out the window—some students flourish their second, third, or even their fourth time around.

Student Sobriety

When Solace Academy opened, all of our students had approximately the same amount of sobriety. They were going through the recovery milestones and pitfalls at the same time. Yes, they were obtaining their medallions or key tags, but then they would question the necessity of having a sponsor or going to meetings. It is difficult to convey the wisdom that comes from varying stages of recovery without having *current* students at various stages of recovery. This was an eye-opening discovery, and since then, we have had students with varying sobriety lengths.

School Name

As mentioned above, Solace Academy was originally called "Dry High." While the name was catchy, during the school's second year, our students felt the name of the school did not represent their recovery. Students also wanted a name they could use in the community that did not scream, "Sober School!" I remember feeling very proud of their ability to recognize that being in recovery was more than being dry or sober and that they wanted the choice of maintaining their anonymity. As a school, we began the process of finding a name that represented them. After a couple months, the students and staff chose "Solace Academy." This process was important for the students because it demonstrated ownership and pride in their community.

Students and Young People in Recovery Are Still Students and Young People

Adolescent students in recovery have unique characteristics, yet they are still similar to non-chemically-dependent students. Students in recovery high schools have the same aspirations for their futures as students in mainstream schools. They are individuals with a variety of needs, which change as they grow and mature. They still need time to be kids. This can be challenging for Solace Academy students, because their experiences can force them to operate in both adolescent and adult worlds. Through their experiences in treatment and 12-step groups, students in recovery are handed many adults skills. However, they have adolescent brains that may be developmentally stunted due to their chemical use.

Through my experiences, I have found students in recovery high schools to be very talented. Solace Academy students usually have a large amount of creative energy, whether it is for the arts or music or theater. During Solace's development, there was a strong push to include art and music as a part of the programming. Thus, since our inception we have had art and music as a part of our program. In the second year, the cooperative received a grant to start a drama troupe. Students from several of the cooperative's programs, including Solace Academy, were trained by professionals to create and perform improvisational skits. The students loved it. Most of the skits that Solace Academy created centered around chemical use and its impact on various life situations. They have performed for local schools, businesses, and community organizations. Each year, a new training takes place for the new recruits. This has been an invaluable outlet for students. It has also been a way for students to give back to their community.

CONCLUSION

When chemically dependent students enter the world of recovery, they are given back the freedom of choice and, once again, all things become possible. Although not all at once, life areas begin to stabilize. Sometimes other issues arise, but recovery high schools like Solace Academy can and do provide an environment that acknowledges the importance of addressing recovery and related issues for students with chemical dependency. Recovery high schools recognize and are equipped to handle their unique needs. They can and do provide a transition for students in recovery to become productive, healthy, and contributing members of society. To me, there is no greater success than when working with students in recovery.

Throughout my career, people have commented on how difficult it must be to work with adolescents with chemically dependency. Yes, at times the work is difficult; but more notably, it is important work that is rewarding and worthwhile. In spite of the difficulties, I get to go to work every day and participate in miracles. Not everyone can say that.

REFERENCES

International Institute for Restorative Practices. (2007). *"What is restorative practices?"* Retrieved May 30, 2007, from http://www.iirp.org/whatisrp.php

Nathanson, D. (1998). *From empathy to community.* Paper presented at the First North American Conference on Conferencing, Minneapolis, MN.

Tomkins, S. (1962). *Affect imagery consciousness (Vol. I).* New York: Springer.

Tomkins, S. (1963). *Affect imagery consciousness (Vol. II).* New York: Springer.

Tomkins, S. (1991). *Affect imagery consciousness (Vol. III).* New York: Springer.

Wachtel, T. (1997). *Real justice: How we can revolutionize our response to wrongdoing.* Pipersville, PA: The Piper's Press.

The Insight Program: A Dream Realized

Traci G. Bowermaster, M.Ed.

ABSTRACT. Traci G. Bowermaster, Lead Teacher and Special Education Teacher at the Insight Program, a recovery high school in White Bear Lake, Minnesota, explains how her school was created and how it has evolved. Using the framework of many recovery stories, she writes about how it was in the early days of recovery schools before special education was emphasized, what happened that lead to the formation of her school, and what her school program is like now. She uses her unique perspective of having taught in a treatment center to explain the importance of incorporating strong special education programming in recovery high schools and illustrates the process her team used to form a recovery school with little financial means. Pitfalls along the way helped the Insight Program find its weak spots, eventually grow stronger, and create an ambitious vision for the program's future.

WHAT IT WAS LIKE...

Recovery high schools are a recent educational option that has emerged from collaboration between secondary schools, treatment professionals,

---

Traci G. Bowermaster, M.Ed, is Lead Teacher/Special Education Teacher at the Insight Program/White Bear Lake Area Learning Center.

parents, and other adults interested in providing a safe school setting for sober teens. Also known as sober schools, recovery schools are distinct in that they specifically serve students who have identified themselves as in recovery from drug and/or alcohol addiction. Typically, such schools provide an educational setting that incorporates a strong sense of community and therapeutic support. The first known recovery school, Ecole Nouvelle, opened in Edina, Minnesota, in 1986 and eventually became Sobriety High, which has grown to five campuses and continues to grow. While the majority of early recovery schools were located in Minnesota,[1] other recovery schools emerged simultaneously in isolation in Arizona, New Mexico, California, Tennessee, and Washington State. The process of starting the Insight Program has paralleled both the recovery story of "what it was like, what happened, and what it's like now" as well as the journey through the 12 steps of Alcoholics Anonymous. This article will tell the story of the Insight Program, a recovery high school within the White Bear Lake Area Learning Center in suburban St. Paul, Minnesota, and the profession journeys of the people who run it.

In 1993, I began working as a teacher at Fairview Recovery Services, an adolescent inpatient treatment center and halfway house in Woodbury, Minnesota, a suburb of St. Paul. I taught social studies and math to the students there and provided special education services to those who needed them. Also, I was part of the clinical team that met daily to discuss the progress of all clients and to create aftercare plans for students getting ready to leave treatment. I first became familiar with recovery schools while employed at this facility.

At that time, there were only a scant few recovery schools in existence and we were fortunate to at least have them within the Twin Cities metro area. While many of our clients came from the Twin Cities, many came from outside the metro area of Minnesota or elsewhere in the country (and some from Canada), where there was little-to-no support for recovering students once they left treatment. Students in those situations were forced to return to their former school environments, which for most were where much of their drug and/or alcohol involvement and contacts were located. As discharge dates loomed, clients who had been successful in treatment often started to unravel a bit, looking ahead to a bleak future where resisting the temptations to use seemed next to impossible in their former stomping grounds. I recall a number of instances in which clients would purposely sabotage their treatment graduation by acting out just before dismissal in an attempt to have their treatment further extended. In processing their intentions afterwards, many admitted not feeling like they would have the support they needed from their schools to stay sober once they returned to their home schools.

What I found back then was that the amount of special education services available to students in recovery schools was limited. Some of the recovery schools had itinerant special education teachers who would come into the recovery schools on a very limited basis, such as once a week to check on the special education students, consult with the school staff, and complete any necessary paperwork. Other schools would actually encourage parents of special education students to sign a form that would discontinue services for students with special needs in order for the student to be eligible to attend the recovery school.

The thinking was that most students in special education who had been in treatment had had a diagnosis of Emotional Behavioral Disorder and that their school problems tended to disappear once they got into recovery. It was also thought that the smaller class size of recovery schools and frequent groups that addressed behavior and attitude would eliminate or at least lessen the need for special education services in most cases. However, this practice was troubling on many levels and created a strong barrier to recovering students with special needs receiving the entire scope of services they needed. To begin with, many recovering students with special needs had disabilities that had surfaced long before their chemical use had become a problem and that would not go away just because they got sober. In the case of students with mild-to-moderate mental handicaps, more severe learning disabilities, and mental health diagnoses such as ADHD, bipolar, and anxiety disorder, being in recovery would not completely cure their school problems.

In my Master's thesis research, it was very clear that students with special needs, especially in the areas of Emotional Behavioral Disorder and Specific Learning Disability, were more prone to drug abuse or addiction than their nonhandicapped peers. In addition, adolescents with mental health disorders had a much higher and quicker rate of relapse than those without mental health disorders. Moreover, adolescents with special needs required more intensive skill training to resist temptation, impulsivity, and peer pressure than their nonhandicapped peers. It was clear that adolescents with special needs who were also chemically dependent required very specialized schooling and therapeutic inter- vention to experience success in sobriety and in life. In other words, recovery schools that were not providing solid special education pro- gramming were turning away those students who were most vulnerable to relapse.

I was eventually transferred out of the treatment center and into a position at a junior high as a teacher of students with Emotional Behavioral Disorders (EBD) and Specific Learning Disabilities (SLD). While I knew that I did not have the desire to continue my position in that particular setting any longer than I had to, I wanted to make the most of the situation and learn all I could from it. Through conversations with Beth Samuelson, chemical dependency counselor and my former colleague at the treatment center, I learned that an alternative school in White Bear Lake was considering starting a recovery school. Beth had been providing services to the high school and the alternative school in White Bear Lake and had been brainstorming ways to start a recovery school in the district with Julia Jilek, the Area Learning Center (ALC) principal. Julia had grown increasingly frustrated with watching her ALC students flounder with their chemical use and get into treatment only to relapse quickly after returning to school. Beth, Julia, and Lyle Helke, the Chemical Health Coordinator for the district, were conducting research and seeking out grants to start up the program. Beth had remembered that I had completed some research on recovery schools and contacted me to assist them with some grant writing. We did not get the grant that we had written, but I did get the special education position with the understanding that I would also start a recovery school as part of my position. Thus, the Insight Program was born.

WHAT HAPPENED...

I visited some of the existing schools to get ideas of policies and procedures I wanted to incorporate; I interviewed directors and took notes on physical details, such as how the rooms were arranged and postings on the wall of rules and recovery slogans. That fall, Julia and I also wrote and received another grant from Education Minnesota for $3000, which was enough to help pay for some fieldtrips and activities specifically for the program, which Julia had named "Insight." Meanwhile, Julia and Beth attended meetings and brainstorming sessions with various members of the education and recovery communities to get ideas and advice.

In early January of 2001, I started teaching at White Bear Lake Area Learning Center. I would spend January getting acclimated to the building, getting to know the students from my special education caseload, and preparing with Beth for the start-up of the Insight Program. It was determined that Insight would exist as a school-within-a-school and that the costs would be absorbed by the existing ALC budget and augmented by grants and subsidies from a local county collaborative. We were aiming to have our first students by the beginning of the second semester, which was at the end of January. I was given a classroom with the typical accoutrements and was encouraged to make it a comfortable, welcoming space for therapeutic groups to occur. A couch, some carpet scraps, and some beanbag chairs were donated or purchased at thrift stores. Posters with recovery themes were purchased and placed on the walls. Catalogs were perused for recovery-related literature and guides about group techniques, which were provided through funds from the collaborative grant.

Crucial steps in creating any school program are to create a mission, belief statements and goals. These steps help to define the perimeters of the program and serve as guideposts for when the program veers off course. We spent a great deal of time and thought on these steps of the process, as we wanted to be sure that we would project a particular image to the community and provide our students with specific services. Our mission gave our program purpose and clarity. It read,

> The Insight Program provides a supportive learning environment for recovering teens that nurtures their mind, body, and spirit, and encourages healthy decision making.

Belief statements explained the underlying philosophies that the staff shared about how best to work with teens in recovery, and helped us shape our policies and practices with students. They read as follows:

We believe that recovering teens need a supportive school community in which to learn and have fun.
We believe that recovering teens can benefit from ongoing skill building in the areas of social skills, relapse prevention, and goal setting.
We believe in providing activities that enhance each student's mind, body, and spirit to encourage complete wellness in recovery.
We believe that recovering teens are motivated by recovery plans and goals tailored to their unique strengths and needs.
We believe that the best way to curb teen drug abuse is by involving positive role models of recovering teens within the community and creating a feeling of "esprit de corps."

Program goals were created to give the program measurable targets of effectiveness that could be charted through time. They read,

To foster healthy choices and to assist the student in maintaining sobriety

To minimize individual and/or group involvement in identified "at risk" behaviors

To support the student in an individual recovery plan

To decrease involvement of participating students in the juvenile court system

To increase school success

Finally, criteria for enrollment were established to attract our target population. To be eligible to join Insight, students must

be between the ages of 16–20,

have at least 1 month of sobriety,

have the desire to remain abstinent, and

have a willingness to complete a UA (*urine analysis*) at their own expense.

The mission statement, belief statement, program goals, and criteria for enrollment along with contact information were formatted into a brochure that served to advertise the program to potential referral sources, interested applicants, and their parents.

In establishing the basic structure of Insight, Julia, Beth and I drew upon what we knew from our own professional experience, what the research taught us, and what resources we had available to us. We wanted to offer Insight students a quality education with classes taught by teachers licensed in their subject area. We also wanted to do what we could to protect the Insight students from temptations to use, as much as possible, because we knew that a large percentage of ALC students were involved in chemical use. While we had put enormous thought into the policies and the day-to-day operations of the school, we learned a great deal from trial and error.

To stagger the start time with the ALC, Insight students would start off each day at 11:00 a.m. with a recovery group. This group, for Insight students only, was meant to help them get into the mind-set of recovery and their goals for the day. I would lead the group most days and would consult with Beth often, who at that time was only at the school once per week. The day that she was there, she would run group. At noon, students would eat school lunch together as a group separate from their ALC peers. The students would then be scheduled in classes in the regular ALC for their academic classes. The ALC has licensed teachers in the following subject areas: English/language arts, mathematics, science, social studies, physical education, health, art and work experience.

At that time, most of the ALC student population attended school in the morning and had jobs or other activities that took them away from the building in the afternoon. It was thought since the building virtually emptied out of students in the afternoon; the Insight students could take classes then without the threat of being tempted or distracted by other students who still might be using. Students would be scheduled in classes based on what credits they needed to graduate, when teachers were available, and what their interests were. I would try to schedule more than one Insight student in each class so that they could rely on each other for support and positive peer pressure. One of my jobs would be to check on the Insight students often in their classes and to be available if a student was in need of emotional or academic assistance.

Beth Samuelson, the licensed alcohol and drug counselor, contributed the following statement explaining her philosophy of how therapeutics and recovery interweave into the Insight Program:

> It was noted in the above that I was only able to be in group about once a week. It was apparent that my services were needed more than once a week. I was also working in the ALC and meeting with students one on one. There was an opportunity for me to work half time in the school district with my main focus being with Insight. I started with my schedule working three mornings a week and two afternoons a week. I would run a recovery group in the mornings I was there and in the afternoons meet with students in Insight and also in the ALC.
>
> In the mornings that I run the group, we focus on recovery and on maintaining positive group dynamics. It is really important to have the group be safe enough to talk and share their pain with one another. I believe you get this by always encouraging honesty and openness in a group and with one another.
>
> Every relapse is looked upon on an individual basis. A huge part in this is if they have come clean about their use before they are caught or "called out" by another member of the group. Often, they are placed on a contract and, if they are unable to follow the contract or use again while on the contract, then we have a meeting with the parents and decide what is to happen next.
>
> When I am in group I always try to have another staff in the group also. Traci and I most often run group together. It is of the utmost importance for the students to have your trust and believe in what you say. I believe you most often get that be leading by example and

really being able to listen well. Teens more often than not have some kind of authority issues and so if you can get them on your side and have them believe in you this really is helpful. You also have to figure out who the leaders of the group are and coach them into taking that role. It is also important to watch for anyone trying to take the power in a negative way. If this happens and you don't let them know that you are in charge of their safety, group chaos can happen quickly and secrets start. It is sort of like a dance where you have to take the lead at times and other times follow.

I believe therapeutics play a very important role in a recovery school and yet the students are there ultimately for their education in a safe environment. This is why we start the day with a group and try to check in with the students at the end of the day also. If you know where they are at before you send them to their classes, you can often ward off trouble with their behavior and find a plan that will help them be successful for that day in school.

When Insight first started, we put the cap at 12 students. Many of the other recovery schools had student populations that were much larger than ours. However, most other recovery schools were housed in a separate building away from other peers, did not share teachers with another program, and had financial reasons for needing to have more students. We looked at the size of our program as a real asset. Fewer students would be more manageable in both groups, and classes and the students would get more personalized attention from all staff. The smaller size of Insight was also a necessity in the building since the students would be spread out into different classes, which would be difficult to manage and supervise. And, of course, there was the conventional wisdom that it was always better to start small. Eventually, as we became more experienced about what worked, we increased our capacity to 15 students.

As our opening day was quickly approaching, we contacted representatives from many different sources for referrals. Beth and I spread the word of Insight's opening at all the adolescent treatment centers in the Twin Cities area, including Fairview, Anthony Lewis Center, Hazelden, HSI, and Dellwood. We also contacted school chemical dependency and guidance counselors from White Bear Lake Senior High School and the surrounding school districts of North St. Paul/Maplewood/Oakdale, Mahtomedi, Stillwater, Roseville, Moundsview, Centennial, South Washington County, and Forest Lake. In addition, we spread the word to various probation officers and juvenile detention centers from Ramsey,

Anoka, and Washington Counties and contacted the Drug Court program in St. Paul. Probably the best networking opportunity we had early on was attending a Recovery Schools Tubing Party at Green Acres Recreational Center in Lake Elmo. At this party, recovering teenagers from various institutions and their adult staff met to go snow tubing in the spirit of "sober fun." Here, we met many of the referral sources we had just contacted, as well as other potential associates that we had not yet considered, such as contacts from halfway homes and therapeutic group homes. We eventually found our first students at this function as a local group home was searching for a nearby recovery school program for its seven clients. While our base has definitely grown, these referral sources have provided us with a consistent flow of students throughout the years.

To establish whether a potential student was a good fit for our program, we carefully considered our enrollment process. Once a referral was made, we would cue the agency to have the parents of the prospective student call us to set up an interview with their student. Beth and I would be present for each hour-long interview, which would consist of three parts. For the first half hour, I explained the components of the program, such as the mission, the schedule, school calendar, how academics worked, and the rules or contract of the program. Then I would explain to the parents how to complete the enrollment forms, health history card, and release-of-information forms. While the parent filled out the paperwork, Beth interviewed the student to get a feel for his or her history in regard to family, school, chemicals and mental health, attitude and commitment toward school and recovery, and tips from the student about what helped him or her through struggle. At the end of the interview, we would invite the parent and student to take the next 24 hours or so to think about whether they thought the Insight Program was a good fit. It was important that the student knew that enrollment at Insight was completely voluntary. Meanwhile, Beth and I would discuss our perception of the student's eligibility for our school and would talk to our principal and other support staff about the student's enrollment. Once our decision was made, I would contact the parent and student to either invite them to start at Insight or to consider other options.

In considering the Insight contract, we strove to keep it simple, connected to the principles of recovery, and broad enough to cover a variety of situations. This way, we were able to keep the contract to one page. We had parents and students sign the contract at the interview to show that they understood the expectations of the program before committing.

We made the first point of the contract about honesty. Since honesty is one of the most important parts of recovery, we emphasized that we expected that students would be honest about their urges to use before it got to the point that they relapsed. If they relapsed, though, coming forward with the relapse right away was always better than waiting to get caught through a drug test, poor behavior, or rumors. Another part of the honesty rule was about not enabling other Insight students to use. To keep the program safe and strong, we told students that they had some options about how to handle a situation in which they knew another student had used and had not shared the information with the group. They could either give the peer who used 24 hours to admit the use to Beth, me, or the group otherwise they would tell us themselves; they could confront the peer directly in group; or they could come to Beth and me privately if they did not know how to handle the situation. We stressed the fact that if we found out that they had known about a peer's use and had done nothing, they could face consequences just as severe as if they themselves had used.

The next point of the contract was about attendance. Because accountability is a big part of recovery, we expected each student to be in attendance every day unless excused by a phone call from a parent or guardian due to illness, appointment, or family obligation. This point was important to spell out because the Insight Program is associated with the ALC, which had a more lenient attendance policy. We assured parents that if a student was not present and we hadn't received a phone call, we would be calling the parents to inform them and there would be strict consequences for missing school.

Working toward earning school credit in each class was our next rule on the contract. Since we were only able to serve a small number of students, and other students might be put on a waiting list if we were full, we expected all the students would be working to their ability in each class. Insight's set-up offered the opportunity for students to get caught up in academic credit if they applied themselves, and we expected students to take advantage of that opportunity.

Next on the contract was our drug test policy.[2] While we did have some money from the collaborative to pay for some urine analysis tests, we wanted the parents to agree to pay for the tests when possible, to help defray the costs to our program and to help promote buy-in to the tests. The rule about drug tests was that if asked, the student would provide a urine sample that day. A staff person of the same gender would monitor all drug tests. Refusal to comply could result in dismissal. If a student were to have a drug test that was positive for a certain chemical, parents would be called for a meeting.

Creating a recovery plan was the next policy on the contract. Once admitted into the program, students would be expected to complete a recovery plan, which would consist of their own perceptions of what they learned about themselves in treatment. They would be asked to share what they do on a daily basis to stay in recovery; which people, places, and things they stay away from to keep themselves safe from using; what triggers could lead them back to using; which people were resources they could rely on to help them make the right choice if they were tempted to use; what they had to gain by staying in recovery; and what they had to lose by going back to using. We told students that we did not dictate what should go on their recovery plan and that we knew that what works for one person might not work for another. As long as they were doing well, staying sober, and seeming serene, we would consider that they had a solid recovery plan. If they were to have a relapse or show poor behavior by repeatedly not following the terms of their recovery plan or the Insight Program contract, we could intervene and help them write a new contract.

The next rule on the contract related to respect. We expected each Insight student to show respect to themselves, each other, Insight and ALC staff, the rules of the ALC, White Bear Lake school district policies and the laws of the community. We pointed out that we were not so concerned with the laws that they had broken in the past (though we expected them to follow through with terms of probation and restitution), but we urged them not to get in further trouble with the law after becoming part of our school. We explained that we were a small school that had a lot of eyes watching us to make sure we were doing what we set out to do, helping students stay sober and also out of further involvement in criminal activity. We also equated being in recovery with having respect for all members of one's community and the law.

The final rule involved students staying within the Insight area at all times unless they had permission from a staff member. In essence, this was our no smoking rule. We expected students not to smoke cigarettes during the hours of school, between classes or during lunch. If caught smoking, they could receive a smoking ticket, which could lead to fines and further court involvement. This rule was also put in place to keep the Insight students apart from influences in the ALC that could be detrimental to their sobriety.

The consequences for violating these rules were progressively more severe, beginning with being verbally warned by the staff, and leading to parental contact, meeting with parents and staff to write behavioral contract, and possible dismissal. Insight staff reserved the right to skip ahead to stronger consequences for flagrant violations of the rules.

Finally, it was explained to students that if they should be asked to leave the Insight Program or if they decided that once they started attending school in Insight that they wanted to be in a different school, our staff would be willing to help them find another school if they would like. However, one option that would not be available to them for at least two quarters would be the ALC. There were two reasons for this policy. First of all, after being in groups where confidential information was shared, it would be awkward for both the student who was leaving and the group members who were staying to be in the same building but not part of the same group. Second, and more important, the Insight staff acknowledged that the student had initially sought Insight as a school setting to get support for his or her recovery, and since the ALC has many students that are still using, we would want to help the student find another school setting that would be more conducive to getting the support he or she needed.

Once I had read through the contract with the parent and the student, I would ask them to sign the contract. Signing the contract signified that the rules and consequences had been explained before a decision being made regarding enrollment.

Running a recovery school within an alternative school within a large school district that had special education as a prominent feature could be quite complicated. The entities of recovery, alternative schools, public schools, and special education can have points of view and philosophies that diverge a great deal. To begin with, the field of recovery itself has a focus on individual accountability, consequences for negative actions, and reliance on the group or on a higher power to help maintain positive change. Treatment centers teach clients to look at the behaviors and attitudes that are detrimental to living life without chemicals, help clients to break through denial and admit to the damage they caused themselves and others, and identify the positive behaviors and resources that are available that will help them stay on track. Alternative schools seek to accept students as they are and help them set and reach the goals they want to achieve through offering a variety of learning experiences. ALCs relish their flexibility in regard to academics, their ability to build relationships with students who are at-risk for dropping out, and their creativity with helping students handle difficult life situations. Not only are public schools required to provide a free and appropriate education to all students within the district, they also must show that all students are progressing academically at a uniform rate and that services are being provided in spite of dwindling financial resources. Last but not least, special education emphasizes that students with disabilities have a right to such practices as educational accommodations and support, adjusted academic expectations, and limitations to disciplinary actions depending on the student's needs. In order for all these entities to work together, it is vital that each consider the multiple perspectives while also making decisions that ultimately complement the mission, goals, and beliefs of the school.

Keeping these varying viewpoints in mind while also staying true to the foundations of Insight meant that my initial beliefs about the students we could serve had to be scaled back. Since we were a small recovery school by design, that provided daily direct services to students with special needs, it followed that sources referring students who received special education and with dual disorders took a keen interest in this school. The fact that Beth had also been a crucial part of starting and providing her services as counselor to a dual-disorders program at Fairview in Forest Lake further strengthened our appeal to such potential students. Therefore, we found that our unique backgrounds and perspectives filled a vital niche in the Twin Cities recovery high school field: that of recovering students with disabilities and/or dual disorders of depression, anxiety, bipolar, ADHD, and so on. However, early on, we learned that there were limitations within our niche to the students we could adequately serve.

Under special education law, students are to be educated in the "least restrictive environment" available to them that can meet their needs. These environments, or Federal Settings, range from being indirectly monitored by a case manager a few times a month on the very low end to requiring education to take place in a hospital setting in the extremely high end, with varying amounts of restrictiveness in between. In other words, if a special education team determines that a student requires that his or her daily instruction take place in a pull-out setting that offers intensive special education support throughout the school day, then the school where the student attends needs to provide that service. Since the ALC and Insight have a "blended model" or have both students with and without special needs in all classes, the school is set up to serve students who require Federal Settings of II or lower. Typically, students who required a higher level of setting in another school could lower their level of service in our school because of our school's lower class sizes, high amount of emotional support available through both staff and other students, and flexibility with methods of offering credit. Sometimes, though, students seeking a recovery school that had more intense needs such as a time out room, token economy behavioral plan, or paraprofessional support in each class might not be able to have all their needs met in our school and would be encouraged to look elsewhere. This always was a difficult call because schools that did have the services available to meet the special education needs of the students still had many students in them that had current issues with using or selling chemicals. We ultimately dealt with this situation by weighing with the team what seemed to be in the best interest of the student and helping the parent in making it possible for them to pursue the setting that best served the student's needs.

Another difficulty in serving this particular niche was determining whether students with dual disorders were emotionally or mentally stable enough to fully participate in the program. Occasionally students came to Insight with their mental health in a fragile state and hadn't yet addressed all their mental health needs. Luckily, we were able to recognize the signs and could intervene to get the students the additional support (either in school or in the community) that they needed so that they could be successful. Occasionally, such students were reluctant to follow through on the suggestions we made for support and continued to cycle downward. In such cases, we would need to look at the behavior of the student and determine whether our program could sustain his or her enrollment based on the student's actions. Also, it sometimes occurred that students with dual disorders stopped taking the medications prescribed to them for their mental health disorders or took them in a way other than prescribed. In these situations, we reminded the students of the need for them to work with their doctors when making decisions regarding their medications and told them that we expected them to follow through with Insight's behavioral expectations regardless of whether or not they were taking their medication.

With both students with a higher need of special education services and students with greater mental health needs, we carefully consider whether we can meet the students' needs without compromising the integrity of the program. In many cases, such students may require additional treatment or intervention before they are ready to enter (or reenter) Insight. Most of the time if we do need to make the decision that enrollment at the school is not a possibility due to special education needs or mental health needs, we are able to let the student or parent know what would need to happen in order for enrollment to be considered in the future.

GROWING PAINS

The Insight Program took its first students in at the beginning of second semester in January of 2001. The first seven students came from a nearby correctional group home for boys, with a recovery focus. We worked closely with the program's director when dealing with student behaviors and issues, which were significant given their background. As word got out to other referral sources, we started taking more students from White Bear Lake district and other surrounding school districts. Those first few months were extremely difficult, as we were in the process of finding our way in the operation of this new school program. Beth was only employed to work in the school one-half day per week and I consulted with her by phone constantly. We struggled greatly with managing student behavior, creating a positive peer culture, and making decisions regarding appropriate enrollment and discharge.

By the end of the school year, Julia, Beth and I made the decision that enrolling all the students from the correctional group home was not a successful practice for a variety of reasons. If the students were placed in the group home, attending Insight was part of the expectations, thus taking the student choice element away from the enrollment. Also, these students had significant criminal backgrounds and their placement in the group home made them part of the correctional system. The presence of these students, many of whom were facing felony charges for violent behavior, detracted other referral sources and parents from sending their students to Insight. Furthermore, with our enrollment cap at 12 and the students from the group home (which was outside of the White Bear Lake school district) permanently comprising over half of our spots, people from within the district cried foul. If our program had been able to serve a larger population and if we were not just starting out with the development of Insight, schooling the students from this group home might not have been as problematic. (It should be noted that the students from this program have since made a similar arrangement with another recovery high school with a larger population. This arrangement has been successful for years.)

For the next couple of school years, through trial and error, we continued to learn about how best to operate the Insight Program. We were able to get Beth hired in the district half time. This way, she was able to conduct group in the morning three days a week and be here in the afternoons twice a week for intake interviews, individual sessions with students and support staff meetings. We began to attract referrals from a variety of treatment programs, school guidance counselors, drug counselors, and probation officers. We upped our enrollment to 15 in our second year and eventually exceeded that number, resulting in our first waiting list. Our parent involvement increased, which brought valuable resources including chaperones for fieldtrips, financial support, and creative ideas for activities. We presented information about Insight to the school board and received unyielding support from them. Beth and I both became involved with the Association of Recovery Schools from its inception and have maintained a significant involvement since.

While we always agreed that it was important to involve parents as a crucial part of our program, we did not formally create a process for parental involvement until the beginning of the second year. At that time, we began Parent Night. This group met once a month in the group room for a potluck supper in the evening. Parents and the Insight staff discussed issues regarding dealing with recovering teens, problem-solved, discussed triumphs and anguishes, and gave the parents a forum of support. Often, Beth or I would have announcements about upcoming events and would ask for volunteers for chaperones, donations, or services, and we would also have special resources or handouts available about specific topics. Occasionally, guest speakers were invited to present on such subjects as college options, support groups for parents, and academics. Always, a phone list of current students and their parents' phone numbers was distributed so that parents could keep in touch with each other as well as be able to contact their child if he or she were with another Insight student. Parent feedback was always quite favorable about this service.

Toward the end of the third year, we experienced some difficulties that placed the future of the program in peril. At the beginning of the fourth quarter of the 2003–2004 school year, we had 17 students enrolled. Throughout the quarter, we had numerous and significant problems with student behavior, including skipping classes, smoking on school grounds, explosive outbursts in class and a great deal of risky behavior outside of school. Teachers reported increasingly alarming "junky talk" (or talking fondly about stories from the past about drug and alcohol use) in class. We began to learn about multiple relapses and had to discharge some students for repeatedly violating the terms of their contracts. Other students ran away from home during that time and ended up in correctional placements or treatments. By the end of the quarter, our enrollment had dwindled from 17 to 7. During the early summer, the news only got worse. We learned that all but one of the remaining 7 students had been actively using chemicals for the last 2 to 3 months and had been going to great lengths to hide their use from their parents and from us. We were devastated and sickened. It was unclear at the time what had gone wrong and even less clear how to fix the problem.

The summer of 2004 brought the opportunity for a great deal of soul searching. Beth and I had plans to attend the Association of Recovery Schools (ARS) Conference at Rutgers University in New Jersey, and I was slated to present on Special Education in Recovery Schools with a special education teacher from another school. We thought that we would look at the conference as an opportunity to learn something from my colleagues, regroup, and get support from others who had been through similar experiences. We gained what we hoped we would gain and more from attending this conference.

Two copresenters at the conference that were particularly inspirational as well as instructional hailed from the Center for the Study of Addiction and Recovery at College of Human Sciences at Texas Tech University; Dr. Kitty Harris, director, and Amanda Baker. Texas Tech had run a collegiate recovery community for several years and is viewed as on the cutting edge of research in the field of addiction and recovery. Their presentation focused on identity and relapse. In Amanda's portion, she emphasized the importance of forging a new identity as a recovering person and discussed how this task is particularly difficult for adolescents and young adults who are already in the middle of their search for self. The temptation for the newly sober young person to revert back to the familiar role of a drug user or drinker, she said, is great. Dr. Harris explained her theory about the cycle of relapse. She said that in looking at relapse in young people, a cycle of four stages tended to occur. First came some type of painful, troubling, or embarrassing event. Next came the residual feelings of shame, pain, or disappointment. After that, a relapse would occur and then more shame about the relapse. Then, the cycle would continue. In her work, she would try to train her students to recognize the trigger feelings and replace the impulse to use with another, more positive and less harmful behavior. This presentation, along with the camaraderie and support of the other ARS members at the conference, gave us the motivation and courage to look at the problems with our program and come up with workable solutions.

Beth, Julia, Lyle Helke and I looked at how the Insight students did not truly have the opportunity to create their own culture of recovery because they spent much of their school day in classes with ALC students who weren't in recovery. While Insight students rarely relapsed with ALC students were rare, Insight students seemed to feel the temptation to fit in with ALC students who talked about partying. Their quest to create an identity of a recovering person was thwarted by too much interaction at a vulnerable time with students who either were still using or never had issues with drugs or alcohol. We deduced that in order for Insight students to be able to have a chance to be successful in recovery, we needed to isolate them from the rest of the ALC; at least until it was clear that recovery had taken root. Julia arranged with contractors to have a wall built across the hallway on the other side of the group room and office. The wall had nonlocking doors so it was not completely blocked off from the rest of the school but it was a symbolic indication that Insight now had its own "space" in the school. Vinyl signs were put up on either entry to the Insight areas, indicating that ALC students were only allowed in the area with Insight staff permission.

Eventually, Insight acquired more rooms in the school that were for Insight only. With Julia's blessing, we reconfigured the schedule so that all Insight students would be in all their academic classes together. These classes would be taught by an ALC teacher in the Insight classroom and no other ALC students would be allowed in the class. This would help students forge their new identity as recovery persons in a safe environment away from nonrecovering peer influence. It would also help create a stronger community culture in which students would learn to be supportive of each other both academically and socially. Most of all, it would help us to be better able to identify when a student was having difficulty so we could intervene sooner and possibly help the student resist relapse.

This change required that we also solicit the teaching staff to get more involved with the operation of the Insight Program. Classroom teachers would go from having a couple of Insight students in their classes at a time to having one class a day with the Insight students exclusively. Each quarter, the Insight schedule would consist of one hour per day of group (run by Beth and Traci) and four different one-hour academic classes. This rearrangement increased the size of the rest of the ALC classes. It also meant that teachers had to deal with the team mentality of the group, which could work in their favor or against it. When the group was functioning well, the team camaraderie of the group would result in better classroom participation and performance overall; however, when the dynamics were off or poor attitudes prevailed among students, the group might "team up" or act out in unison in class. Beth, Julia, and I met with staff during the week of workshops before the start of the school year to talk about our reasons for the change, to get feedback and concerns, and to problem-solve potential trouble spots ahead of time. This helped build rapport among staff and ownership in the new-and-improved Insight Program.

Incorporating a phase system was another change we made to the Insight policy. A common wisdom in the addiction world says that emotional growth and maturity stops at the point at which a person starts using heavily. Most teenagers in recovery started using heavily in their early teens, which means that even 17- or 18-year-old newly sober addicts are "stuck" developmentally at 13 or 14 years of age. One developmental milestone is the ability to be motivated by nontangible or intrinsic rewards rather than token or extrinsic rewards. It had been our experience that the students we worked with in the Insight Program needed more motivation to stay sober and make good choices in their lives than just the good feelings they got from doing the right thing. They seemed to need incentives to earn privileges along with additional responsibilities. With this in mind, we created the phase system. Students would start out as Phase I, which meant one of three things:

they were new to the program and had the same privileges or responsibilities as everyone else,
they had been with the program for a while and had hadn't yet progressed to the next phase, or
they had lost their Phase II status through a relapse or poor behavior choices.

Students could earn Phase II status by accomplishing the following:

enrolling in Insight for at least 2 months;
remaining continuously sober for at least 3 months;
demonstrating positive behaviors in all classes for at least 2 weeks as indicated by classroom teachers;
absolutely not enabling Insight peers;
being caught up on all current school work;
not being tardy for at least 2 weeks or not missing school unexcused for at least 1 month;
showing evidence of attendance of at least two meetings a week, one of which could be a therapy session but the other of which had to be some sort of 12-step meeting;
acquiring either a sponsor or a therapist;
demonstrating recovery behaviors at home as reported by parents; and
showing leadership in the program in some capacity.

Students would present their proposal for Phase II in group with signatures they had obtained from parents and teachers signifying their agreement. Then the group and the staff would discuss whether or not they agreed with the Phase and state why. The rewards for Phase II were being able to take a non-Insight class in the regular ALC, being eligible for overnight fieldtrips, and being able to take Fridays off as long as the student remained caught up in all classes and didn't otherwise miss any school (even excused) for the week. If school were missed within the week for any reason, a student with Phase II would be required to come on Friday. Also, Phase II students were considered the leaders of the program and were expected to act accordingly by giving extra effort to help new students or others who were struggling.

With these changes in place, we felt we had successfully responded to the lessons we had learned from the profoundly disappointing events of the spring of 2004 and the inspiration we had received from the ARS conference. We emerged stronger and confident that the adjustments we made would result in a higher quality, more efficient recovery school program.

WHAT IT'S LIKE NOW...

The fall the 2004–2005, school began with the changes in place to the structure of the school and the new school schedule. Staff was very supportive of the changes with Insight and seemed to respond well to working with the students as a group. Referral sources responded that they were relieved about the changes and we earned a few more referral sources who wouldn't recommend us previously when we had recovering students mixed with nonrecovering students in classes. Students also seemed motivated by the new phase system. One of the students, who had relapsed during the spring of 2004, returned to treatment and successfully completed a month later. He reinterviewed and was accepted back into Insight for the fall and was asked to give some feedback on the proposed changes. Interestingly, he thought that the criteria for Phase II was too easy and that we should increase the numbers of meetings required per week from one to two. His involvement in the creation of the phase system seemed to make it much more palatable for the other new students. Not surprisingly, this young man became one of the program's strongest leaders and was the first to earn Phase II.

The phase system, the physical changes to the structure by adding the doors and adding the classroom, and keeping the Insight students together for all classes all day have resulted in the program becoming more cohesive and more functional overall. We continue to grow and change and have incorporated new practices along the way. As another motivator for classroom performance, we began a Student of the Month award.

More Insight graduates are going on to college or have aspirations to continue their education past high school. We received a grant through a local foundation and used the funds to pay for college preparatory curriculum materials and pay expenses. As part of this project, we have incorporated college visits to multiple local college sites (including Augsburg's StepUP Program) and a college mentor reading group program. Feedback from this project has been overwhelmingly positive from both the college students and the Insight students.

All of what we are able to do at Insight would not be possible in just any school district. White Bear Lake School District had the belief and trust that Traci, Beth, Julia and the rest of the ALC staff could make this "experimental" program work. Our superintendent, Dr. Ted Blaesing, has made it a point in a number of his August staff convocations to mention Insight and the successes of the small program to district staff. School board members recognize and support the importance of having a recovery school within the district. Special education and regular education administration have both been very flexible and supportive with assisting us with navigating through tricky aspects of school policy. In spite of the current climate of budget cuts and increased national mandates, White Bear Lake School District has sent a clear message that they value the presence of a recovery school within the district and will continue to allow it to thrive.

Still, there will always be challenges. While running the program is mostly rewarding, dealing with student behavior, lack of motivation, or relapse can be grueling. There is also the pressure from outside referrals to take students that might not be appropriate for our school because it is thought that their enrollment in Insight is the lesser of evils. Budget and staff cuts threaten to make all of our loads heavier and make it necessary to continue to seek out other sources such as grants for funding of extra costs of fieldtrips and activities. In addition, shortened treatment stays and cuts in insurance benefits mean that students are being sent back to school (and into schools such as Insight) before they may be completely stable. These difficulties will need to be met with confidence and optimism to insure that Insight will continue to be successful.

NOTES

1. PEASE or Peers Enjoying a Sober Education opened in Minneapolis in 1989; the Gateway Program opened in St. Paul in 1992; the Arona Campus opened in St. Paul in 1995; Y.E.S. or Youth Education Sobriety, now closed, opened in Hopkins in 1997; ExCEL, now closed, opened in New Hope in 1998; and Aateshing opened in Cass Lake in 1998.

2. Through associates in the field, we found a company in California called Redwood Toxicology, which was able to test urine samples for five different chemicals for $6.00 a sample. They would also provide the sample cups for free, provide free airmail service if five or more samples were sent at a time, and were able to give technical and expert information about any of the test results through their toll-free phone line. Results were faxed to the school within 24 hours of the lab receiving the samples.

REFERENCES

Alcoholics Anonymous. (2001). *The Big Book, 4th Edition*. New York: Alcoholics Anonymous World Services, Inc.

Bowermaster, T., & Finch, A. J. (2003). *Post-treatment educational considerations for adolescents with chemical dependency*. Paper presented at the Annual Meeting of the American Education Research Association, Chicago.

Finch, A. J. (2005). *Starting a recovery school: A how-to manual*. Hazelden, Center City, MN.

Finch, A. J., & White, W. L. (April 2006). The recovery school movement—its history and future. *Counselor: The Magazine for Addiction Professionals, 7*(2), 54–57.

Harris, K. S., & Baker, A. K. (2004). *The process model of recovery and its impact on young adult programming in recovery schools*. 3rd Annual Association of Recovery Schools Conference, Rutgers University, NJ.

Teas, T. G. (1998). *Chemically dependent teens with special needs: Educational considerations for after treatment*. St. Paul, MN: Bethel College.

Achieving Systems-Based Sustained Recovery: A Comprehensive Model for Collegiate Recovery Communities

Kitty S. Harris, PhD, LMFT
Amanda K. Baker, MS
Thomas G. Kimball, PhD, LMFT
Sterling T. Shumway, PhD, LMFT

ABSTRACT. The Center for the Study of Addiction and Recovery (CSAR) (a Center within the College of Human Sciences at Texas Tech University, TTU), has developed a comprehensive Collegiate Recovery Community (CRC). This community provides a model of support and relapse prevention for college students recovering from addictive behaviors—primarily alcohol/drug addiction. This model is specifically targeted for implementation

Kitty S. Harris, PhD, LMFT, is an Associate Professor, College of Human Sciences, Department of Applied and Professional Studies, Addictive Disorders and Recovery Studies Program at Texas Tech University. Dr. Harris is also the Director of the Center for the Study of Addiction and Recovery.

Amanda K. Baker, MS, is an Assistant Director of Grants and Special Projects, Center for the Study of Addiction and Recovery, Texas Tech University.

Thomas G. Kimball, PhD, LMFT is an Associate Professor, College of Human Sciences, Department of Applied and Professional Studies, Addictive Disorders and Recovery Studies Program at Texas Tech University.

Sterling T. Shumway, PhD, LMFT, is an Associate Professor, College of Human Sciences, Department of Applied and Professional Studies, Addictive Disorders and Recovery Studies Program at Texas Tech University.

in the college/university setting and has been used at TTU for 20 years. The purpose of this paper is to briefly review the literature related to substance use among college-aged individuals, discuss the challenges of recovery within this population, describe existing collegiate programs, and provide an extensive description of the CRC model. The CRC model specifically incorporates recovery support, access to higher education/educational support, peer support, family support, and community support/service in an effort to help individuals attain what we describe as systems-based sustained recovery. Preliminary evidence of success indicates that support services offered by the CRC work for the current population as evidenced by an average relapse rate of only 8%, a graduation rate of 70%, and an average GPA of 3.18 among members. Limitations of the model and plans for future research are also discussed.

INTRODUCTION

The Center for the Study of Addiction and Recovery (CSAR) (an autonomous unit within the College of Human Sciences at Texas Tech University, TTU), has developed a comprehensive Collegiate Recovery Community (CRC). This community provides a model of support and relapse prevention for college students recovering from addictive behaviors—primarily alcohol/drug addiction. This model is specifically targeted for implementation in the college/university setting and has been used at TTU for 20 years. The CRC is a program that has maintained one primary focus: the creation of a comprehensive recovery support, education, and prevention network for students.

The purpose of this paper is to briefly review the literature related to substance use among college-aged individuals, discuss the challenges of recovery within this population, describe existing collegiate programs, and provide an extensive description of the CRC model. Within this model/community, individuals are given the opportunity to develop key characteristics that further their individual development while they interact with both recovering and nonrecovering communities. The CRC model specifically incorporates recovery support, access to higher education and educational support, peer support, family support, and community support/service in an effort to help individuals attain what we describe as systems-based sustained recovery.

LITERATURE REVIEW

The consequences of alcohol and drug use/abuse and addiction affect virtually all college and university campuses. Recent national surveys have identified the misuse of alcohol as a major social and health concern for colleges in the United States (O'Malley & Johnston, 2002; Wechsler, Kuo, Seibring, Nelson, & Lee, 2002). In addition to academic problems, college students' misuse of alcohol is associated with health problems, suicide attempts, unsafe sex, vandalism, and property damage (Hingson, Heeren, Zakocs, Kopstein, & Wechsler, 2002; Wechsler et al., 2002). Compared to all other age groups, young adults aged 19 to 24 reported the highest prevalence of heavy and high-risk drinking defined by five or more drinks in a row within the past two weeks (Johnston, O'Malley, & Bachman, 2001). In addition, young adults enrolled full time in college are more likely to engage in heavy or binge drinking when compared to their noncollege peers (O'Malley & Johnston, 2002). These findings suggest that specific factors exist within the collegiate environment that influence student drinking behaviors.

As a result of the prevalence of alcohol abuse and addiction among college-aged individuals, many colleges/universities have begun to implement strategies for assessing, treating and preventing alcohol and drug abuse and addiction within the collegiate setting. Recognizing the complexity and seriousness of alcohol and drug misuse, many colleges/universities have acknowledged the need for multidisciplinary efforts toward prevention and intervention that include both research-oriented and campus-based approaches. As well, the federal government has identified binge drinking among college students as an important public health concern. In an effort to address this ongoing problem, the U.S. Surgeon General and the U.S. Department of Health and Human Services have included the targeted reduction of college students' binge drinking among public health goals in a plan entitled, "Healthy People 2010" (USDHHS, 2000).

Although increased awareness and understanding of the problem has made treatment more accessible for college students, little attention has been given to posttreatment concerns of recovering students. The transition to the college or university environment poses significant risks to the recovering student. The heavy drinking and drug using subcultures of most college/university campuses suggest that the environment is not welcoming to students recovering from addictive disorders. For recovering students, the primary challenges may come from the lack of a supportive recovery system within the college or university environment. With the unique risks and challenges recovering students face, there is a clear need to provide special recovery support programs for these students. Colleges and universities should be aware of this population and be prepared to respond to their special needs.

Individual Development and the Challenges of Recovery within the Collegiate Environment

The extension of adolescence and the prevalence of the collegiate experience in American mainstream culture has extended the period of development for individuals ages 18–25. This period of life, often termed emerging adulthood, "should be a time of increased growth, when young adults begin to develop stable identities and take on adult responsibilities." (Gotham, Sher, & Wood, 2002, p. 40). The move from adolescence to emerging adulthood often involves a move to a different geographical region, the transition to a college/university, and/or a change in socioeconomic status. Unfortunately, the outcomes for individuals in the collegiate setting are often mediated by alcohol/drugs and other addictive behaviors (e.g., eating disorders, gambling, sex).

The pervasiveness of alcohol and other drug use among 18–25 year olds, many of whom are attending a college/university, makes it difficult for recovering individuals in this age range to locate peer support and find an environment in which recovery from addictive disorders is valued and rewarded. Lack of social and peer support can make it extremely difficult for college students, especially recovering young adults, to complete the developmental tasks of this time period without being immersed in alcohol/drug use and/or relapse (Schulenberg & Maggs, 2002). The juxtaposition between the need for finding a social support mechanism while attending a college/university and the need to remain abstinent prevents many recovering young adults from pursuing higher education and thus, from fulfilling their personal and professional potential. Some of the barriers encountered by students in recovery are discussed below.

Finding a network of social support. A component of young adult development involves finding a social support network of peers who support an individual's identity and the values and beliefs that accompany it. The identity of recovering students and the choice to remain abstinent in the college environment are not often rewarded by the majority of young adults. Because of this lack of social support, students in recovery may find it difficult to access the activities necessary to grow and maintain their recovery. They may have difficulty resisting social pressures toward group conformity in what appears to be an alcohol-saturated environment (Perkins, 2002). In addition, young adults in recovery are often a minority population in 12-step groups. The adult composition of most groups may prevent young adults from finding support, identification, and a sense of commonality in 12-Step meetings (Harrison & Hoffman, 1987).

Learning to live outside of a parent/guardian's supervision. The transition from adolescence into young adulthood involves the process of achieving autonomy from an individual's family of origin. This usually necessitates moving out of a parent/guardian's home and thus, moving away from their direct supervision. For recovering students, this developmental milestone can be difficult to surmount. Many recovering students may be moving from an alcohol/drug free environment into an environment in which exposure to drinking/drug use is the norm (Woodford, 2001). This expanded environment with increasing pressure to drink/use, combined with less accountability, offers challenges to those in recovery attempting to make healthy decisions.

Setting and attaining educational and career goals. Alcohol/substance use disorders are related to lower educational and occupational attainment (Gotham et al., 2002). Often young adults in recovery have spent the majority of their adolescence under the influence of chemicals. Their educational backgrounds may have been affected by their drinking/drug use. In the attainment of educational goals, adolescent drinking/drug using can impact development in two important ways: (1) recovering young adults may not have demonstrated academic accomplishments that warrant admission to a college/university and (2) recovering young adults may need extra academic support when they enter, or return to, the college/university setting due to the lack of basic educational knowledge that would normally be attained in high school.

Developing healthy peer relationships. During young adulthood, the formation of close friendships and adult sexual relationships is vital to healthy development (Dworetzky, 1996). Available data suggests that those students who have positive peer relationships have positive behaviors and outcomes in school. These positive relationships shape the way they view their entire school experience. Research findings also indicate that friendships are associated with the psychological, social, and academic adjustment of students across groups (Feldman & Elliott, 1990). Students in recovery, without a community that supports abstinence, may find it difficult to negotiate the formation of these close bonds. The development of peer relationships and/or romantic relationships is complicated by the fear of self-disclosure and the seeming impossibility of finding someone who they could identify with or relate to in regard to their recovering self.

Purpose of a Recovery Community

The primary purpose of a recovery community is to create, implement, and maintain peer-to-peer support services that promote a culture of abstinence from alcohol and other drugs and that extend the continuum of recovery. This is accomplished by offering strength-based services that emphasize social support as a factor in initiating positive lifestyle changes. One of the factors that assists people in moving along the change continuum is social support. According to White (2001), ongoing support from a community of peers is critical to sustaining recovery over long periods of time. The creation of collegiate recovery communities is an accessible and potentially effective method for enhancing recovery outcomes of young adults struggling with addictive disorders.

Recovery Communities on College/University Campuses

Moving away from home is stressful to many college students. For students in recovery, this transition may provide not only much desired personal independence, but also independence from familiar support systems of their particular program of recovery. The primary benefit of collegiate recovery communities is establishing a system of support within the students' new environment that can enable them to continue their recovery and access mechanisms of social support that enhance their quality of life. Collegiate recovery communities provide active support for a program of recovery and allow for healthy social interactions with recovering peers that further students' educational, personal, and professional goals.

Collegiate recovery communities blend abstinence with higher education. Thus, social support must exist on two levels: (1) students must feel supported in their decision to remain abstinent from alcohol and other drugs and must have access to an environment that reinforces the decision to remain in recovery and (2) students must feel supported in their decision to pursue a degree in higher education and must have access to an environment that rewards academic achievement.

Existing Programs

In the existing body of literature, there is little information about collegiate programs targeted at supporting recovering students. Based on information provided by the Association of Recovery Schools (ARS), there are three collegiate recovery programs that have been in existence for over five years (e.g., Texas Tech University's CRC at the Center for the Study of Addiction and Recovery, Rutgers University's Alcohol and Other Drug Assistance Program for Students Recovery Housing, Augsburg College's StepUP program). Replication efforts are under way to expand collegiate recovery community programs across the country. This effort is being spearheaded by TTU through a Federal grant funded by SAMSHA and the U.S. Department of Education to develop replication curriculum based on the CRC model. Pilot programs informed by this curriculum are currently being implemented on three campuses (e.g., University of Colorado—Boulder, University of Texas—San Antonio, and Tulsa Community College).

All the programs listed above are important and make significant contributions to their respective campuses. However, our objective is to provide information regarding the development of the CRC program and the comprehensive model that emerged from our extensive and long-term work with recovering students.

The Creation of the Collegiate Recovery Community

The CSAR opened in 1986 as a program to educate chemical dependency counselors in the state of Texas. Initially, it existed only to manage an 18-hour substance abuse studies curriculum within the Department of Human Development and Family Studies at TTU. Given its focus, the 18-hour curriculum attracted a large number of recovering individuals who began to construct a peer support system that shared a common experience and a desire to maintain abstinence from alcohol and other drugs. Through their choice of study and their willingness to disclose their recovery status, this group of students developed into a visible population at TTU. As this population emerged, professionals associated with the CSAR saw the need to provide increasing structure and guidance that initially took the form of 12-Step meetings held on campus. Over the past 20 years, the CSAR has increased its support of the recovering student population to develop the CRC.

A SYSTEMS-BASED COMPREHENSIVE MODEL
OF COLLEGIATE RECOVERY

The CRC at TTU provides recovery support services within the context of a comprehensive model that seeks to nurture systems-based sustained recovery within a collegiate community. According to our experience with this population, systems-based sustained recovery incorporates individual development within the context of a multitiered social system. "Systems-based" refers to the interdependent relationships and mutual influences of the interrelated parts or elements of an individual, family, or in this case a support community. The CRC model facilitates systems-based support in a collegiate environment by utilizing a series of five components that build on individual and contextual experiences of recovering students in higher education. These components include: (1) recovery support, (2) access to higher education and educational support, (3) peer support, (4) family support, and (5) community support/service (see Figure 1).

Within this social system, individuals are given the opportunity to develop key characteristics that include hope/purpose (Ridgeway, 2001), positive identity development (White, Boyle, & Loveland, 2005), reclamation of agency (Ridgeway, 2001), a sense of achievement/accomplishment (White, Boyle, & Loveland, 2005), a capacity for stable interpersonal relationships (White, 2000), and healthy coping skills (Ridgeway, 2001).

The CRC is a peer-driven community where program components have been developed according to student needs throughout the history of the community. Figure 1 represents both the historical development of the CRC program (beginning with education) and the movement of recovering students through their individual development within the program.

Recovery Support

The CRC was established to focus exclusively on supporting recovering students who have made a choice to stop using alcohol and other drugs. While initial support focused on educational interventions, the need for recovery support services became evident early in the formation of the CRC. At its inception, recovering students and faculty secured an on-campus location for 12-step and other support group meetings. Subsequently, recovering students organized a meeting in "celebration" of all 12-Step programs that was, and remains, open to members of the TTU campus and broader community regardless of their recovery status.

FIGURE 1. Comprehensive Model for Collegiate Recovery.

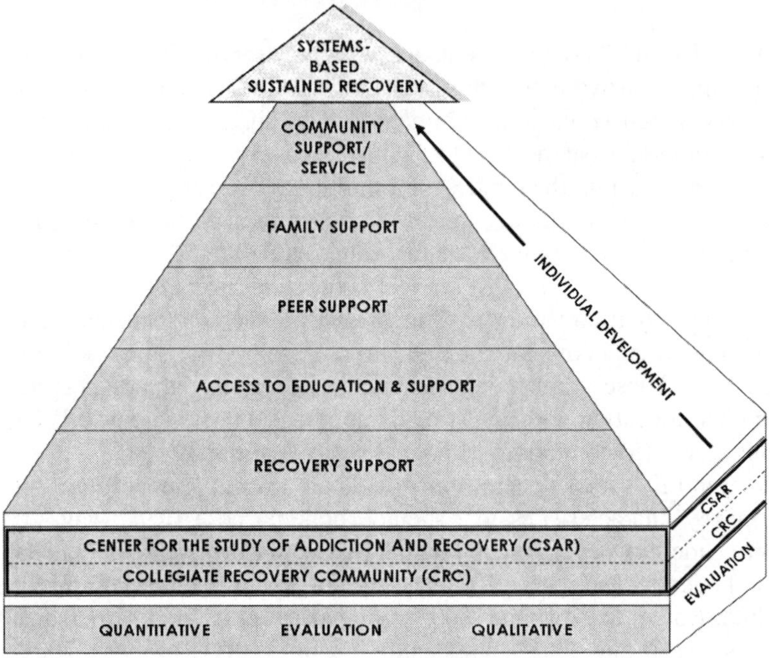

12-Step meetings and other support groups. According to White (2001), ongoing support from a community of peers is important in maintaining long-term abstinence from alcohol and other drugs. A critical component of collegiate recovery is providing students with a peer group that supports their decision to make positive changes in addictive behavior patterns. The CRC has found support groups and 12-Step meetings to be highly effective in creating a community for students attempting to recover from chemical dependency. These groups provide a safe, anonymous place for students to express their struggles with alcohol and other drugs and to find peer support for behavior change. The CRC hosts 12-Step meetings and/or support groups that provide recovery support on the TTU campus seven days a week. Current meetings include Alcoholics Anonymous, Narcotics Anonymous, Sex and Love Addicts Anonymous, Eating Disorders/Self-Harm Groups, and CODA groups.

Celebration. Besides traditional 12-Step meetings, the CRC created a weekly meeting called *Celebration of Recovery*. Though the format of the meeting is similar to a 12-Step group, *Celebration of Recovery* is designed to provide continued support to the CRC and also to educate the campus community about the reality of addiction and the opportunities for recovery. At this meeting, recovering students celebrate milestones of recovery, share their experiences, and offer public support to other addicted and recovering individuals. *Celebration of Recovery* is facilitated by recovering students in conjunction with the staff and faculty of the CSAR. Weekly attendance at this meeting usually exceeds 100 individuals and is regularly attended by members of the Texas Tech faculty, staff, administration, and the broader community.

Access to Higher Education and Educational Support

Access to higher education. The need to provide services that increase access to education for recovering individuals at TTU developed as a result of the Addictive Disorders and Recovery Studies (ADRS) curriculum, formerly called Substance Abuse Studies. In 1986, the ADRS minor began offering coursework to the students of TTU for the purpose of providing educational training for individuals seeking licensure as chemical dependency counselors in the state of Texas. These classes drew a high concentration of students with substance abuse problems and students in recovery from addiction. As these individuals interacted, a community of recovery began to form on the TTU campus. The formation of this community increased faculty awareness of the unique educational needs of recovering students. Thus, the CRC program began to develop around providing educational support services to this population.

Educational support. Often students in recovery have spent the majority of their adolescence under the influence of chemicals. Their educational backgrounds have been affected by their drinking/drug use. In the attainment of educational goals, drinking/using can impact recovering students' educational development in two ways: (1) lack of confidence in their ability to successfully navigate within academic settings and (2) lack of financial resources needed to achieve their educational goals.

A college/university campus can be a web of forms, papers, online submissions, and identification numbers. In addition to the peer-facilitated assistance within the CRC (see Peer Support below), the program provides a full-time staff member who assists students in completing the university admission process, overviews basic orientation information to the CRC and TTU, helps develop individual plans of study, and provides general academic advising (e.g., completing forms, paying tuition, registering for classes, developing study skills). Educational support services provided by peers and staff of the CRC are designed to teach recovering students the skills needed to be successful in higher education and to engender confidence in their academic abilities.

It is also critical to mention the financial difficulty that recovering students face when attempting to pursue higher education. Many recovering students have used college savings for treatment, have been ineligible for federal financial aid due to prior felony drug convictions, or cannot afford higher education due to financial responsibilities. Assistance with scholarships and financial aid applications is essential to the CRC model. Specific assistance includes filling out FAFSA forms for federal financial aid, searching for scholarships available through TTU and other sources, and providing financial assistance in the form of direct scholarship awards. The CRC program has developed an endowment for the specific purpose of awarding scholarships to recovering students. The scholarship endowment fund has been part of the CRC program since its inception. All scholarship accounts are managed by the CSAR and are funded through private donations from individuals and foundations. On average, this endowment allows the CRC to award $80,000 annually to students who demonstrate quality recovery, academic success, and community service.

Peer Support

Students' decisions about alcohol and other drug use are intricately linked to their experiences on a college campus. Early in its formation, members of the CRC recognized the dangers inherent in the campus culture that promote heavy drinking and drug use. In an effort to mitigate these dangers, the CRC created peer support mechanisms that include seminar classes in addiction and recovery and a peer mentoring system.

Seminar classes in addiction and recovery. The CRC has developed a specific course for students who wish to maintain recovery, provide and receive support, and engage in campus and community service. This course, titled *Seminar in Addiction and Recovery*, is a college credit course offered at TTU through the Department of Applied and Professional Studies. Classes are facilitated by faculty and staff associated with the CSAR and focus on (1) relapse prevention, (2) methods for building a positive social support network, (3) healthy decision-making and conflict resolution skills, (4) spiritual issues in a collegiate environment, (5) time management, and (6) general health and wellness.

Peer mentoring system. The peer mentoring system designed by the CRC addresses both recovery and educational issues. Individuals who are new to the community are assigned a peer mentor before their enrollment in classes. These peer mentors assume responsibility for helping new students choose classes, locate their classrooms on the TTU campus, and create a schedule for recovery support group attendance. In addition, new students are advised to contact these peer mentors should extenuating circumstances arise in which they need educational and/or recovery specific support.

Family Support

The families of college students are often-overlooked partners in supporting students in their recovery. Learning to live outside of a parent/guardian's supervision is one of the greatest stressors for a college student. In addition, a student's arrival on a college campus is one of his or her greatest times of risk for developing or relapsing into alcohol or other drug problems (Schulenberg, Maggs, Long, Sher, Gotham, Baer, et al., 2001). Yet, parents and recovering students are offered few means of education and support in helping make this critical transition. Beginning in 2004, the CRC began hosting parent and family weekends. This component of the CRC is still in the pilot stages and continues to be an evolving process.

Family programs. The CRC currently hosts one family weekend per year during which parents can visit the campus and participate in recovery programs. During this weekend, they are also able to ask questions of the CRC staff and gain needed support from one another. Topics covered include how to offer support to students during academic breaks (e.g. holidays, spring break, etc.), how to offer support when students transfer or graduate, and the overall organization, services, and resources available through the CRC model. Parents/family also have expressed interest in participating more fully in programs of support and considered how they could be more supportive of other TTU parents.

Community Support/Service

To give back to TTU and the overall Lubbock community, the students associated with the CRC are encouraged to be part of a student organization sponsored by the CSAR, which assists students in their broader community involvement and in increasing their level of community service. In addition, students affiliated with the CRC are expected to provide a minimum of 6 hours of documented community service every semester they are enrolled.

ASAS. The Association of Students About Service (ASAS) is a critical component of the CRC and is recognized by the TTU Student Government Association. While this organization is facilitated by a faculty supervisor affiliated with the CSAR, it is a student-led and student-funded association. The primary focus of this organization is to give back to the community through service projects. In addition, ASAS is responsible for organizing substance-free, recovery-oriented recreational activities, assisting in National Recovery Month efforts on the TTU campus, and sponsoring speakers that provide alcohol education and other drug education for the campus community. Every year for the last ten years, ASAS has hosted a convention for the campus and local community to learn more about recovery from alcohol and other drug addiction. ASAS members meet weekly to ensure members are working to better themselves, their campus, and their community.

Required community service. As a requirement of the *Seminar of Addiction and Recovery* class (see above), students are expected to perform 6 hours of service to the community every semester they are enrolled. While some of these hours may come from ASAS-sponsored events, many students choose to fulfill this requirement at an agency or organization that is important to them (e.g., Rape Crisis Center, Ronald McDonald House, Habitat for Humanity). In addition, each semester, the CRC selects one service project that the entire community, including faculty and staff, completes together.

DISCUSSION

While colleges and universities have begun to recognize the need for effective prevention, intervention, and treatment programs, most have failed to see the importance of supporting these students who have chosen to discontinue their alcohol/drug use. Through implementation of the services outlined as part of the CRC's comprehensive model, individuals are given the opportunity to develop systems-based sustained recovery. The CRC model accomplishes this by utilizing a series of five systemic components of support including recovery support, access to higher education and educational support, peer support, family support, and community support/service (see Figure 1). These interconnected components work together to create an environment that values recovery from addictive disorders and provides a safe foundation for individuals to pursue their own developmental pathway. The experience of the CRC at TTU suggests that recovering students who embrace the community and actively participate in the systemic components of the CRC model develop key characteristics that include hope/purpose, positive identity development, reclamation of agency, a sense of achievement/accomplishment, a capacity for stable interpersonal relationships, and healthy coping skills. These characteristics are the individual hallmarks of systems-based sustained recovery.

Preliminary Evidence of Success

The research part of the CRC is in its formative stages and all components have University Institutional Review Board approval. However, the faculty and staff involved in these efforts recognize the urgency and importance of documenting and further evaluating the services that comprise the CRC model. The CRC faculty and staff have identified three measures that provide anecdotal evidence of success. These include (1) the incidence of relapse, (2) academic success as determined by GPA of enrolled students, and (3) the graduation rate of students affiliated with the CRC. The table below shows the incidence of relapse in the collegiate recovery community program along with the average GPA of students each semester (see Table 1). Relapse rates were calculated by taking the total number of students who relapsed in a given semester and dividing by the total number of students served in that semester. Students who relapsed, returned to the program, and relapsed again were counted for each instance of relapse for this statistic. In addition, students associated with the CRC community have an average graduation rate of 70%.

To give meaning to the numerical representation above, it is important to compare them with other samples. Because collegiate recovery support

TABLE 1. CSAR Outcomes

	Number of Enrolled Students	Number of Relapses	Relapse Rate	Recovery Rate	Average GPA
Spring 2002	36	3	8%	92%	3.224
Fall 2002	44	3	7%	93%	3.340
Spring 2003	63	5	8%	92%	3.023
Fall 2003	63	5	8%	92%	2.916
Spring 2004	72	0	0	100%	3.097
Fall 2004	75	0	0	100%	3.445
Spring 2005	66	4	6%	94%	3.084
Fall 2005	81	4	5%	95%	3.321

programs are virtually nonexistent, comparisons to other programs with similar population parameters is appropriate. For the 18-to-25-year-old demographic, the Hazelden Center for Youth and Families posts a recovery rate of 54% after one year away from the facility (Hazelden, 2006). While this is not a direct comparison, these numbers do suggest that the CRC may be effective in supporting sustained recovery among this population. In addition, the average GPA (2002–2005) of students affiliated with the CRC (3.181) is consistently higher than the overall TTU student average (2.926).

It is important to note that one of the criteria for admission into the CRC is that students must document 6 months of recovery. Though exceptions to this rule have been made (some students having less than 30 days of recovery), most have a track record of abstinence and evidence of sustained recovery before entering the CRC. As a result, anecdotal evidence regarding the success (e.g., relapse, GPA, and percent of graduation) of the CRC model may be a product of the admission criteria and not a direct result of CRC support.

Research and Evaluation

The CRC provides an opportunity to participate in research that can impact the way recovery is viewed from an individual, familial, and social perspective. In the spring of 2002, faculty associated with the CSAR began to examine the collegiate recovery program by collecting preliminary research data with approval of the University IRB. Initial research has focused on describing the population accessing recovery support services through the CRC. The CRC has collected three waves of data that provide information on demographics of the population, family of origin information, age on onset of first use of tobacco, alcohol, and other drugs, length and intensity of use, and the prevalence of co-occurring disorders (Cleveland, Harris, Baker, Herbert, & Dean, 2007). As a follow-up to this data collection, the CRC is piloting a diary study with its members in which they record their daily access of social support while monitoring their physical, mental, and emotional states simultaneously. This study is expected to show significant predictors of alcohol/drug cravings and, consequently, relapse.

Replication. The CSAR has also received federal earmark funds to document the community support and recovery support programs it offers to the CRC. The documentation of this program provides an opportunity for other institutions of higher education to implement recovery support and relapse prevention programs for recovering students. This documentation follows a curriculum format integrating literature, the experiences of the CRC in program development and administration, and recommendations for program evaluation in an effort to create a step-by-step guide for implementing and maintaining a collegiate recovery community (Harris, Baker, & Thompson, 2005).

Family. Although the CRC programs are comprehensive in nature for the college student, parents and families who wish to stay involved and active in the recovery of their college-aged students must typically do so with few formal guidelines and over long distances. In a recent pilot study conducted by the CRC ($N = 52$), it was found that the more the student identified his or her family members as part of the social support network, the more the student reported experiencing support in decisions to abstain from substance use. However, students who identified a greater proportion of family members in their social support network also reported that explicit discussions of their recovery occurred less. These findings suggest that family members may be providing much needed general support but may not have the know-how or the guidance to provide greater levels of recovery-specific support and relapse prevention for their student.

Little is known about family members' experiences and the potential effectiveness of their involvement and support in a collegiate recovery community. Thus, the CRC has planned to increase its interaction/research with parents and to expand current offerings to include additional family members and more frequent interactions. This will give the CRC an opportunity to conduct more extensive research regarding family interaction and its impact on sustained recovery.

Future Direction and Conclusion

Future research includes the formation of an extensive data set specific to adolescent and young adult recovery and a better understanding of family involvement in the process of preventing alcohol and other drug-related problems in their adolescents and assisting families in providing more effective recovery support. In addition, the CRC is currently evaluating the impact of its college curriculum on prevention and recovery and is creating a more extensive program evaluation and outcome data set to evaluate the effectiveness of the CRC.

This paper is an initial attempt to introduce and document the CRC model. In short, the CRC is a model that has maintained one primary focus: the creation of a comprehensive recovery support, education, and prevention network for students. This model highlights the opportunities that may exist on all college/university campuses to establish communities of recovery that are viable and to promote a culture of systems-based sustained recovery.

REFERENCES

Cleveland, H. H., Harris, K. S., Baker, A. K., Herbert, R., & Dean, L. R. (2007). Characteristics of a collegiate recovery community: Maintaining recovery in an abstinence-hostile environment. *Journal of Substance Abuse Treatment, 33*(1), 13–23.

Dworetzky (1996). *Introduction to child development.* Belmont, CA: Wadsworth Publishing.

Feldman, S. S., & Elliot, G. R. (1990). *At the threshold: The developing adolescent.* Cambridge, MA: Harvard University Press.

Gotham, H. J., Sher, K. J., & Wood, P. K. (2002). Alcohol involvement and developmental task completion during young adulthood. *Journal of Studies on Alcohol, 63,* 32–42.

Harris, K. S., Baker, A. K., & Thompson, A. A. (2005). *Making an opportunity on your campus: A comprehensive curriculum for designing collegiate recovery communities.* Funded by the Center for Substance Abuse Treatment and the U.S. Department of Education. Center for the Study of Addiction and Recovery, Texas Tech University, Lubbock, TX.

Harrison, P. A., & Hoffmann, N. G. (1987). *CATOR Report: Adolescent residential treatment, intake and follow-up findings.* St. Paul: Ramsey Clinic.

Hazelden. (2006). *Why choose Hazelden?: What is Hazelden's "success rate"?* Retrieved August 2006 from http://www.hazelden.org/servlet/hazelden/cms/ptt/hazl_7030_shade.html

Hingson, R. W., Heeren, T., Zakocs, R. C., Kopstein, A., & Wechsler, H. (2002). Magnitude of alcohol-related mortality and morbidity among U.S. college students ages 18–24. *Journal of Studies on Alcohol, 63,* 136–44.

Johnston, L. D., O'Malley, P. M., & Bachman, J. G. (2001). *Monitoring the Future National Survey Results on Drug Use, 1975–2000. Volume 1: College Students and Adults Ages 19–40.* Bethesda, MD: National Institute on Drug Abuse.

O'Malley, P. M., & Johnston, L. D. (2002). Epidemiology of alcohol and other drug use among American college students. *Journal of Studies of Alcohol Supplement, 14,* 23–29.

Perkins, H. W. (2002). Social norms and the prevention of alcohol misuse in collegiate contexts. *Journal of Studies on Alcohol, 14,* 164–72.

Ridgeway, P. (2001) Restorying psychiatric disability: Learning from first person recovery narratives. *Psychiatric Rehabilitation Journal, 24*(4), 335–43.

Schulenberg, J. E., Maggs, J. L., Long, S. W., Sher, K. J., Gotham, H. J., Baer, J. S., et al. (2001). The problem of college drinking: Insights from a developmental perspective. *Alcoholism: Clinical and Experimental Research, 25*(3), 473–77.

Schulenberg, J. E., & Maggs, J. L. (2002). A developmental perspective on alcohol use and heavy drinking during adolescence and the transition to young adulthood. *Journal of Studies on Alcohol, 14,* 54–70.

U.S. Department of Health and Human Services. (2000, November). *Healthy People 2010. 2nd ed. With Understanding and Improving Health and Objectives for Improving Health. 2 vols.* Washington, DC: U.S. Government Printing Office.

Wechsler, H., Lee, J. E., Kuo, M., Seibring, M., Nelson, T. F., & Lee, H. P. (2002). Trends in college binge drinking during a period of increased prevention efforts: Findings from four Harvard School of Public Health study surveys, 1993–2001. *Journal of American College Health, 50,* 203–17.

White, W. L. (2000). *Toward a new recovery movement: Historical reflections on recovery, treatment, and advocacy.* Paper presented at the meeting of Recovery Community Support Program Conference. CSAT, SAMHSA, Working Together for Recovery, Arlington, VA.

White, W. L. (2001). A lost vision: Addiction counseling as community organization. *Alcoholism Treatment Quarterly, 19*(4), 1–30.

White, W., Boyle, M., & Loveland, D. (2005) Recovery from addiction and from mental illness: Shared and contrasting lessons. In R. O. Ralph & P. W. Corrigan (Eds.), *Recovery in mental illness: Broadening our understanding of wellness.* Washington, DC: American Psychological Association.

Woodford, M. S. (2001). *Recovering college students' perspectives: Investigating the phenomena of recovery from substance abuse among undergraduate students.* Unpublished doctoral dissertation. The Curry School of Education, University of Virgina.

The Need for a Continuum of Care: The Rutgers Comprehensive Model

Lisa Laitman, M.S.Ed., LCADC

Rutgers University

Linda C. Lederman, PhD

Arizona State University

ABSTRACT. College drinking has been a concern of college administrators, parents of college-age students and health care professionals for some time. Over the last few years an increasing number of institutions have begun to understand that the problem is complex enough that it warrants attention and that a variety of strategies are necessary to attempt to reduce dangerous drinking and the unwanted attendant consequences (for example, Berkowitz, 2005; Berkowitz & Perkins, 1986; Burns, Ballou & Lederman, 1991; Burns & Goodstadt, 1989; Knight et al., 2000; Lederman & Stewart, 2005; NIAAA, 2002; O'Malley& Johnston, 2002; Perkins, 1997; 2002; 2003; Weschler & Kuo, 2000.). While some institutions have looked for a silver bullet that would serve as a cure all, over time it has become clear that institutions of higher education need to have comprehensive plans designed to address drinking behaviors and provide a continuum of care.

The purpose of this article is to describe the Rutgers Program, a comprehensive model addressing the continuum from prevention to recovery support that can meet the complex needs of a college community who are involved in a wide spectrum of alcohol and other drug use from nonuse, social/recreational use, dangerous use, abuse, addiction, and recovery. The paper begins with a description of the problem of college drinking, which is presented as the backdrop for the Rutgers Model. We have combined the experience of the second author as a research scholar and the first author as a practitioner to create the description of the continuum. The differences in the voices of the researcher and practitioner we believe reflect the collaborative approach that this continuum requires to embed itself into the campus culture (Lederman & Stewart, 2005).

THE CONTEXT: COLLEGE DRINKING AS A NORMATIVE IMAGE

College drinking has often been portrayed by the media as out of control, excessive, and essentially a one-dimensional phenomenon. As a result, it is difficult to think of drinking on college campuses today without imagining excessive drinking. Thus, the image of excessive drinking becomes intertwined with the popular conception of college life in America. This perception is reinforced through various mediated messages including television, films and the news (Lederman, Lederman, & Kully, 2004; Lederman & Stewart, 2005).

In many ways, college culture itself vigorously communicates and perpetuates the myth that this type of behavior is the norm and that excessive drinking is an integral part of every college student's life (Lederman, 1993; Lederman & Stewart, 2005). Unfortunately this means that it often seems as if the popular view of the college student is somehow incomplete without a reference to the "typical" alcohol-doused, rowdy college party. This creates, in a sense, an image of a culture of college drinking. According to Lederman (1993), the *culture of college drinking* is the shared images, behaviors, attitudes, and perceptions that create a culturally specific sense that drinking heavily in college is an inherent and inevitable part of the college years. In the culture of college drinking, heavy drinking is viewed as a rite of passage rather than a health issue or social concern. In this view, drinking excessively is simply something that exists, has existed, and will always exist as part of growing up. The question is: how to teach students that they don't have to drink dangerously. To answer the question it is important to examine how this culture is created and transmitted.

Lederman and Stewart (2005) argue that much of the answer lies in what they refer to as *socially situated experiential learning (SSEL)*. SSEL is the experience-based process of acquiring and interpreting social information (and misinformation) received from peers and other sources within the context of direct learning experiences. The process of learning through socially situated experiences is complex and multifaceted. Many factors (e.g., other students, friends, family, faculty, law enforcement) influence students' perceptions of their role in the culture of college drinking as well as their perceptions of the behavior of others. For example, on many contemporary college campuses Thursday is party night. How and why this becomes the night to party, and even the meaning of the word "party" to indicate drinking together, is a product of the local culture. It is possible to understand any college drinking culture if we get to know the ways in which students (and other campus constituencies) talk about drinking. It is that talk that creates a reality, or perception of reality, that drinking is a rite of passage. Thus social norms regarding college drinking are created by individuals' attitudes, beliefs, and behaviors in relation to one another and the interpretive processes of the individual within the sociocultural community. Workman (2001), for example, studied the narratives students used to describe their drinking-related behaviors as part of their college experience.

CONTINUOUS DATA COLLECTION AT RUTGERS

Years of data collected regarding the culture of college drinking at Rutgers painted a complex picture of the socially situated experiential learning in that cultural scene. In these studies, students reported that their perceptions of college drinking results from their own experiences and the ways in which they learn by trial and error (Burns, & Goodstadt, 1989). Regardless of how much they drank, students reported that they believed that drinking dangerously is a "learning experience" (Burns, Ballou, & Lederman, 1991; Cohen & Lederman, 1998; Lederman, 1993; Lederman, Stewart, Goodhart, & Laitman, 2003; Lederman & Stewart, 2005). This learning takes place within a social context, and the interpretations and the behaviors to which it leads are a product of both the experience and the social context. Included in the social context are the student's comparison of self with others and the student's own individual's own sense of self. Attitudes toward alcohol use grow out of both the student's own first-hand experiences with alcohol and his or her perceptions (based on firsthand experiences or observations of others' behaviors) of the apparent benefits and costs (i.e., expectancies) of performing this behavior weighted by the importance he or she places on each of these positive or negative outcomes (Fishbein & Ajzen, 1975). A strong positive attitude toward alcohol use will predict a strong likelihood of engaging in drinking behavior, while a strong negative attitude will significantly reduce this possibility.

Students' comparisons of themselves with other people often include perceptions that are inaccurate. These mistakes or "misperceptions" (Berkowitz, 2005, 2003, 1997; Hanson, 1984; Haines & Spear, 1996) increase as social distance increases (Yanovitzky, Stewart, & Lederman, 2006). In the college environment this means that most individuals perceive that their friends drink more than they do and that students in general drink more than their friends (Berkowitz & Perkins, 1986; Bourgeois & Bowen, 2001). If college students routinely misperceive how much others are drinking, they are measuring their own drinking behavior against a misperceived norm. The most disturbing consequence of these misperceptions is the pressure that students then experience to increase their drinking in an effort to fit in with their social group by drinking more. A person's motivation to rely on normative judgments when making behavioral decisions is a key element in many social influence theories (for a review, see Petty & Cacioppo, 1986).

Rutgers' researchers have been collecting both quantitative and qualitative data on students' alcohol use and consequences since the early 1990s. Rutgers students tend to feel that it is permissible to drink alcohol because "others" expect that they will drink. The "others" who contribute to the norms that create the perception that everyone is drinking are the media and advertisers, other students, parents, university faculty and staff, residents around campus, police and security personnel, and anyone else who believes that college students drink and will continue to drink regardless of the policy or law.

DRINKING BEHAVIORS DIFFER FROM PERCEPTIONS OF DRINKING BEHAVIORS

Along with the misperception of what is normative, those students who actually do drink excessively often do not recognize their drinking or other drug use as problematic. Many students believe themselves to be more interpersonally competent and communicative when drunk (Cohen & Lederman, 1998). Drinking is treated as a particularly social experience, always done in public and with groups of friends, fostering the notion that it is "what you're supposed to be doing." And those college organizations, such as fraternities and sororities, for whom the overuse of alcohol has "historically" been an integral part of the organization's function can have a greater impact in prompting students to develop habits of alcohol abuse (Bourgeois & Bowen, 2001). Whereas the need to belong to a peer group is very strong among young people, especially as they enter college, the need for acceptance by one's peers becomes so strong that it helps students accept a view of reality prescribed by their targeted peer group. Students can learn to see and accept the world through the eyes of a group they desire to join. Thus, as counselors, parents, and school administrators repeatedly experience, students are more willing to heed the advice of friends and schoolmates than adults.

THE REALITY ON MOST CAMPUSES IS COSTLY AND DANGEROUS

Unfortunately, the reality of dangerous drinking is often far more costly and dangerous than the romanticized narratives enacted in the residence halls or fraternity/sorority culture (Workman, 2001). In contrast to the tales of harmless, youthful brawling, too often the result of dangerous drinking is very real and very destructive. In colleges across the country, dangerous drinking is repeatedly associated with serious physical injuries resulting from either fighting or motor vehicle accidents (Wechsler,Davenport, Dowdall, Moeykens, & Castillo, 1994; Weschler & Kuo, 2002). The reckless overconsumption of alcohol also claims many ancillary victims. The orbit of dangerous-drinking college students includes their nondangerous drinking peers who experience "secondary dangerous effects," such as getting insulted, humiliated, hit or pushed; having their property damaged; becoming sleep- or privacy-disturbed; or being sexually assaulted or raped (Perkins & Wechsler, 1996).

The culture of college drinking is an experience-based, socially situated set of attitudes, beliefs, and behaviors. It is the product of what students talk about, what they see around them, how they interpret the behaviors of themselves and others, and the socially and experientially constructed filters that shape those interpretations and beliefs about what is socially acceptable and attractive and what is simply required of them to fit into the college social scene.

While the image of a culture of college drinking in which everyone drinks to excess creates a one-dimensional view of college life and the role of drinking in it, researchers and college professionals understand that college drinking is far more complex and varied. There are students who are nondrinkers and low-risk drinkers. Even among the group of students abusing alcohol there is variety, from regular abuse that occurs in the first year of college but tapers off, to abuse that worsens with age and time and moves into the area of dependence (Lederman & Stewart, 2005). It has become far more productive to understand these distinctions and develop a variety of strategies rather than the one-size-fits-all strategies of the past, which have proved to be ineffective (NIAAA report, 2005) roads have been made in focusing on developing different strategies to address different drinking patterns that have withstood the scrutiny of research such as Brief Intervention Models (Dimeff, Baer, Kivlahan, & Marlatt, 1999; Marlatt & Baer, 1997).

At Rutgers University the various prevention and treatment strategies over more than 25 years has led to an insight and approach that has been combined into what we refer to as the Rutgers Comprehensive Model.

THE RUTGERS COMPREHENSIVE MODEL

In 1979 the president of Rutgers, President Edward Bloustein, formed the Presidential Committee on the Use of Alcohol. In 1981 a report was completed by the committee, which became the basis for the Universities first Alcohol Policy. Along with being one of the earliest such policies at a university is was also progressive for recognizing the continuum of the complex drinking patterns in our student population. (Goodhart & Laitman, 2005) In 1983 a prevention/education coordinator and an alcohol counselor were both hired to implement the recommendations of the 1981 report by the presidential committee. The mission of the Alcohol Assistance Program for Students, coordinated by an alcohol counselor, was to provide counseling services to high-risk students and adult children of alcoholics and to provide recovery support to students in recovery from addictions on all three Rutgers campuses (New Brunswick, Newark and Camden), which have a total of 50,000 students. The program was expended within the first few years because drug abuse was identified as a problem area in the college population. The name was also changed to Alcohol and Other Drug Assistance Program for Students (ADAPS) to reflect this change in focus. In the 24 years since the implementation of these programs on the Rutgers

University campuses, the original commitment to alcohol/drug prevention, education, intervention, treatment and recovery support remains a model for a comprehensive campus community-based approach to addressing the complex array of campus alcohol/drug related issues.

When we look at the use of alcohol in American culture most of the research consistently shows that most young people have their first drink by age 13. Data over the years contributed by the Monitoring the Future Study from the University of Michigan have given prevalence rates for 8th, 10th and 12th graders use of tobacco, alcohol and other illicit drugs (Johnston, O'Malley, Bachman & Schulenberg, 2006; O'Malley & Johnston, 2000). These annual assessments show patterns of alcohol and illicit drug use behaviors of incoming first-year students. As the study also gives college data we can compare college students to national norms. The College Alcohol Program at the Harvard School of Public Health published a frequently cited study in 2002 estimating the prevalence of college students meeting DSM IV criteria for alcohol abuse and alcohol dependence at 31% and 6% respectively. While the same data was not as available for drug abuse and dependence, the authors speculated that adding other drugs of abuse would increase those numbers. (Johnston, O'Malley, Bachman, & Schulenberg, 2006).

The experience of many addiction treatment professionals is that most adults in treatment programs report their teen years or early adulthood as the time when their drinking problems accelerated. While we know that the alcohol abuse of many first-year college students does often lessen from first year to second year and with each successive year as well as when students graduate from college and enter the "real world" of work, marriage, and parenthood we also know that a steady significant percentage do not. Anecdotal sources include the clinical information of those who have sought treatment as adults, from family histories and from Alcoholics Anonymous meetings. However, the experiences of students who have either come to college in recovery from high school or started recovery in college have offered another perspective on the benefits of early intervention. Laitman, Lederman, and Silos (2005) compiled fifteen autoethnographic stories of recovering alcoholics whose recovery began while in college, and other research (Ridgeway, 2001; Workman, 2005) reports that the lived experiences of recovery evidence a sense of vital, positive self-related feelings and images that are echoed in the recovery stories of many young adults.

Rutgers students in recovery often go to 12-step meetings and get support from older members who express the sentiments that they did not access to recovery earlier in life (or in college) and continued their addictions far longer (and with more destructive consequences) and wished they had received help far earlier in their lives.

The mission of higher education is to prepare young people for the intellectual and emotional demands of a productive adult life. Therefore, institutions of higher education need to make a commitment to remove the widely known obstacles that alcohol and other drug abuse and dependence can create by institutionalizing intervention services and recovery support services seem logical and cost effective for our society.

BENEFITS OF EARLY INTERVENTION

When working to engage clients in treatment, professionals have historically analogized addiction to other medical conditions for which early intervention improves the prognosis for recovery. However, in part due to the negative stigma associated with addiction, many clients resist diagnosis and miss the opportunity for early intervention. Providing intervention services for college students would prevent some of the problems associated with carrying an addiction into adulthood or later.

Clients with substance abuse problems are often the last to acknowledge these problems. Much of the work of the last 15 years in the prevention and addiction fields has centered on improving the likelihood that clients will be receptive to the interventions provided. Brief intervention models, motivational enhancement therapy, and motivational interviewing assist and support clients to begin the process of making changes with their substance use and abuse.

Intervention with the college population does not assume that we are intervening with only a diagnosed dependence. Intervening can be assisting students engaged in high-risk behaviors to reduce use, or abstain from alcohol and other drugs for short or longer periods. In addition, teaching skills to manage stress, relationships or other life events without making substances the primary method may allow young people to learn a wider range of strategies to halt the pattern of developing dependence. Intervention can also be the more traditional form of identifying dependence or addiction and trying to halt the progression.

To their credit, young people are often more open and impressionable than older adults. Though being more open can be a negative with peer influences to drink, it can also be an asset in an intervention or a counseling relationship.

FINDING THE AT-RISK COLLEGE STUDENT

There are many ways that are used to describe addiction as well as diagnostic criteria that help professionals determine abuse and dependence. One of the simplest definitions has at times been the most useful:

Addiction or dependence occurs when an individual experiences a pattern of problems, over time, related to alcohol/drug abuse that interferes in any or several different areas of life. These can include, academic, social, psychological, legal, health or occupational. Addiction is characterized by the repeated use of substances or behaviors despite clear evidence of dysfunction related to such use.[1]

If we want to be able to find the at-risk student on a college campus, we need to develop a community of people who regularly interact with students having problems in any area of their life. That is a tall order on a college campus because it involves, faculty, residence life staff (both professional and student staff), enforcement, judicial officers, academic deans, health services, local emergency rooms, students clubs, counseling centers. It can also include families, local bars, local law enforcement and municipal court judges. AOD training must be institutionalized at a college or university and include not only front line staff working directly with students but also upper administrators and faculty.

For front line staff turnover is annual (sometimes more frequent) as student staff and students graduate every year. Training staff, developing referral procedures (both voluntary as well as involuntary or mandatory) are all responsibilities of alcohol/drug professionals on a campus and must be done more than once a year during National Collegiate Alcohol Awareness Week in October. Alcohol/drug use and abuse in our culture reflects many ambivalent beliefs and attitudes. Professionals working on a college campus are reminded to respect the complexity of the problems and stay clear of giving information and simplistic solutions in exchange for an approach that recognizes the perspectives of students, faculty and staff and engages them in the development of solutions.

Other potential obstacles that exist on a campus (or perhaps in our culture at large) include the personal, family or student experiences with addiction that are part of the personal and professional experiences of faculty, staff and students. Despite the advances made in intervention and treatment many people have deeply personal experiences that affect their approach to this pervasive problem negatively.

In the process of training and educating members of our educational community we must accept that stigma regarding addiction still exists.

Without exposure to recovery most people working on a college campus see only the dangerous drinking culture. Changing this view has been part of many recovery movements such as the *Association of Recovery Schools, the Faces and Voices of Recovery, and Friends of Recovery.*

Campus professionals are often frustrated by students with alcohol/drug problems, who often are not forthcoming with information regarding their alcohol/drug abuse. The problems presented by these students to professionals without adequate training can often be confused with other diagnoses or problems and can fail. To have success working with people with alcohol/drug problems, individuals need to understand how to effectively assess and intervene. Special training in this area is what makes the difference and leads to successful interventions, even for the well-trained general therapist. Alcohol and drug counselors also need adequate supervision and administrative support.

When a campus does not embrace a comprehensive AOD approach, policies tend to be limited to a legal or enforcement perspective issue (i.e.; no-tolerance approaches). Without balancing enforcement with health and wellness perspectives we lose the opportunity to engage young adults in learning to make life long healthy decisions about alcohol/drugs as enforcement is externally driven. Alcohol interventions that are predominantly punitive on a college campus are incomplete.

Working with College Students with Alcohol/Drug Problems

Engaging young adults in a process of change can be productive and rewarding for both the student and the therapist. However, the therapist working with this population (as well as families and adult community) must appreciate the difficulties of addressing substance issues in a college environment. It is critical to have an understanding of the developmental stage of this age group to have success. The struggles and the norms of a college population are unique. The experienced college therapist has developed an extensive understanding of separation struggles that young adults and adolescents have with the parents/guardians/ and other authority figures in their lives. Separation is rarely completed by the time a young adult goes to college. During this time of life young people learn to develop many of the skills and competencies that they need to move into the workforce and become financially independent. Learning their relationship with alcohol and other drugs is a developmental task of this age group and the skilled therapist knows that simply offering a "just say no" message is not only ineffective but does not engage the young adult in a relationship of respect and support to make changes.

Appreciating the goals and difficulties of this age include understanding their limited life experience associated with relationships especially in a new setting, loss of external structure imposed by parents and family life combined with the natural excitement of leaving home and being "on your own" (which occurs even for commuter students) and includes structuring time to study and play and sleep and eat!

Additionally, in their academics they experience the dramatic change from the structure of secondary education having an eight-to-four type schedule to a much wider variation of time in class and out of class, the expectations of college professors that students manage their work as adults. Other challenges for the first-year student are the lack of privacy and quiet space for most resident college first-year students, the "drama" of being a young adult (in part due to lack of life experience).

For parents and campus officials it is critical to realize that telling an inquisitive young adult to just stop their use of alcohol/drugs will not automatically change behavior and is not respectful of the developmental stage.

What are the difficulties that challenge young adults beginning college to make healthy decisions about their relationship with alcohol/drugs?

The pervasiveness of the drinking culture on a campus and in the media
The lack of privacy and private space in most residence halls
The difficulty of finding friends who do not drink
The difficulty of finding friends who drink moderately (not because they
    are rare, but because they are not always as obvious as heavy drinkers)
Ambivalence regarding making changes and being uncertain if these
    changes are the right move for them

The following are difficulties for the college student in recovery from addiction:

Thinking they are too young to stop using "the rest of my life"
Fear of missing out on all the fun perceived to be involved in a using
    lifestyle
Access to intensive outpatient treatment off campus without transportation
    and the difficulty of finding campuses with on-campus intervention or
    recovery support services

Lack of adequate health insurance that covers addiction treatment
Finding a young support network for recovery on the campus
Lack of campus support professionals who are knowledgeable about the
range of alcohol/drug problems, addiction and the needs for successful
recovery

Recovery for the College Student

"AA is a cult."

"Twelve-step programs are not for everyone."

"AA is a White male–oriented program."

"Twelve-step programs are religious."

"People in AA tell you that you have to go to meetings for the rest of
your life."

Most people who have worked with individuals and families living with
addictions have heard all these statements regarding 12-step programs
and probably more than once or twice. Twelve-step meetings are not for
everyone. Just as was discussed earlier in this article, there are many
variations of alcohol/drug problems and many people have successfully
resolved abuse and addiction with other methods. For others, even AA
acknowledges in the text *Alcoholics Anonymous* (most commonly referred
to as the "Big Book") the possibility that there are some who cannot get
sober with AA or any other program.

Support for Early Recovery

Twelve-step programs, however, have a great deal to offer a young
addicted college population. The benefits are not always obvious on the
surface. The problem for a young adult in recovery on a college campus
is often the lack of support for abstinence in early recovery; a particularly
fragile time. Students (and adults in general) who do not exhibit problems
with alcohol and other drugs often do not understand someone who
cannot have "just a couple." While this may not be considered active peer
pressure, for the person in early recovery it only serves to make them feel
deficient or misunderstood in most cases. The expectation in our culture

is to be able to "handle your drinking" and there are those individuals who are not able to drink moderately (and have often failed repeatedly). In a comprehensive treatment model, young college students should have access to assessment that would include harm reduction approaches both as a method of assuring accurate diagnosis as well as to develop a therapeutic alliance based on trust and a sense of partnership rather than perpetuating adult/adolescent dynamics.

This early time in recovery is the time to adjust to living without alcohol, developing coping strategies and coming to terms with the losses incurred during an active addiction. Twelve-step programs often do a great deal to educate, help heal emotionally and aid in the transitions into a sober life. Comfort in finding others who have had the same problems and emotional support are universally healing. Social support is also critical for the young person in recovery. Having fun not drinking and using drugs, feeling a part of a same age peer group and feeling the comfort of being with others in the same situation are especially important components of a recovery program for college students as this age group tend to be very peer oriented.

Campus Recovery Communities also provide the vehicle for entry into treatment, recovery, close access to 12-Step programs and peer support networks for students in recovery. In a comprehensive campus program there are many entry points for a high-risk alcohol/drug dependent student to eventually reach the people on campus who have an expertise in alcohol/drug problems.

Goals of Recovery

As young people feel more comfortable being in recovery and develop a solid base of recovery support, they can then develop other relationships and activities. Often these relationships are not alcohol/drug centered but based on common interests and intellectual experiences. As people begin to feel more comfortable with themselves, and are not seeking out drinking friends and using environments, they are far less likely to put themselves in risky situations and at risk for relapse. However, this takes time to accomplish and the 12 steps can support this self-actualizing process within a safe and supportive process.

Recovery from addiction for a college student is providing them an opportunity to have a full and productive life without the limitations and losses that life with an active addiction often cost an individual. Developing the skills and strategies to stay in recovery at a young age to enjoy a full life are the essential goals of a Campus Recovery Community.

A Recovery Story: Mary[2]

Mary is a 19-year-old sophomore who was referred for an alcohol/drug evaluation by her therapist at the university counseling center. The therapist became concerned with Mary's use of alcohol when during the course of more that one session in discussing the problems with her current boyfriend, Mary stated that he didn't like it when she drank at parties where his friends were present. He found her very flirtatious to a point where his friends were uncomfortable with her behavior.

When Mary's boyfriend told her about her behavior the next day (on more than one occasion), she was also upset both at how upset he was when he described the behavior but also because it embarrassed her. She considered the relationship a good one and was quite serious about him. The therapist discussed the alcohol/drug referral with Mary and she came soon after for an appointment.

During the course of the alcohol/drug evaluation Mary got very emotional. She told the alcohol/drug counselor that what she had told her therapist about her present boyfriend was true but she had not told the therapist that she had lost a previous boyfriend due to the same circumstances: her behavior when she drank became intolerable to her last boyfriend and he had ended the relationship of 2 years.

What is not described in the details of Mary's presenting problem is how the alcohol/drug counselor talked with Mary about her history and the way questions were framed. From the beginning it was obvious that Mary was very ashamed about her drinking and subsequent behavior, in verbal and nonverbal ways. As she revealed more details the alcohol/drug counselor was able to intervene sometimes with statements indicating that these were universal feelings and common problems related to heavy use of alcohol, and particularly to women. Mary appeared to feel relief that she was not alone and asked more questions about other women with alcohol problems. As Mary became more comfortable in the session she was able to reveal more negative consequences she had experienced.

Over time, she was able to talk about her abuse of other drugs and extended family history. A commitment to abstinence was made within one to two sessions. As she moved away from her blackout behavior and her sober behavior was more consistent with her values she started to feel better about herself. When old friends tried to pressure her to drink with them, she was able to stand up to the pressure because her self esteem had improved. Support from other women in recovery and attendance at AA meetings also provided her with a support network and an ongoing way to continue to move away from an alcohol-centered social world.

The Recovery House at Rutgers

Rutgers University has offered a special housing opportunity for students who are in recovery since 1988. Students, if eligible, are able to live with students like themselves and receive emotional, social and environmental support in maintaining their sobriety. Students in Recovery Housing socialize together as well as with other friends. There is an emphasis on doing well in school and having a fun sober time in college.

Recovery Housing is just one of many special housing options available to students at the University that includes language houses, housing for women in science majors, and so on. Recovery Housing has several distinctive features:

It is a strictly confidential housing option.
Anonymity is protected.
It is a smoke-free environment.
There are house meetings monthly.
It has a supportive, community environment.
Students are motivated and have maintained sobriety for at least several
    months.

Selection. To quality for Recovery Housing the student is required to interview either on the phone or in person with a counselor in the Alcohol and Other Drug Assistance Program for Students. If the student is meets the eligibility requirements then the student will then be assigned housing.

Most interviewing and selection of prospective students occurs in the fall semester and spring semester of the academic year before the student's matriculation. However, due to the nature of recovery from addictions, admission to the Recovery House can be made at other times during the academic year as long as space is available.

Supervision. There is a housing contract that all resident students are required to sign and written guidelines specific for the Recovery House that students agree to abide by in writing. The Alcohol and Other Drug Assistance Counselors have regular meetings with students and have individual sessions as needed. For those new to recovery the student meets with a counselor through the first year of recovery. Other new students to the Recovery House but not to recovery meet with a counselor during an adjustment period. In addition, Resident Advisors who are in recovery live in the house with the students and have close communication and supervision from the ADAPS staff.

History. Rutgers University has supported students in Recovery Housing successfully since 1988. Students in recovery have been instrumental in developing this program with the University. The University is nationally known for its innovative campus-based treatment of alcohol/drug problems. Students who have participated in this program have this to say about their experience:

"College is a place to party. The Recovery Housing is an oasis for us."
"We have bundles of energy that we used to channel in our addictions."
"The urge to drink still surfaces but is no longer a compulsion."
"You can't fool anyone here."
"It is a place to live with people I like which is no different from any other dorm."

CONCLUSIONS

The college years present a difficult transition for young people through the final stages of adolescence (Schulenberg, & Maggs, 2002). A very important goal of higher education is to help young people learn critical thinking skills. We need to be willing to engage in an honest, informed dialogue with young people who are learning how to make complex decisions. Many young adult's use and abuse of alcohol/drugs is causing interference with this development of critical thinking skills, as well as in the pursuit of an expertise and passion for a course of study that leads to a career. Effective techniques that respect the integrity of college students while reducing the harm and damage caused by alcohol/drug abuse need to be part of the campus culture and mission.

The Rutgers Model presents an exemplar of a continuum of care that takes into account the variety of needs that students have in relation to alcohol and the different ways that are needed to address this variety. Rather than a silver bullet the Rutgers Model is an umbrella under which students' needs can be understood and addressed.

NOTES

1. A compilation of several common definitions.
2. Mary is a pseudonym used to protect her identity. In any recovery stories cited in this article, the identities of individuals have been protected.

REFERENCES

Berkowitz, A. D. (2005). An overview of the social norms approach. In L. Lederman & L. Stewart (Eds.), *Changing the culture of college drinking* (pp 241–60). Cresskill, NJ: Hampton Press.

Berkowitz, A. D., & Perkins, H. W. (1986). Problem drinking among college students: A review of recent research. *Journal of American College Health, 35*, 21–28.

Bourgeois, M. J., & Bowen, A. (2001). Self-organization of alcohol-related attitudes and beliefs in a campus housing complex: An initial investigation. *Health Psychology, 20*(6), 1–4.

Burns, W. D., Ballou, J., & Lederman, L. (1991). *Perceptions of alcohol use and policy on the college campus: Preventing alcohol/drug abuse at Rutgers University.* Unpublished conference paper, U.S. Department of Education Fund for the Improvement of Post Secondary Education (FIPSE).

Burns, W. D., & Goodstadt, M. (1989). *Alcohol use on the Rutgers University campus: A study of various communities.* Unpublished conference paper, U.S. Department of Education Fund for the Improvement of Post Secondary Education (FIPSE).

Cohen, D. J., & Lederman, L. C. (1998). Navigating the freedom of college life: Students talk about alcohol, gender, and sex. In N. Roth & L. Fuller (Eds.), *Women and AIDS: Negotiating safer practices, care, and representation* (pp. 101–26). New York: Haworth Press.

Dimeff, L. A., Baer, J. S., Kivlahan, D. R., & Marlatt, G. A. (1999). *Brief Alcohol Screening and Intervention for College Students (BASICS): A harm reduction approach.* New York: Guilford Press.

Fishbein, M., & Ajzen, I. (1975). *Belief, attitude, intention and behavior: An introduction to theory and research.* Reading, MA: Addison-Wesley.

Goodhart, F. W., & Laitman, L. (2005). An integrated environmental framework: Education, prevention, intervention, treatment, and enforcement. In L. Lederman & L. Stewart (Eds.), *Changing the culture of college drinking* (pp.). Cresskill, NJ: Hampton Press.

Haines, M., & Spear, S. F. (1996). Changing the perception of the norm: A strategy to decrease binge drinking among college students. *Journal of American College Health, 45*, 134–40.

Hanson, D. J. (1984). College students' drinking attitudes: 1970–1982. *Psychological Reports, 54*, 300–302.

Johnston, L. D., O'Malley, P. M., Bachman, J. G., & Schulenberg, J. E. (2006). *Monitoring the future national survey results on drug use, 1975–2005. Volume II: College students and adults ages 19–45* (NIH Publication No. 06-5884). Bethesda, MD: National Institute on Drug Abuse, 302 pp.

Knight, R., Wechsler, H., Kuo, M., Seibring, M., Weitzman, E. R., & Schuckit, M. A. (2002). Alcohol abuse and dependence among U.S. college students. *Journal of Studies on Alcohol, 63*(3), 263–70.

Laitman, L., Lederman, L. C., & Silos, I. (2005). *Voices of recovery: Stories of recovering from alcoholism in the college years.* New Brunswick, NJ: CHI Prevention and Educational Series.

Lederman, L. C. (1993). Friends don't let friends beer goggle: A case study in the use and abuse of alcohol and communication among college students. In E. B. Ray (Ed.), *Case studies in health communication* (pp.). Hillsdale, NJ: Lawrence Erlbaum.

Lederman, L. C., Lederman, J. B., & Kully, R. D. (2004). Believing is seeing: The co-construction of everyday myths in the media about college drinking. *American Behavioral Scientist, 48*(1), 130–36.

Lederman, L. C., Stewart, L. P., Goodhart, F. W., & Laitman, L. (2003). A case against "binge" as the term of choice: Convincing college students to personalize messages about dangerous drinking. *Journal of Health Communication, 8*, 1–13.

Lederman, L. C., & Stewart, L. (2005). *Changing the culture of college drinking.* Cresskill, NJ: Hampton Press.

National Institute on Alcohol Abuse and Alcoholism (NIAAA). (2002). *A call to action: Changing the culture of drinking at U.S. colleges.* Washington, DC: National Institute on Alcohol Abuse and Alcoholism/National Institutes of Health.

Marlatt, G. A., & Baer, J. S. (1997). Harm reduction and alcohol abuse: A brief intervention for college student binge drinking: Results from a two-year follow-up assessment. In P. G. Erickson, D. M. Riley, Y. W. Cheung, & P. A. O'Hare (Eds.), *Harm reduction: A new direction for drug policies and programs* (pp. 245–62). Toronto: University of Toronto Press.

O'Malley, P. M., & Johnston, L. D. (2002). Epidemiology of alcohol and other drug use among American college students. *Journal of Studies on Alcohol, Supplement No. 14*, 23–39.

Perkins, H. W. (1997). College student misperceptions of alcohol and other drug norms among peers: Exploring causes, consequences, and implications for prevention programs. *Designing alcohol and other drug prevention programs in higher education: Bringing theory into practice* (pp. 177–206). Washington, DC: U.S. Department of Education.

Perkins, H. W. (2002). Social norms and the prevention of alcohol misuse in collegiate contexts. *Journal of Studies on Alcohol, Supplement No. 14*, 164–72.

Perkins, H. W., & Berkowitz, A. D. (1986). Perceiving the community norms of alcohol use among students: Some research implications for campus alcohol education programming. *International Journal of Addictions, 21*, 961–76.

Perkins, H. W., & Wechsler, H. (1996). Variation in perceived college drinking norms and its impact on alcohol abuse: A nationwide study. *Journal of Drug Issues, 26*, 961–74.

Petty, R. E., & Cacioppo, J. T. (1986). *Communication and persuasion: Central and peripheral routes to attitude change.* New York: Springer-Verlag.

Ridgeway, P. (2001) Restorying psychiatric disability: Learning from first person recovery narratives. *Psychiatric Rehabilitation Journal, 24(4)*, 335–43.

Schulenberg, J. E. & Maggs, J. L. (2002). A developmental perspective on alcohol use and heavy drinking during adolescence and the transition to young adulthood. *Journal of Studies on Alcohol, 14*, 54–70.

Wechsler, H., Davenport, A., Dowdall, G., Moeykens, B., & Castillo, S. (1994). Health and behavior consequences of binge drinking in college. *Journal of the American Medical Association, 272*, 1672–77.

Wechsler, H., & Kuo, M. (2000). College students define binge drinking and estimate its prevalence: Results of a national survey. *Journal of American College Health, 49*, 57–64.

Workman, T. A. (2001). Finding the meanings of college drinking: An analysis of fraternity drinking stories. *Health Communication, 13*, 427–47.

Workman, T. A. (2005). Drinking stories as learning tools: Socially situated experiential learning and popular culture. In L. Lederman & L. Stewart (Eds.), *Changing the culture of college drinking* (pp.). Cresskill, NJ: Hampton Press.

Yanovitzky, I., Stewart, L. P., & Lederman, L. C. (2006). Social distance, perceived drinking by peers, and alcohol use by college students. *Health Communication, 19*(1), 1–10.

An Exploratory Assessment of a College Substance Abuse Recovery Program: Augsburg College's StepUP Program

Andria M. Botzet, MA
Ken Winters, PhD
Tamara Fahnhorst, MPH

ABSTRACT. Objective: To describe the academic, life functioning, and drug use outcomes of students who participated in the StepUP recovery program, a college program designed to support sobriety for students recovering from substance abuse. Method: Eighty-three StepUP program students (46 current students and 37 alumni) participated in a survey using a slightly modified version of the Global Appraisal for Individual Needs (Dennis, 1998), which assesses drug involvement, mental health, and other life-functioning domains. In addition, a subset of 20 current students completed a second assessment approximately 6 months after the first. Results: The large majority of both current students and alumni reported that they abstained from alcohol and drug use, and that they regularly attended self-help groups. Perceived personal assets and social support were endorsed at high levels by the respondents, as were screens for mental health problems. Conclusions: Students involved in the StepUP program either currently or

The authors wish to thank Patrice Salmeri and David Hadden, StepUP program, as well as their staff, for their assistance with this project.

Andria M. Botzet, MA, Ken Winters, PhD, and Tamara Fahnhorst, MPH are in the Department of Psychiatry at the University of Minnesota, Minneapolis, MN 55455.

in the past were largely able to maintain sobriety, as well as a favorable GPA. StepUP students also endorsed a sizeable amount of assets and social support, which espouse the maintenance of sobriety.

INTRODUCTION

The use of chemical intoxicants has been present for centuries and exists among people of many continents, cultures, and religions. The cultivation of cannabis, for example, was first recorded as early as 28 BC, and THC, nicotine, and cocaine have been identified in Egyptian mummies dating as early as 950 BC (Kuhn, Swartzwelder, & Wilson, 2003). Health and social problems from the use of these drugs have also existed for centuries, and recovery from these problems is seldom achieved in a vacuum. Rather, people in recovery seek strength and hope through healthy relationships and within environments that support abstinence. Thus was born the roots of modern recovery programs: the Temperance Movements of the early to mid 1800s, including the American Temperance Society and the Christian Women's Temperance Union, among others ("Temperance Movement," 2007). As these movements proliferated, other coalitions or movements were born, including Alcoholics Anonymous (AA) in the 1930s. Recovery programs have continued to expand and adjust to clinical needs, as currently indicated by the birth of recovery schools on college campuses.

Current research reveals that the rates of binge drinking (defined as consuming five or more drinks in one sitting or in a single occasion) are highest among college-age individuals, peaking at age 21 (SAMHSA, 2004). Approximately one fifth (21.4%) of college-aged people (ages 18–25) are estimated to meet DSM-IV criteria for substance abuse or dependence (SAMHSA, 2004). Furthermore, college students who are enrolled in full-time classes are significantly more likely to engage in alcohol use, binge drinking, and heavy alcohol use (five or more drinks in one sitting on 5 or more days in the past month) than are their same-age peers who are not enrolled in full-time classes (SAMHSA, 2004). These rates suggest that the college environment is not conducive to recovery from drug addiction and would not provide the peer support that is critical to maintaining a sober lifestyle. Thus, a college student working to overcome substance abuse may be facing more recovery challenges from the environment compared to a similar-aged person in recovery who is not attending college.

In response to this situation, the first recovery-based school services in the United States were developed roughly 30 years ago at Brown University (1977; White & Finch, 2006) and Rutgers University (1983; White & Finch, 2006). These services were incorporated as a program within the larger school with the intention of providing confidential and emotionally healthy environments for students experiencing drug use recovery issues and offering social support necessary to sustain sobriety while students continue their higher education (McSharry, 2007). In 1986, Texas Tech University joined this recovery college movement, which was then followed by Rutgers' expansion of the "Recovery College" notion by becoming the first to incorporate recovery housing in 1988, which offered dormitory options exclusively for the students in their recovery program. Since the inception of these pioneering recovery college programs, 11 such programs, as well as 14 recovery high schools, have been developed in the United States.

The StepUP program at Augsburg College became part of the recovery college movement in 1997 (White & Finch, 2006), promoting the sense of "recovery college" by expanding the number of students served and providing holistic services, including not only the maintenance of recovery and peer support, but also general life skills, spirituality, and recreation. Key features of the StepUP program include: (1) drug- and alcohol-free living options, (2) weekly one-on-one and group meetings to discuss recovery and school-related issues, (3) individual sobriety contracts, and (4) drug-free social activities. Four full-time staff members have daily contact with the nearly 60 students served each school year and enrollment in the program is voluntary. Most students choose to enroll in the program for 1 to 2 years and then transition elsewhere as they finish their degrees.

Behavioral contracts are an integral part of the StepUP program, as they promote individual recovery and group cohesiveness. These contracts serve as the foundation of the program and incorporate 17 key behavior requirements, such as attending all AA/NA and mandatory meetings, refraining from visiting high-risk environments (e.g., bars), being a punctual and responsible student, and avoiding gambling. StepUP has also established a student government in which staff-selected members are responsible for reviewing the relevance of contracts, recommending necessary changes, and enforcing violations of student contracts. This type of government allows for peer-initiated accountability and the assurance of a safe and healthy environment.

Despite the existence of recovery schools for nearly three decades, no methical scientific evaluation has been published. Recognizing the need for a more thorough and scientific measurement of their recovery school, the Augsburg College StepUP program recruited the Center for Adolescent Substance Abuse Research (CASAR), a research unit within the Department of Psychiatry at the University of Minnesota, to assist in the development and execution of a descriptive study. The aims of this preliminary study were to assess and describe current students and alumni of the StepUP program pertaining to recovery attitudes and progress, mental health, school adjustment, and perceptions of the StepUP program.

METHOD

Participants

A summary of participant characteristics is presented in Table 1. Both current students ($n = 46$) and alumni ($n = 37$) were recruited to participate in this study, resulting in a total sample of 83 participants, nearly all of whom identified themselves as Caucasian (97.6%). Enrollment in the StepUP program required a previous drug treatment experience, a motivation to maintain sobriety, a strong academic record, and favorable entrance exam scores to gain initial acceptance into the greater college. Roughly 65% of the sample was male, and ages ranged from 18 to 32 years, with a mean age of 22.5 years (mean age of current students = 20.8 years, range 18–27; mean age of alumni = 24.5 years, range 19–32). Among current students, 44% were freshmen. Alumni had been enrolled in the StepUP program for an average of 3.8 semesters; 16% did not complete their undergraduate program.

MEASURES

The tool used to evaluate the current and alumni StepUP students was adapted from the existing and psychometrically sound Global Appraisal for Individual Needs (Dennis, 1998). The GAIN, a highly structured interview, is a well-established instrument developed to assess youth drug involvement, mental health and other functioning domains. Added to the study instrument were new items related to perceptions of the StepUP program and to recovery behaviors and attitudes. Measures of recovery assessed perceived personal assets or strengths, as well as relapse-risk associated with work and social environments. Relapse-risk variables were computed

TABLE 1. Background Characteristics of the Study Samples

	Current Student ($n = 46$)		Alumni ($n = 37$)	
Item	n	%	n	%
Male	30	65.2	24	64.9
Caucasian	44	95.7	37	100
Highest Level of Education				
Currently enrolled undergrad	45	97.8	11	29.7
Did not graduate from college	1	2.2	6	16.2
Graduated from college	0	0	13	35.1
Enrolled in post-baccalaureate	0	0	6	16.2
Graduated post-baccalaureate	0	0	1	2.7
Married	1	2.2	3	8.1
Employment Status				
Full-time student	23	50.0	3	8.1
Part-time student	2	4.3	0	0
Full-time work	0	0	17	45.9
Part-time work	0	0	4	10.8
Student & work	20	43.5	12	32.4
Stay-at-home parent	0	0	1	2.7
Missing	1	2.2	0	0
In your lifetime, have you:				
Received treatment tor a mental/behavioral problem?	32	69.6	29	78.4
Been stopped by police/arrested 5+ times?	17	37.0	11	29.7
	Mean (sd)	range	Mean (sd)	range
Age	20.8 (2.4)	18–27	24.5 (2.9)	19–32
GPA	2.90 (0.8)	.05–4.00	3.40 (0.5)	2.00–4.00

by summing the "most" or "all" responses on a 4-point Likert scale for a set of seven work or social environment variables that measured the frequency of contact with others who use drugs or the frequency of stress-inducing situations that may trigger an urge to return to drug use. For example, items in the work environment scale include, "Of the people with whom you work regularly, how many: (1) were employed or in school full-time; (2) were involved in illegal activity; (3) got drunk weekly or had 5 or more drinks in a day; (4) used any drugs in the past 90 days; (5) shout, argue, and fight most weeks; (6) have ever been in drug or alcohol treatment; and (7) would describe themselves as being in recovery." Parallel questions were asked for the social/peer relapse-risk environment. Perceived personal assets were measured by computing a count of positively endorsed items when asked, "Which of the following areas do you consider to be your strengths?" Respondents were shown a list of 10 topics to which they could reply "yes," this area is one of my strengths, or "no," it is not. The areas of strength included "doing well" at work, at school, with family, with friends, at sports or a physical activity, at music or performing arts, at drawing or visual arts, at listening or communicating with others, at problem solving, and at working with computers.

Current students had the opportunity to complete the adapted GAIN during both the fall and spring semesters. All items on the GAIN were modified so they could be completed as a self-administered questionnaire. The fall session questionnaire included a detailed evaluation of current (prior 12 months) level of functioning, mental health, alcohol and other drug use, as well as a history of these same variables. Though the mode of administration of the GAIN was changed to ease the administration process with this sample, the highly structured interview format of the GAIN lends itself to a face-valid adaptation of a self-administered format. Inquiries were also made in regard to challenges and successes with recovery and expectations about the StepUP Program. The spring session version for the current students was similar to the fall assessment except that the time frame for many questions was changed to the prior 6 months.

The alumni questionnaire was retained as structured interview. Items closely followed the fall questionnaire for current students. Additional items were added to assess the alumni's perception of strengths and weaknesses of the StepUP Program.

PROCEDURE

The current students were initially assessed in September 2005 at the conclusion of a regularly scheduled monthly meeting of StepUP students and program staff. CASAR research staff introduced the study and administered the consent form and questionnaire, in accordance with the Augsburg College Internal Review Board (IRB) procedures. Students were reminded that participation was voluntary, that there was no penalty if the student chose not to participate, and that their answers would remain anonymous. Students did not record their names on the questionnaire; rather they recorded a code that was most likely unique to the person but would not disclose their identity (e.g., first portion of home phone number, month of mother's birth, month of father's birth). In April 2006, current students were again invited to complete the spring questionnaire at the conclusion of the monthly StepUP meeting. For some students, this represented their second (prospective) administration, while for other students this was their first administration of an evaluation questionnaire (i.e., newer students and those who were absent at the fall meeting).

Alumni students were mailed an introductory letter, consent form, and a stamped return envelope by StepUP staff during the fall semester. A volunteer called those who returned their signed consent forms and the interview was administered via telephone. Due to a relatively low response to the first mailing, two additional reminders were sent (one in late fall and the other in early spring). Thus, administration of the alumni interview was conducted over the course of the school year.

STATISTICAL ANALYSES

Because the study's main purpose was to provide a description of current StepUP students and alumni, basic descriptive statistics were primarily used. ANOVA was used to compare the current students with the alumni on various measures to see if the two groups differed and as an initial measurement of program impact (i.e., have alumni remained sober and academically successful in comparison with those still participating in the program?). Finally, a brief prospective analysis was conducted to explore the level of change occurring from the fall assessment to the spring assessment.

RESULTS

The results of the evaluation are organized around two sets of data: the combined baseline sample of current and alumni students ($n = 83$); and the prospective sample ($n = 20$), which comprised the subset of current students who completed both a fall and spring assessment.

BASELINE SAMPLE

Responses to questions related to health and well-being are detailed in Table 2. The overall sample also reported having approximately 3.5

TABLE 2. General Health and Well-Being

Variable	Current Students (n = 46)		Alumni (n = 37)		
	Mean	sd	Mean	sd	F
# of Sources of Stress (range 0–9)	3.9	2.6	3.4	2.5	1.36
# of Physical health problems (range 0–7)	1.0	1.1	1.0	1.7	.03
# of Psychological distress symptoms (range 0–3)	0.4	0.6	0.3	0.6	.17
# of Eating Disorder symptoms (range 0–3)	0.2	0.6	0.1	0.3	2.28
# of Gambling symptoms (range 0–3)	0.9	1.0	0.4	0.8	8.00**
# of Depression-related symptoms (range 0–5)	1.9	1.7	1.0	1.4	6.46*
# of Suicidal symptoms (range 0–3)	0.2	0.4	0.2	0.5	.05
# of Anxiety symptoms (range 0–3)	1.0	1.1	0.7	1.1	2.50
# of Post-traumatic Stress symptoms (range 0–4)	1.3	1.2	1.1	1.2	.73
# of Attention-deficit symptoms (range 0–6)	3.4	1.8	1.7	1.5	21.74***
# of HIV-risk symptoms (range 0–3)	0.7	0.8	0.8	0.8	.01
Total symptom count (range 0–40)	8.7	4.6	5.0	4.8	12.70***

*$p < .05$; **$p < .01$; ***$p < .001$.

(of 10 possible) sources of stress in the past 6 months, with current students reporting slightly more sources of stress (3.9 versus 3.4). Although severe physical health problems were not frequently reported, symptoms of mental health problems were prevalent among the sample, with anxiety, depression, posttraumatic stress, and attention-deficit problems being the most frequently endorsed mental health categories. MANOVAs were conducted to correct for multiple-comparison error, and results indicated that current students reported higher symptom counts than alumni students across all mental health problem screens (F [1,82] = 12.70, $p < 0.001$), though the rates for the individual mental health screens were significantly higher for current students only on the gambling problem screen (F [1,82] = 8.00, $p < 0.01$), the depression-related screen (F [1,82] = 6.46, $p < 0.05$), and the ADHD screen (F [1,82] = 21.74, $p < 0.001$).

A summary of responses to the items pertaining to substance use is presented in Table 3. Only nine students (11%) reported using alcohol or other drugs during the prior 6 months, and only two students (2%) met DSM-IV criteria for a current substance use disorder. Among current students, only one student reported using alcohol and other drugs and no student had a current substance use disorder. Current and past students endorsed roughly the same number of substance use disorder symptoms, though current students reported using tobacco significantly more often

TABLE 3. Substance Involvement Data

Variable	Current Students ($n = 46$)		Alumni ($n = 37$)		
	n	%	n	%	$?^3$
Used any alcohol or drugs in past 6 months	1	2.2	8	21.6	7.42**
Meets criteria for Substance Abuse in past 6 months	0	0	1	2.7	1.26
Meets criteria for Substance Dependence in past 6 months	1	2.2	1	2.7	.02
	mean	sd	mean	sd	F
# of Substance Abuse symptoms (range 0–4)	0.1	0.4	0.1	0.4	.04
# of Substance Dependence symptoms (range 0–7)	0.2	1.0	0.2	1.2	.00
# of days tobacco was used over past 3 months (range 0–90)	75.7	29.6	40.6	43.9	10.82**

*$p < .05;$** $p < .01;$*** $p < .001.$

than the alumni (76 days and 41 days, respectively, out of the past 90 days).

We also examined data related to recovery, as shown in Table 4. Current students attended self-help groups more frequently than the alumni (30 days and 17 days, respectively, out of the past 90 days), but reports of assets or personal strength were high for both past and current students, with a mean number of seven assets (out of 10). In addition, both groups of students reported high levels of social support (mean = 7.2 and 7.8 of ten possible support sources, respectively). Alumni reported facing a slightly greater rate of relapse-risk in their present social and work environments than the current students, though this difference was not statistically significant using a MANOVA [F (1,82) = 0.72, $p > 0.05$ and F (1,82) = 2.32, $p > 0.05$, respectively].

Open-ended questions were posed to participants to gain a broader understanding of their reasons for attaining sobriety, as well as the ways the StepUP program assisted in that attainment (as shown in Table 5). Participants were allowed to list multiple reasons, which were then categorized and tallied by two research staff who were blind to the respondent's school grouping (current student or alumnus). Categories were then compared between the two researchers, and any discrepancies were discussed and categorized upon mutual agreement.

TABLE 4. Recovery-related Data

Variable	Current Students (n = 46)		Alumni (n = 37)		
	mean	sd	mean	sd	F
# of Days attended self-help group (AA/NA) over past 3 months (range 0–90)	29.7	19.5	17.0	14.5	10.56**
# of Relapse risk factors at work (range 0–10)	4.2	2.5	3.6	1.9	2.32
# of Relapse risk factors in peer/social environment (range 0–10)	4.7	2.7	5.5	1.8	.72
# of Personal assets/strengths (range 0–10)	7.2	1.7	7.4	1.7	.09
# of Social support (range 0–10)	7.2	2.2	7.8	1.3	.39

TABLE 5. Summary of Motivation for Sobriety and Benefit of StepUP Program

Variable	Current Students (n = 46)		Alumni (n = 37)	
	n	%	n	%
Primary reasons for getting sober				
Improved Quality of Life	29	63.0	30	81.8
Interpersonal Reasons	8	17.4	15	41.5
To Avoid Further Negative Otucomes	12	26.1	7	18.9
Personal Quest	9	19.6	6	16.2
Other	2	4.3	2	5.6
Ways StepUP assists in sobriety				
Interpersonal Support	37	78.7	25	67.6
Safe/Healthy Environment	27	58.7	18	48.6
Educating/Counseling	11	23.9	15	40.5
Accountability	18	39.1	7	18.9
Other	2	4.3	0	0
Did not help	0	0	2	5.6

The primary reason for attaining sobriety among this sample was to improve quality of life, which categorized responses such as "my happiness depended on sobriety," "to attain a better future," or "I was too depressed when I was using." Likewise, interpersonal support (e.g., support from peers, positive staff communication and relationships, advice and direction from staff and alumni) was the most prominent way that the StepUP program assisted in sobriety.

TABLE 6. Demographics of Prospective Sample ($n = 20$)

Variable	n	%
Gender		
Male	13	65.0
Female	7	35.0
Race		
Caucasian	19	95.0
Current Level of College		
Freshman	8	40.0
Sophomore	7	35.0
Junior	2	10.0
Senior	3	15.0
Employment Status		
Full-time student	8	40.0
Part-time student	1	5.0
Full-time student & full-time work	0	0
Full-time student & part-time work	11	45.0
Part-time student, part-time work	0	0

PROSPECTIVE SAMPLE

Table 6 provides a summary of the demographic variables for the prospective sample ($n = 20$); these students completed both a fall and spring questionnaire. Responses to items inquiring about health and well-being are summarized and compared in Table 7. Sources of stress increased from the first assessment to the second assessment, though this increase was not statistically significant. Physical health slightly declined at the second assessment, and symptoms of recent (prior 6 months) mental and behavioral health problems showed a slight decrease from the fall to the spring assessment on four of the five mental health screens: (1) depression-related problems (mean symptom counts of 2.4 and 1.7, respectively), (2) anxiety problems (1.4 and 1.1, respectively), (3) posttraumatic stress problems (1.5 and 1.1, respectively), and (4) attention-deficit problems (3.5 and 2.9, respectively). Furthermore, a paired-samples *t* test was conducted to measure differences over time among rates of risk within the aforementioned mental health screens, which indicated that the individual mental health variables did not significantly change over time. The count of total mental health symptoms (an aggregate symptom count of aforementioned mental health screens) significantly decreased (paired sample $t = 2.49$, $p < 0.05$); however, when corrected for multiple-comparison error using

TABLE 7. Analysis of Change for Mental and Behavioral Health Outcomes in Prospective Sample

Variable	1st Assessment		2nd Assessment		Paired-Sample t-test*
	Mean	sd	Mean	sd	
In the past 6 months.......					
# of Sources of Stress (range 0–9)	3.9	2.5	4.6	2.6	.88
# of Physical health problems (range 0–7)	1.1	1.0	0.5	1.0	1.60
# of Gambling symptoms (range 0–3)	1.0	0.9	1.0	1.1	.00
# of Depression-related symptoms (range 0–5)	2.4	2.0	1.7	1.7	1.76
# of Suicidal symptoms (range 0–3)	0.2	0.4	0.2	0.5	.00
# of Anxiety symptoms (range 0–3)	1.4	1 2	1.1	1.2	1.45
# of Posl-traumatic Stress symptoms (range 0–4)	1.5	1.1	1.1	1.1	l.51
# of Attention-deficit symptoms (range 0–6)	3.5	1.2	2.9	1.6	1.55
# of HIV-risk symptoms (range 0–3)	0.8	0.8	0.8	0.9	.24
Total symptom count (range 0–34)	9.9	4.3	7.9	4.2	2.49
Grade Point Average	2.86	0.9	3.05	0.6	.71

*All paired-tests were corrected for multiple-comparison error using Bonferroni correction, and all variables were non-significant at the $p < .05$ level.

Bonferroni correction ($p = 0.05/\#$ of tests [11] $= 0.005$), this difference was no longer significant.

We also analyzed change with respect to the substance use and recovery variables. There were no significant changes across time for all these variables.

DISCUSSION

The overwhelming majority of current StepUP students is not using drugs, is maintaining a favorable GPA, is functioning quite well socially, and perceives the StepUP program as vital to their overall well-being. A considerable number of students screened positive for a variety of mental health problems, but this number is not surprising, considering other reports of college-age mental health problems (see Benton et al., 2003; Kadison & DiGeronimo, 2004) and the frequency at which mental health disorders co-occur with substance use disorders (i.e., Clark et al., 1999; Costello et al., 1999). Students' responses infer that they are vested in a successful recovery, as shown by their involvement in self-help groups, their reasons for getting sober, and their avoidance of situations that may increase the risk of relapse (i.e., living where people use drugs/alcohol, socializing with people who use drugs/alcohol). Current StepUP students also endorsed a sizeable number of assets and social support, which is an encouraging factor in maintaining sobriety.

Most StepUP alumni are also successful with recovery, function well in the academic and work worlds, are not suffering from significant physical health problems, and perceive the StepUP program as vital to overall well-being. Again, screens for mental health problems were endorsed at a considerable rate, though reports of personal assets and social support were pronounced. Overall, the results suggest that StepUP is a beneficial experience for past and present enrolled students, facilitating the maintenance of sobriety while simultaneously promoting academic success.

IMPLICATIONS

The study findings suggest that many students enroll in this program early in their college experience (nearly half of the current students were freshmen and half of the alumni were still enrolled in some type of college program). Thus, the StepUP program may serve for some students as an effective transitional program, in which young adults in recovery use the program as a stepping stone to help them adjust to academic life while maintaining sobriety in a high-risk college environment. The value of this program is also indicated by the open-ended responses referring to the ways StepUP assists in sobriety (e.g., support received from peers and staff, the structured community and safe environment, the tools and resources gained, and the accountability established by the program). The prospective data suggest that many students gained additional over the course of the school year. Whereas we did not find statistically significant changes from fall to spring, many variables did show a trend toward improvement, especially pertaining to mental health symptoms.

LIMITATIONS

Since little scientific research has been conducted on the efficacy and outcome of recovery schools, we feel this study was an important initiation of a research-oriented examination of these programs. However, limitations existed in this study, such as the small sample size and the restricted sampling area (students were recruited from only one recovery college). These factors result in inadequate generalizablility, in addition to the inability to conduct more sophisticated statistical analyses. Future research on college recovery programs should include a control sample to better determine the efficacy of these programs, including a sample of students in recovery who have enrolled in the traditional college setting, as well as a matched sample of nonrecovery students from the same college (i.e., Augsburg). Gender-specific statistical analyses are also an important area for future study (our sample was too small to conduct a gender analysis). Results from these types of samples may provide a better measurement of progress and program value, including the ascertainment of a needs assessment to identify program strengths and areas in need of enhancement.

REFERENCES

Benton, S. A., Robertson, J. M., Tseng, W.-C., Newton, F. B., & Benton, S. L. (2003). Changes in counseling center client problems across 13 years. *Professional Psychology: Research and Practice, 34*(1), 66–72.

Clark, D. B., Parker, A. M., & Lynch, K. G. (1999). Psychopathology and substance-related problems during early adolescence: A survival analysis. *Journal of Clinical Child and Adolescent Psychology, 28*, 333–41.

Costello, E. J., Erkanli, A., Federman, E., & Angold, A. (1999). Development of psychiatric comorbidity with substance abuse in adolescents: Effects of timing and sex. *Journal of Clinical Child and Adolescent Psychology, 28*, 298–311.

Dennis, M. L. (1998). *Global Appraisal of Individual Needs (GAIN) manual: Administration, scoring and interpretation* (Prepared with funds from CSAT TI 11320). Bloomington, IL: Lighthouse Publications.

Kadison, R., & DiGeronimo, T. F. (2004). *College of the overwhelmed: The campus mental health crisis and what to do about it.* San Francisco: Jossey-Bass.

Kuhn, C., Swartzwelder, S., & Wilson, W. (2003). *Buzzed: The straight facts about the most used and abused drugs from alcohol to ecstasy.* New York: W. W. Norton.

McSharry, K. (2007, February). *Issues of chemical dependency: Brown University.* Retrieved February 6, 2007, from http://www.brown.edu/Administration/Dean_of_the_College/resources/?id=256

Substance Abuse and Mental Health Services Administration (2004). *The 2003 national survey on drug use and health: national findings (NSDUH Series H-25, DHHS Pub No. SMA 04-3964).* Rockville, MD: Office of Applied Studies.

Temperance Movement (2007, January). Retrieved January 29, 2007, from http://en.wikipedia.org/wiki/Temperance_movement

White, W. L., & Finch, A. J. (2006). The recovery school movement—its history and future. *Counselor: The Magazine for Addiction Professionals, 7*(2), 54–57.

Reflections on Chemical Dependency in a College Setting and Its Intersection with Secondary School Programs

Bruce Donovan, PhD

ABSTRACT. For more than 25 years, I served Brown University as Associate Dean with Special Responsibilities in the Area of Chemical Dependency, a long title, but one in which, in those early days, each word had its own political value: the idea of this deanship was without precedent, and questions of turf were a big concern. The status of "associate," for example, made clear that others of higher rank exercised some authority. (Happily, over the years, my supervision was always supportive, trusting and even distant.) "Special" suggested that my responsibilities did *not* include medical matters addressed in the Brown Medical School and that still other departments had responsibilities in the alcohol and drug area. "In the area" made clear that my own purview had considerable range—academic affairs, athletics, faculty matters, personnel, student life—and was not merely clinical.

At the outset, few—locally or nationally—were paying attention to alcohol and other drug issues on campus. I was a full professor in Classics and an alumnus familiar to and with my institution. I was also five years sober. Brown had welcomed a new president that year, an experienced college administrator from Minnesota, Howard Swearer, who, eager

Bruce Donovan, PhD, is Professor of Classics, Emeritus and Associate Dean of the College and Associate Dean for Problems of chemical Dependency (Retired), Brown University.

Remarks delivered at the Annual Conference of the Association of Recovery Schools July 10, 2004—with references and a postscript added for publication, April 2007.

to create a program to assist alcohol-troubled faculty, initiated the Associate Deanship/Chemical Dependency. This was a quarter-time position with a modest budget; the additional three-quarters involved responsibility for more strictly academic issues, for example, advising, monitoring academic honesty. From the start I broadened Swearer's mandate to include work with members of the staff and especially graduate and undergraduate students, who were to become my most numerous clients. I assumed the Associate Deanship in 1977, retiring in July 2003.

In this presentation I will limit my remarks to interactions with students, and place particular emphasis on the use of alcohol, although other drugs were surely prominent in my work. "Student" here includes both undergraduate and graduate students, individuals of very different ages and of all races and sexual orientations. Most undergraduates matriculated immediately after high school, although some had been away from college for as long as twenty years when they returned to complete degree requirements. I emphasize counseling and leave to one side, for example, bibliotherapy and generally leave unremarked commentary on interactions with other individuals and offices on campus—chaplains, health educators, members of the faculty, psychologists, security officers—with whom I developed networks for information and support.

THE DEANSHIP FOR PROBLEMS OF CHEMICAL DEPENDENCY AT BROWN UNIVERSITY

The Setting

The President and I determined to house the new position in the academic deanery, *not* the office of student affairs, even now a fairly unusual but highly significant setting for a program of this sort. We chose to identify my work with the central educational purposes of the University in order to give the issues and the position greater prestige and to earn greater influence. The location also seemed to help curb the stigma associated with drug addiction. Were the position to be located in Student Affairs, the public could assume we were most concerned with broken windows and broken noses and not a broader spectrum of individuals. In fact, not all of my clients were miscreants; many were of high accomplishment who nonetheless ran afoul of alcohol and other drugs. Too, interactions were easier with faculty members who more easily made referrals to an academic officer than to those responsible for non-academic discipline. Additionally, my position allowed me easier access to students whose academic difficulties might indicate addiction, whether or not they had disciplinary problems.

Procedures

I was neither a clinician nor counselor, but rather someone who in his day-to-day life demonstrated incidentally that abstinence from drugs could be combined with a happy, productive personal and professional life and who acted as a special breed of academic advisor. Ferdinand Jones, who was at one time the Director of Brown's Psychological Services and an early ally as a provider of support services to addicted students, observed in another context that Brown was neither a treatment center nor a holding tank: to remain enrolled, students must be capable of at least 'passing' academic work. Student addicts were thus subjected to a high standard: they must maintain sobriety *and also* meet the usual academic expectations of the university. In this insistence Brown anticipated unwittingly what was to become the recovery schools movement.

Over the years, gradually and somewhat hit-or-miss, I developed my own style and procedures, basing my work firmly on the Twelve Steps, supplementing those principles with insights gleaned at seminars, institutes and summer schools. In those early days little was available in the literature, helpful as it could be otherwise, about problems in the academic setting. Along the way I was reassured to learn that I had devised serendipitously, and with Twelve Step help happily acknowledged, procedures proven appropriate by the research and experience of others. I approached addiction chiefly as a matter of health, essentially a medical challenge, although I recognized that others—including colleagues paid to enforce these other views—saw it primarily as a moral *or* legal *or* educational *or* reputational matter.

Because of my non-clinical background, I never made formal diagnoses but, when a formal assessment was deemed necessary, relied on diagnosticians in the community. This was *not* a handicap: most individuals who elected to utilize my services were demonstrably experiencing significant difficulties with drugs. Abstinence always seemed an appropriate suggestion, if only as a short-term remedy: abstaining from chemicals never hurts and, even if not a final prescription, can be a useful moment for introspection. And abstinence was a requirement, if consultations were to continue. I might add that on this matter of diagnoses, I often wonder, still, how firm and final a diagnosis can or should be with the young, who have relatively short drug histories and for whom the evidence for diagnosis can be significantly limited.

In this matter of diagnoses, I was happy not to step beyond my own capabilities. It was also important to maintain clear professional boundaries, a critical necessity in a university, where credentials carry so much weight. This attention to boundaries was also significant as offices with different overlapping turfs to my own, for example, health education, developed in the course of my tenure.

All of my clients received, deservedly, my positive regard: I sought always to distinguish between any misbehavior and the agent thereof. It was my son who articulated for me the credo that all folks have a right to a life of joy and dignity—and for me this belief applied especially to the recovering, who perennially felt that joy and dignity were not characteristics to which they were entitled. Students also claim to have benefited from my positive, optimistic outlook and my abiding faith in their progress, which was not always easy to maintain.

Additionally, if they could accept the label of alcoholic or addict, labels that had to be substantiated through formal assessment if this option were to be exercised, students were apprised of their coverage under the Rehabilitation Act of 1973 and the Americans with Disabilities Act (ADA) of 1990. They learned that the University had enacted the possibility of special accommodations, provisions rooted in the ADA, to ease their academic progress in recovery: ultimate degree requirements were not affected, but a student's pace towards that goal might be relaxed. They were also reminded that Brown did not routinely notify parents of drug-related incidents, even though an exception to the Family Educational Rights and Privacy Act (FERPA)—the Buckley Amendment—allowed such notice: my conversations with students would be confidential and subject to their express written release. However, I reserved the right to contact parents in extreme situations and did on occasion exercise that prerogative.

Students are all different, and I individualized my approach to each one in a way that respected the unique qualities and issues they brought to their addiction. Still, I observed certain rules that I made clear to the students with whom I worked, which were designed in part to assign them maximum respect and responsibility:

All conversations were to be confidential. My colleagues—let alone parents—would learn nothing about my interactions with addicted students without their written permission. No record of our conversations would be placed in University files. This was a particularly significant matter because of my concomitant chairmanship of the Committee on Academic Standing, a committee of faculty members and administrators that monitored students' academic progress and applied sanctions of Warning, Serious Warning and Dismissal. It was no irrational apprehension on the part of students that I might divulge their histories, even inadvertently. I am proud to say that this never occurred: I managed throughout my tenure to keep my roles separate and distinct, even though with some students my involvements were lengthy and much of it informal.

Students were not to use drugs prior to an appointment in order that they not be radically drug-affected during our consultations. They were to be as clear as possible in our discussions, both mentally and emotionally.

Students were asked to speak only the truth. Rather than deceive, they were asked to decline to answer any of my questions. Were their choice silence, however, they were advised that I would probably lobby them for a response. Rarely, in fact, did students refuse to respond to a well-phrased inquiry.

I explained that I had no butterfly net to drop over students to rescue them from their own baser impulses. If students told me that they would never smoke, drink or *whatever* again, and I subsequently spotted them on campus hugging a bong and a bottle, I would not intervene. Further, I asked them not to bother to attempt to hide their behavior from me. However, the incident would clearly be the topic of discussion in a subsequent appointment.

As I have mentioned, students could always expect to be treated respectfully. This did not mean, however, that I accepted without affect any unacceptable behavior. Only rarely did I express anger for special—and memorable—effect. I believe that, in the vast majority of instances, students felt genuine warmth, concern and support for right behavior, that is, behavior targeted towards sobriety.

From the start, intuitively—as I suspect was the case with many other practitioners—I observed what I was to learn much later were the tenets of motivational interviewing (Miller and Rollnick, 1991).

Additionally, although I conducted no formal drug assessments, I routinely threaded through my initial conversation with any student the four CAGE questions, the acronym derived from the key term in each query (Ewing, 1984). I often used my own words and phrasing, but the acronym always proved to be a helpful aid. The questions proved helpfully and unobtrusively—if informally—diagnostic: Have you ever felt you should *cut* down on your drinking? Have people *annoyed* you by criticizing your drinking? Have you ever felt bad or *guilty* about your drinking? Have you ever had a drink first thing in the morning to steady your nerves or get rid of a hangover (*eyeopener*)?

At the end of introductory first visits—if students did not grasp the apparent seriousness of their condition—I would propose a variation of the Mann Test, named for Marty Mann who, to the best of my knowledge, first articulated the proposal that a likely alcoholic try for as long as possible to drink only two drinks daily, strictly defined, and to observe and record the outcome (Mann, 1958, pp. 83–85). Addicts find this test extraordinarily difficult, if not impossible, to pass.

I particularly liked the CAGE and MANN devices: students, whether or not they returned to me, would at least have in their possession for their own use evidence on the nature of their drinking, a tactic that clearly recognized and emphasized a student's responsibility.

My advising usually focused on the student as a productive member of the university community, academically and socially, albeit a student with a unique set of challenges. Were medical assistance or extensive counseling necessary at any point, and they frequently were, I made appropriate campus or community referrals.

In addition to one-on-one counseling I also monitored the availability of meetings on or immediately adjacent to campus of Alcoholics and Narcotics Anonymous and, similarly, meetings of Al-Anon and Nar-Anon. In some instances I established such meetings; sometimes I encouraged and supported others in that task. Two of those that I established were special meetings held on Homecoming and Commencement/Reunion weekends at which students could meet alumni and see the tradition of which they were a part.

On campus I facilitated a weekly discussion session, The Early Sobriety Group, an alternative to 12-step meetings for the rare students who found AA not to their taste and a supplement for the rest. As things developed, few were the students who chose not to affiliate ultimately with AA. The Early Sobriety Group, however, provided a helpful transition while students learned more about 12-step programs, killed off their pre-conceived and erroneous impressions of AA and/or came to grips more significantly with their addiction. Such a group was especially helpful and comfortable when a student wanted to discuss matters peculiar to college or university life. Even the most self-absorbed student understood, at a community 12-step meeting, the distinction between lamenting homelessness and worrying over a grade on an examination. The latter might be labeled a problem of abundance, the former not. Finally, the Early Sobriety Group played an enormous role in forging strong bonds among recovering students themselves: some of the Group's greatest benefits were found not in group sessions but in the mutual support offered member-to-member through the week.

For students, as well as recovering members of the faculty and staff, I sponsored a "no-host" Lunch Bunch six or seven times each academic year, an opportunity for kindred folks to meet and broaden their on-campus network and, not so incidentally, to ease the demands on me for casual support. Additionally, the lunches provided those in recovery with less anonymous associations than those afforded by AA: in the "check-in" that was a feature of each luncheon, individuals were asked to identify themselves by first and last name. Even though security and access were always carefully guarded, such a procedure helped with the gradual return of the participants to a 'normal' way of life. The Lunch Bunch also allowed participants, often unawares, to practice social skills in sobriety. Too, the multi-generational, multi-class mix of students and members of the faculty and staff, from full professors through lawn cutters or security officers proved salutary—a modest dose of "the real world" amidst the groves of academe. Such diversity allowed students to learn from older community members how and why parents acted as they did when ensnared in addiction, just as members of faculty and staff learned much about their own children from the students with whom they ate their lunch. Finally, Lunch Bunch members often cited the value of simply being able to spot recovering colleagues going about their business and sometimes to engage in conversation.

Language

For students who learn daily in their classrooms the value of careful research and appropriate citations of evidence, 12-step programs, which eschew these procedures, can be puzzling. Consternation multiplies when members are urged to accept information from strangers whose mere names they may never know. To grant, perhaps in a minor way, greater legitimacy and respectability to addiction as a topic of intellectual merit, as a subject which has its own history and literature, I chose my words carefully and sought to avoid the 12-step vernacular. This strategy seemed to cast greater seriousness over my work. The more formal diction also provided students with correct vocabulary and, because it avoided the colloquial and thereby seemed somewhat novel, tended to catch their attention. They soon learned that my attitudes—even my language—might be different from what they were used to in their dormitories or with their friends.

For example, I chose to speak of "tolerance" rather than "capacity," a term which in campus parlance can escalate to a primary virtue an individual's ability to 'hold' large amounts of alcohol. I similarly tried to eliminate "drunkenness." "Drunkenness," with its connotations of grossness and excess, tends to narrow the focus of perceived alcohol-related difficulties: those whose lives were impaired by less extreme and rowdy drinking behavior, however constant and troubling their use might be, might more easily escape notice and the opportunity for aid. I chose instead "intoxication," a term which has the added attraction of introducing quite naturally the idea of "toxicity." I also tried to stamp out "substance abuse" as being counter-productive. "Substance" has always struck me as overly general and perhaps unhelpfully euphemistic—and I know no individual who would choose to be guilty of "abuse" of *anything*. "Chemical dependency" is more direct and can more easily be worked into ordinary conversation.

I want to add another, odd note. Despite my aversion to colloquialisms in drug-related conversations, I found it important to use language with which I was comfortable and which felt and sounded genuine rolling out of my mouth. Curiously, I found myself always asking, ungrammatically, "Do you do much drugs?" Somehow this grammatically incorrect phrasing 'worked' and many seemingly impervious addicts would respond fully and openly to my direct question, however inelegantly phrased.

Again, as part of this *pot pourri* of self-conscious diction, I used liberally the various slogans of the 12-step world and catchy formulations perhaps inspired by them: "You may not get into trouble every time you drink, but have you been drinking every time you get into trouble?" "You don't have to be a problem drinker to have a problem with your drinking."

A final comment on language. The care which I exercised in my own diction was something I also encouraged in students themselves. I asked that they use, outside of 12-step meetings, non-12-step language, to get used to discussing their condition, whenever necessary, in an appropriate, commonly understood way.

Humor

Addiction, to be sure, is no laughing matter, but it *is*, as I was reminded early on by a physician friend, one of the few diseases that can be *treated* with laughter; and so my students and I laughed a lot. This was their life, after all, whatever its particulars, and needed full acceptance—and if humor helped, good enough! As a wise and witty colleague once opined, memorably, "If you take life seriously, you needn't be serious about it twenty-four hours a day."

An Endnote

This detail deserves a rubric of its own. I always traveled with two handkerchiefs, one for my use and another, carefully stored in a pocket, available if a student broke into tears. Many accepted the offer of my handkerchief, assuring me that they would return it cleaned. I have often wondered how many realized that, in addition to my sincerity in being helpful, the return of the laundered handkerchief assured a follow-up visit.

THE INTERSECTION OF THE BROWN PROGRAM WITH PRE-COLLEGE EXPERIENCES

As Associate Dean, I was always conscious of the attitudes and behaviors which students (as well as their parents and guardians) brought with them to college.

The Coherence of a Student's Experience

Although their perspectives may differ depending on whether they work at the secondary or post-secondary level, practitioners will agree that time spent in secondary school and college forms an unbroken continuum, periods discrete but integrally related: for maximum effectiveness the first must anticipate the latter, and the latter must build on what precedes.

To argue the essential coherence of a student's experiences may seem unnecessary, yet many observers seemed to assume college to be a "fresh start," an event that bursts full-blown from a student's life as did Athena from the head of Zeus: drug problems which occur on campus, these observers might argue, are unrelated to influences from secondary school or home. Brown's University Chaplain, Janet Cooper-Nelson, has observed with insight and no small irony the 'Cinderella moment,' that instant when secondary students—at graduation, now 18 and legally "adult"—are transformed magically and immediately into agents prepared to assume full responsibility for their lives. Such a moment is, of course, illusory. The transition is more intricate and students more complex than such a construct requires: the transition from secondary school to college is virtually seamless and, to mix metaphors, pre-collegiate experiences cast a long shadow.

Correctly Perceiving the Pre-College Experience

Those in higher education must understand accurately the essential facts of what a student's prior history has *actually* been. Too many of us—and especially the addicted—have more good memories than we had good times.

I was always curious with what experiences and pre-conceived notions students entered college. I recall an orientation meeting where the entering class learned about the University's attitudes and policies toward alcohol and other drugs. Facilitators at one point asked the group if their secondary schools had policies governing alcohol and other drugs. Almost all students answered affirmatively. Students were then asked if they knew colleagues penalized for violating these rules. Most students knew of such instances.

Another more important question—at least in my estimation—was never asked, despite my annual entreaties. I was anxious to know whether incoming students knew instances where wrongdoers in high school, well known to their peers, had broken rules and yet "escaped" scot free. It was and is my belief that *these* situations do more than published policies (often unobserved in the breach) to establish strong, if implicit, cultural norms. My goal was—and would be—to reveal a secret we were all keeping. Common acknowledgment of this darker side of things, as opposed to wishful thinking, is important if all parties are to share a common understanding.

Honesty

It may seem odd to stress truth-telling. My emphasis on veracity stems directly from the American drug story, so rife with avoidance and denial. Somewhat paradoxically, those in recovery, usually deep in *self*-denial as they consider sobering up, often have the keenest sense of how society *actually* deals with drug issues, what the *real* policies and risks are. I think, in this connection, of a student apprehended for carrying a keg into a fraternity house in the clear light of day, although he must surely have been aware of the prohibition against kegs on campus. "Did you not know such behavior was illegal?" I asked with feigned incredulity. The response came: "I knew it was illegal, but I didn't know it was *illegal* illegal." This response suggested to me that this student was no fool and had learned over time that the institution had not infrequently winked at infractions of the keg ban. I was glad we had a common understanding.

Such shared awareness restores a measure of self-respect to clients, in that their perception of reality is recognized and validated. Informational equality between addict and advisor also initiates trust between the two parties, a vital pre-condition for success in counseling and progress in recovery.

Truth-telling also comes into play in the providing of data on individual drugs and the portrayal of current laws and enforcement. What are the pragmatic as opposed to the merely ethical advantages? One example may suffice. Aaron had been told in secondary school that grim sequelae would ensue, were he to smoke marijuana. He took this warning to heart and avoided use; as a trained peer advisor he also passed the information on to elementary school youngsters. When he arrived at college, he was stunned to find peers who smoked pot occasionally and without incident and who, indeed, prospered. As his college years went by, Aaron himself experimented with drugs and settled on Robitussin—a sort of 'socially acceptable' non-drug drug, not one commonly discussed as problematic— and it was dependency on this over-the-counter drug that led him to me. It was not easy to establish trust with one who had been misinformed, whose trust had once been casually abused.

Law and Regulation

The law and college/university regulations present a far more complex challenge.

Over the length of my tenure, no issue engaged me so steadily on intellectual, moral and pragmatic grounds as did questions of law and obedience to them, both a student's obedience and my own. I knew well first-hand, from experience in the 1960s, distinctions between good laws and bad, of disobedience (including civil disobedience) and its penalties. I found it difficult, therefore, to confront stiff jail sentences for possession of marijuana, especially when sanctions manifestly varied on racial and class grounds and when penalties shifted from state to state, including at least two in which marijuana had been decriminalized by the electorate. How did one represent such complex issues to students? How did one respond when a campus arrest made a jail term likely? More difficult than articulating a credible theoretical position was taking action when a student violated either a federal or state law, university regulation or probationary stipulation.

Another complexity arose when campus disciplinary agents stipulated that a student on probation for a first drug-related offense be separated automatically from the university for a second infraction. For many of us working with addiction, this was tough stuff, as we had come to—almost—anticipate relapse and to understand its unexceptional role along the path to long-term recovery. These situations provoked various questions. Were all instances of relapse to be treated alike—or were some appropriate for stiff sanction, while others might be the moment when true recovery would begin? In such instances, rather than separation from the institution, might a quasi-therapeutic response be more appropriate, for example, mandated treatment, coupled with a disciplinary penalty? Other examples will suggest themselves, instances where an advisor might pause and see the complexity in a moment of illegality and seek to leverage it most effectively to the student's ultimate advantage.

A wise and seasoned president of a not-so-competitive college provided a slightly different and broader acknowledgment of these same issues. At a national conference, where presenters urged stern measures for fairly minor drug offenses, this chief executive confessed with astonishing and refreshing candor: "All well and good for the rest of you to cast out these students. I cannot afford that route. My campus is peopled with your cast-offs."

A firm yet sympathetic approach to a student's drug use frequently raised these thorny questions and also led to open if difficult and challenging conversations with the young. It was always my view that a student should be well aware of my perspective, my decisions and the risks I was prepared to take in his or her service. I am happy to say that my judgments generally yielded positive results.

Abridgement of the Truth and the Matter of Anonymity

Despite my general and overwhelming belief that truth is crucial, in rare and clearly defined instances I reminded clients that the truth need not be complete. I think of when a student seeks admission to an academic institution and, again, the matter of résumés. In both instances—especially given the protections of the Americans with Disabilities Act—I counseled recovering students carefully, clarifying that less than full disclosure was in no sense an indication of personal shame but a matter of strategy in a society where views of addiction are often inaccurate, prejudicial and apt to do unfair and unmerited harm. In many instances a student and I salvaged for a résumé inclusion of activities which (by their standard names) might prove harmful: we avoided drug-related terms and carefully described an activity in vague if nonetheless essentially honest language, e.g., not "peer *drug* counseling" but simply "peer counseling." In a word, I advised students to disclose their addictive histories cautiously, with an eye on legal protections and only after carefully assessing the need and considering their motives.

A footnote: Twelve-step programs operate anonymously, and it is crucial to preserve the essential anonymity of AA and similar programs, both because of their spiritual underpinnings and also because of the protections which anonymity affords both the organization of AA and its members, especially as they ease into early sobriety. An unintended consequence of anonymity, however, may be students' feelings of shame and occasionally an irrational fear at disclosing their condition. It is important to confront these feelings directly and to help addicts accept their condition without remorse or shame.

And perhaps it is necessary to note the valid distinction, often muddied, between an AA member's need to protect through anonymity an affiliation with AA, even as the same individual may feel wholly at ease in disclosing personal alcoholism. A certain measure of forthrightness is vital if we are ever to win the battle that seems eternal against the stigma generated by alcoholism and other drug addiction, even as membership in a 12-step program goes unmentioned.

A final comment. Some have thought that anonymity might be less necessary on campus, given the usual guarantees of academic freedom. This was not my experience. Particularly on small campuses personal privacy is greatly valued. And on any campus, although a faculty member's job security may be assured, all of the false information and misimpressions that fuel stigma remain securely in place.

The Integrity of the Student

Early in my sobriety a counselor-friend remarked that those in recovery must retain or perhaps *regain* a sense of their own integrity. It must be clear to the reader that I always sought to assure students that they "mattered" and had my full regard.

Most students, as they move from the secondary to the collegiate level, become adult before the law. They must now be considered partners in their own affairs. I suspect there may be something of a disjunction here with procedures at the secondary level, given a student's different legal status and developmental stage.

Vital, too, is respect for students, whatever their level and immediate situation. This is true, of course, for all students, yet positive regard seems somehow to slip away easily—sometimes precipitously—when students run seriously afoul of drug regulations. Young people in college, even when found guilty of significant offenses, are still our students and must be treated with respect. Even moments of crisis are educable moments.

A final point: I always emphasized that, whatever help I might provide, the responsibility for success or failure would be the student's—perhaps the ultimate acknowledgment of the student's integrity.

Parents

Almost every time a drug problem erupts, a parent is hurt, generally angry, almost always confused and often, though perhaps not truly *surprised*, embarrassingly ignorant of the nature of their child's behavior, problem and challenges. A wise parent in another context opined, where expectation did not match an outcome: "What a discrepancy between the dreams of a twenty year old and my twenty year old dreams." One must sympathize and try hard to enlist as allies these disappointed and vulnerable individuals, even when they are abrasive, misguided, ashamed—and sometimes strong, powerful and manipulative.

The involvement of a parent was not always a positive experience. Occasionally a parent—and two parents (or more) do not always constitute a united front—argued strenuously for a student's enrollment when it was otherwise universally agreed that a leave of absence would be the best option. In another instance a parent succeeded in pushing for transfer admission of a child with a severely troubled drug history before the young woman was "ready." In yet another instance a therapist seemed to have been encouraged to understate the seriousness of a student's addiction and to prettify the prognosis of the student, who had been on medical leave and who now sought readmission.

On the other hand some parents accepted the University's recommendations and yet lovingly supported their children, fully cognizant of the circumstances—when the situation was mild, when the student ran afoul of university regulations and needed in-patient treatment, when a child turned to thievery to support a habit, even when a child was imprisoned for use-related dealing. In these instances parents embraced, however sadly, the necessity for punishment, the need for time out in the progress of their son's or daughter's life—and nonetheless at the same time maintained a supportive stance.

I sometimes think that my work with parents was merely the sharing of common sense:

- Do not confuse a child's behavior with the child herself/himself: children are larger than their drug activity.
- Take a long view and realize that the current crisis is a small part of a whole life.
- Why do you want your child drug-tested? What will you *do* with that information?
- Try to save your anger for another day.
- Pick your battles. Is this really the time to criticize your child's taste in music or style of dress?
- Choose language that your child can hear.
- Try to remain optimistic, hopeful.

The sooner we all help parents to face these issues, the more helpful and supportive they may be when a problem arises. To prepare them for the possibility of serious drug-involved difficulties is an important task throughout the educational process.

Before I move along and leave the subject of parents, let me note that I also provided support for individuals whose parents were themselves drug addicts, including, of course, alcoholics. This is a separate tale that I mention here simply for the sake of completeness.

Difficult Situations

I must note that things did not always go smoothly with all those I worked with. Some simply chose not to alter apparently dangerous use of alcohol and other drugs. Some students with dual diagnoses had to overcome special challenges in reaching a drug-free lifestyle, and some-times the attempts were many. Others would arrest addiction to one drug yet fall prey to another. Sometimes shame for drug-related behavior led to frequent relapse. And sometimes parents fueled a student's unrealistic ambitions, setting unattainably high expectations. In many of these in-stances dismissals and academic or medical leaves—and sometimes more than one—were in order. Fortunately, most students with whom I worked eventually attained their goals. Each instance proved the value of never giving up on an individual, especially young people whose lives stretch out before them full of promise.

The Need for Support for Those Working with Students in Recovery

Isolation and Support of Practitioners

To deepen understanding of shared drug-related problems for practitioners at the secondary and collegiate levels, I sponsored for a decade, through the great generosity of an anonymous donor, an annual day-long conference of practitioners, parents and students. The day featured a keynote talk, panels and workshops, as well as luncheon and free time for informal discussion. Attendance was strong for all ten years. My clearest, most sobering finding was not that individuals valued new information—though they did—but rather that practitioners in particular valued the simple opportunity to speak frankly about their daily challenges with knowledgeable peers. (A procedural note: although we tape-recorded and transcribed the proceedings for publication, in an effort to encourage open dialogue we never identified speakers by name or institution.) The New England Collegiate Alcohol Network (NECAN) for many years sponsored a similar regional opportunity.

It seems to me vital that all of us involved in drug-related work, whether at the secondary or post-secondary level, maintain contact: our work is integrally related. Additionally, our work is lonely and stressful, and recognition and thanks are not common. However, when a crisis develops, we are expected to devise an acceptable solution—and fast. Our mutual association allows the possibility of easing the stress that such a situation produces. I am glad that such a possibility is provided these days by The Association of Recovery Schools.

Postscript

I am pleased to report that, at the time of this publication, the position in chemical dependency which I held at Brown has been maintained. For one who in large measure designed the position, it is gratifying that transition to my successor was highly effective and that the work continues under an endowment which was created at my retirement and which bears my name. It is also reassuring to note that, despite what a few generous souls said about my own person's being necessary for success, such is not the case.

Unsurprisingly, the need continues for the services that I once provided, which are now provided by an individual for whom I have high regard. She is carving her own path in her own way, relying on her own ingenuity, yet striving to meet the same goals that I identified over the years—and clearly a few of her own.

REFERENCES

Ewing, J. A. (1984). Detecting Alcoholics: The CAGE Questionaire. *Journal of the American Medical Association, 65,* 1905–1907.

Mann, M. (1958). Marty Mann's New Primer on Alcoholism. In *Who Is Not An Alcoholic* (pp. 78–93). New York: Holt, Rinehart and Winston.

Miller, W. R., & Rollnick, S. (1991). *Motivational Interviewing: Preparing People to Change Addictive Behavior*. New York: Guilford.

Twelve Step Meeting—Step Twelve

Recovery School Students

Welcome to the Young Peoples Twelve Step Meeting
Step Twelve-Part I 041507
Andrew has entered the room "Young Peoples Twelve Step Meeting"
s_k_011 has entered the room "Young Peoples

Twelve Step Meeting"
s_k_011: hey so do you think more people will come this time?
Andrew: I hope so but it's already 10 and there's just the 2 of us
s_k_011: Yeah I know. I don't understand why no
one has been showing up.
Andrew: me neither, not only do they not come but I haven't heard back from most people
s_k_011: Yeah i know. When I sent out the email for tonights meeting nobody replied to me.
s_k_011: Is jeffery suppose to be here too?
Andrew: they may not have computer access but most people got back to me once or twice along the line
Andrew: I thought he would be here but if not I can email him the transcript

s_k_011: ok cool. just wondering
s_k_011: should we start or do you want to wait and see if anyone else comes?
Andrew: I don't know, what do you think?
s_k_011: I mean we can have a meeting, but it is a

Andrew made two attempts to organize a meeting on Step Twelve. Each meeting attracted one other member; the first meeting included Stef who had attended the first two meetings, and the second meeting included Ryan, who attended for the first time.
The initial conversation expresses their concern about this lack of participation. Typical for the process of recovery from addiction, these concerns are openly expressed and then surrendered for the purpose of moving on with the task.

The group acknowledges my having been present as an observer at previous meetings. Again, discussion of my role is open and explicit, and once addressed, the process moves on.

Decisions continue to be made with the benefit of input from both members of the meeting.

288

bummer that there is no one else. Cause Im sure our meeting would only last 20 minutesor so, I guess I really don't know what to do..

Andrew: yeah i agree

Andrew: well we could wait a while or just get started

s_k_011: well we can start if you want.. I mean if anyone else shows I am sure that it would probably be soon. you want to?

Andrew: sure

s_k_011: alright well Welcome to the young peoples 12 step meeting. Tonight I believe we are on step 12, would anyone like to start?

Andrew: !

s_k_011: Hi andrew

Andrew: Well my experience with step 12 is somewhat limited because in working through the steps with my sponsor I have not yet reached step 12

Andrew: but as for a spiritual experience, I had more of a gradual spiritual experience than a sudden one

Andrew: more of an evolution of my understanding of my higher power and realizing its presence

Andrew: I do try to help other alcoholics in some

small way

Andrew: whether it's helping a friend from the program move or giving people rides or making or taking phone calls

Andrew: even just talking to new people at meetings, because these are the kinds of things that people did and still do for me and they were so helpful

Andrew: I also try to help out by sharing my story through "leading" (speaking at) a meeting or taking on service positions at meetings

Andrew: I have not sponsored others, and I don't feel I'm ready to yet, but I know the value of sponsorship because it helped me out a lot

Andrew: And as for the last part of step 12, practicing these principles in all our affairs, It's something I work on and I certainly see progress rather than perfection, but often

Stef "steps up" to take the position of chairing the meeting. Even though only two members are present, the formal structure of the meeting is maintained.

Many addicts in recovery experience working the twelve steps in the order that they are given. Even so, from the very beginning of the process of recovery, most addicts are able to identify with working each of the steps in some fashion. Hence the notion of a gradual spiritual experience.

Carrying the message of recovery is also referred to as service. This service to others is often very simple, as Andrew describes. Indeed, participating in these on line meetings might be considered a form of service in carrying the message of recovery from addiction to professionals in the community.

times I have a whole lot of improvement to do, because how well I'm working a program depends not on how I am in a meeting, it's the other 23 hours of the day that are a reflection of my spiritual condition or lack thereof.
Andrew: Thanks for listening, I'll pass.
s_k_011: Thanks andrew
s_k_011: !
s_k_011: Hi im stef i am sn alcoholic and addict Andrew: Hi stef
s_k_011: Well Step 12 "Having had a spirtual awakening" I can't say that there is one moment that I recall. I do believe that I have had glimpse and little bits of spirtual awakenings. like you had mentioned coming to really unstand my higher power and put trust that my high power is there and what not

Stef joins Andrew in the experience of spiritual awakening being a gradual process. The gradual nature of these changes is consistent with providing support over extended periods of time in structured programs of the type that are described in this book.

s_k_011: I have had many small spiritual awakenings, just by being a part of the program. And by starting to understand what its all about
s_k_011: Carrying the message and service work is something that I always try to do
s_k_011: as you said giving people rides to meetings, making coffee, chairing a meeting, speaking opportunities such as at schools or other meetings (sharing my story)

Carrying the message entails actions that are taken in addition to words that are spoken.

s_k_011: I also try to reach out to new comers because I know how I felt when I was first introduced to the program. Through my experience I feel that you are spreading the message and carrying it by just talking in meetings and sharing your experience strength and hope.
s_k_011: Though one thing i need to mention is
when working step 12 and trying to help other alcoholics from my experience can also be hard. I can become co dependant and start to care so much about a person and end up getting dragged down. I need to be careful that I don't become to attached when working with alcoholics/addicts because we are all still sick and have things to work on
s_k_011: I need to make sure that I am still working my program and not trying to work theirs

Carrying the message also entails attaching to other people. This attachment benefits the person who is carrying the message; the primary purpose of each of the Twelve Steps, especially Step Twelve, is to strengthen and safeguard the individual's sobriety.

Stef underscores the importance of maintaining one's sense of self in carrying the message. Working with those who still suffer needs to be an uplifting experience. When Stef refers to the need to avoid becoming attached, she is probably referring to not becoming attached to outcomes, and in particular, not becoming attached to the addiction of another person.

s_k_011: I completely agree with you andrew on what you said about practicing the principles in all our affairs. there is no better way to say it then how you put it

s_k_011: Step 12 is important because someone 12 stepped me by carrying the message to me and I need to make sure that I am doing the same because the program saved my life and I know that it can do the same for others. I need to try and give back what it has given to me.
s_k_011: Well thanks for letting me share and listening. I will pass.
Andrew: Thanks Stef
s_k_011: anyone else have anything to share?
s_k_011: I guess we are still the only 2 in here
s_k_011: lol
Andrew: yep
s_k_011: so.. what now? =)
Andrew: Well, I have nothing else to share that I can think of on this topic
s_k_011: me either
Andrew: well, should we just close?
s_k_011: I am thinking so. I don't see that anyone would come if they haven't already?
Andrew: probably not
s_k_011: well then i guess we are done. Is there
anymore meetings after this or was this the last one?

Andrew: I think this is the last one
Andrew: there's no more time anyway
s_k_011: Yes true
Andrew: we were supposed to be done about a month ago
s_k_011: Yeah I just found out and filled in last minute so I didn't even know that
Andrew: Well, I can email the transcript to Jeffrey
s_k_011: were there any meetings that were done about a month ago
Andrew: hah nope
s_k_011: crazy
s_k_011: haha
Andrew: I was supposed to be setting it up but nobody got back to me and showed up

This principle, which applies to all Twelve Step programs, has been clearly described in another Twelve Step program, Al-Anon, for the families and friends of alcoholics. Al-Anon calls this attitude "detaching with love."

With both members having shared, discussion now centers on how to proceed.
Lol= laugh out loud
=) may represent a smiley face, indicating a light-hearted move towards closure.

Stef and Andrew share information that would help both of them make a decision on closure.

With the meeting about to end, my presence (and implicitly the presence of the readers of the book) is acknowledged.

it was pretty bad
s_k_011: Thats crapy
s_k_011: so are you going to be in DC
Andrew: yeah, I'm flying in wed. night
Andrew: you?
s_k_011: alright. Yes Ill be there. I am pretty excited it is an amazing opportunitie that I was given
Andrew: agreed, I'm really looking forward to it.
s_k_011: Yes it should be really neat. So where exactly are you coming from?
Andrew: well I live in New York but I go to school in Cleveland so I'm coming in from Cleveland
s_k_011: Oh ok, cool. I am coming in from Minnesota, the st. paul area
Andrew: nice
s_k_011: Yeah
s_k_011: Well.. I guess ill be seeing you in DC you have a wonderful nigh
Andrew: you too
Step Twelve-Part II 052007
dryry, "Hello!"
dryry, "Who else is out there?"
Andrew, "Andrew"
Andrew, "Is this Ryan from D.C.?"
dryry, "yup, how you doing?"
Andrew, "pretty good"
Andrew, "enjoying summer"
Andrew, "how have you been?"
dryry, "not bad, i was a good day today did some area service and some meditation"

Andrew, "nice"
dryry, "do you think anyone else will sign onto the chat?"
dryry, "I've never had a meeting like this before"
Andrew, "In the past, all our meetings were small, but our last meeting was just two people."
Andrew, "This was supposed to " "replace" that meeting and get everyone to join, but that doesn't look promising."
dryry, I guess we'll see. How does it work? I guess there's no "speaker" (ha ha). Do people just share, or just chat about

Andrew and Stef were two of eight student participants in a national meeting of JMATE on treatment of adolescent addiction. Their interaction after the formally structured part of the meeting is typical of social exchanges that occur outside of the boundaries of the meeting. These interactions are called "fellowshipping," and contribute to the formation of a tightly knit social network that supports sobriety. Engaging in these social exchanges may therefore also be considered part of carrying the message of recovery.

In this second meeting on Step Twelve, Andrew and Ryan meet. Since Andrew is the experienced member in this online format, his welcome to Ryan reflects the theme of the meeting, carrying the message of recovery. As in the prior meetings, the interchange before the meeting starts is an important part of the process. Note how naturally Ryan volunteers his service activity (Step Twelve) and time spent in meditation (Step Eleven).
Note how quickly Ryan engages in examining the process in the here and now. This sensitivity is a major signal of recovery. He also is alert to the presence of a task for the meeting, and asks Andrew for help in understanding this task.

recovery related issues?

"Andrew," Well the topic is supposed to be Step 12 and we usually just took turns sharing anything we felt like about step 12

"dryry," nice, I'm just finishing going over that step

with my sponsor

"Andrew, "do you think we should go ahead with the meeting or not?

dryry, "Well, good question, I think it'll be a miracle if anyone else joins us at this point. I'm up for just sharing a little bit about the 12th step and then calling it a night, what do you think?

"Andrew," sounds good

"dryry," Maybe I'll share some of my experience with the 12th step:

"dryry," Step 12, having had a spiritual awakening as a result of these steps, we tried to carry the message to addicts and practice these principles in all our affairs. I think for me what's been tough

about the 12th step is to be totally open to helping someone even when they releapse or don't want to take suggestions. Recently, I meet a newcomer in a meeting who I tried to help by taking him to meetin

"dryry," ings and calling him on the phone. He seemed to be doing really good, until he suddenly drank one day. It didn't make sense but I know I'm only responsible for carrying the message, not the addict."

dryry, "What's your experience with the 12th step?"

Andrew, "Well I am currently making my list of amends to make (Step 8) so I don't have lots of experience with the 12th step. I try to practice the principles of the program in all my affairs but I have good and bad days."

Andrew, "Prayer certainly helps with this as well as acceptance, but I still have lots of progress to look forward to."

Andrew, "As for helping people, one thing I found very helpful this past school year was the reliance of my fellow Recovery House residents on me for rides to meetings."

Andrew, "It was nice to be able to help them and also to have a sort of" "commitment" "to get to a meeting every day."

That Ryan has a sponsor with whom he works the steps is an indication that he brings some direct experience with that step to this meeting.

Having asked Andrew about the agenda, Ryan jumps in and appears to assume the role of chair for this mini-meeting; those who chair the meeting often starts their comment by reading the step they are talking about.

Ryan's leadership style is more directive than Andrew's style, as we see from the previous meeting. Ryan asks Andrew to share rather than waiting for Andrew to indicate an interest in speaking. The structure of Twelve Step meetings is open enough to embrace a rather wide variety of leadership styles.

Andrew's example shows an advantage to living in a collegiate recovery community. He also demonstrates his understanding that his performance of service to others has the immediate benefit of leading him to attend meetings himself.

Andrew, "One issue I'm currently having that sort of relates to step 12 is at home with 2 of my brothers. I used with both of them, getting them into drinking and smoking weed. Now that I'm home from college, I am in an environment where they are still using."

Andrew, "I cannot say whether they are addicted or not, but it is difficult to simply stand by and watch them do what I did, knowing all I can do is be an example to them and to be there if they need help."

Andrew, "I know I can't try to force anything on

them, and I definately wasn't open to things like that when I was still actively using, but I'm just dealing now with accepting what they are doing and trying not too feel to guilty for starting them using. I also have to know that at some point, even if it wasn't me, someone would have introduced them to drugs/alcohol."

Andrew, "But i know now that I am a good example, at least most of the time, for them and I try to be of maximum service to god and my fellows. Progress, not perfection though, that's for sure."

Andrew, "I guess that's all I really have on step 12 tonight."

Andrew, "Is there anything else you want to say?"

dryry, "Well, I just wanted to say that's rough about

your brothers, I mean living with them now that schools out. My stepbrothers were some of the first people I used with and it was really hard to be

around them in early recovery. But, once they understood what I went through (out patient and going to meetings) they had a lot of respect for me."

dryry, "I think that's about all I have for now"

Andrew, "Well thanks for sharing, this was good for me"

Andrew, "I'll email a copy of the transcript to Andy and Jeffrey"

dryry, "Yeah, same here, this is interesting and i'm glad to know it exists. Thanks for sharing too. I still have your number from DC, so I'll text mine to you. Keep in touch!"

Andrew, "Sounds good, take care Ryan, enjoy your summer"

dryry, "Thanks man, you too! Peace"

Andrew's relationship with his brothers is a poignant example of addiction being a family disease. Often recovering addicts face the challenge of maintaining their own sobriety in the face of family members continuing to become intoxicated. Sometimes the recovering addict shoulders responsibility for introducing other family members to alcohol or drug use, and then ironically becomes the family member to introduce others to a process of recovery.

Ryan's identification with Andrew supports the common occurrence of addiction in other family members.

Index